# Textbook of
# Vascular Anesthesia

With  containing video files of Chapter 7

# Textbook of
# Vascular Anesthesia

*Editor*

**Usha Kiran** MD

Professor and Head
Department of Cardiac Anesthesia
Cardio-Thoracic Centre
All India Institute of Medical Sciences
New Delhi

*Coeditors*

**Sandeep Chauhan**          **Minati Choudhury**          **Vishwas Malik**

**Neeti Makhija**          **Sambhunath Das**          **Suruchi Hasija**

**Poonam Malhotra Kapoor**          **Parag Gharde**          **Arindam Choudhury**

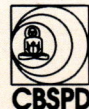

CBSPD

## CBS Publishers & Distributors Pvt Ltd

New Delhi • Bengaluru • Chennai • Kochi • Kolkata • Lucknow • Mumbai
Gujarat • Hyderabad • Jharkhand • Nagpur • Patna • Pune • Uttarakhand

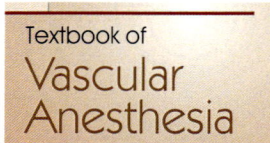

ISBN: 978-93-85915-40-6

**First Edition: 2017**
**Reprint: 2025**

Published by Satish Kumar Jain and produced by Varun Jain for

**CBS Publishers & Distributors** Pvt Ltd

4819/XI Prahlad Street, 24 Ansari Road, Daryaganj, New Delhi 110 002, India.
Ph: 011-23289259, 23266838          Website: www.cbspd.com
                                                  e-mail: delhi@cbspd.com
*Corporate Office:* 204 FIE, Industrial Area, Patparganj, Delhi 110 092, India.
Ph: 011-49344934          Fax: 011-49344935          e-mail: publishing@cbspd.com; publicity@cbspd.com

## Branches

- **Bengaluru:** Seema House 2975, 17th Cross, K.R. Road, Banasankari 2nd Stage, Bengaluru 560 070, Karnataka, India
  Ph: +91-80-26771678/79          Fax: +91-80-26771680          e-mail: bangalore@cbspd.com
- **Chennai:** 18/8B, Subbarayan Street, Shenoy Nagar, Chennai 600 030, Tamil Nadu, India
  Ph: +91-44-42032115, 26681266          e-mail: chennai@cbspd.com
- **Kochi:** 42/1325, 1326, Power House Road, Opposite KSEB, Power House, Ernakulum 682018, Kochi, Kerala, India
  Ph: +91-484-4059061-65          Fax: +91-484-4059065          e-mail: kochi@cbspd.com
- **Kolkata:** 147, Hind Ceramics Compound, 1st Floor, Nilgunj Road, Belghoria, Kolkata 700 056, West Bengal, India
  Ph: +91-33-25330055/56          e-mail: kolkata@cbspd.com
- **Lucknow:** Basement, Khushnuma Complex, 7 Meerabai Marg (behind Jawahar Bhawan), Lucknow 226 001, UP, India
  Ph: 0522-4000032          e-mail: tiwari.lucknow@cbspd.com
- **Mumbai:** PWD Shed. Gala no. 25/26, Ramchandra Bhatt Marg, Next to JJ Hospital Gate no. 2,
  Opp. Union Bank of India, Noorbaug Mumbai 400009, Maharashtra, India
  Ph: 022-66661880/89          e-mail: mumbai@cbspd.com

## Representatives

| • **Gujarat** | 0-9879558667 | • **Hyderabad** | 0-9885175004 | • **Jharkhand** | 0-9811541605 |
|---|---|---|---|---|---|
| • **Nagpur** | 0-8692091830 | • **Patna** | 0-9334159340 | • **Pune** | 0-9664372571 |
| • **Uttarakhand** | 0-9716462459 | | | | |

*Printed at* HT Media Ltd., Sector 63 Noida, UP, India

_to_

_Almighty Supreme Being_
_God Father Shiva and_
_Brahma Kumaris_
_who empower me as well to my teachers and predecessors in cardiac anesthesia_
_who sustained me and to cardiac anesthesia colleagues_
_who supported me all the time_

**Akshay Kumar Bisoi**
Professor
Department of CTVS
All India Institute of Medical Sciences, New Delhi

**Arindam Choudhury**
Associate Professor
Department of Cardiac Anesthesiology
All India Institute of Medical Sciences, New Delhi

**Arun Subramanium**
Consultant
Department of Cardiac Anesthesiology
Lourdes Hospital, Cochin

**Balram Airan**
Professor and Head
Department of CTVS
Chief CTC
All India Institute of Medical Sciences, New Delhi

**B Uma**
Senior Resident
Department of Cardiac Anesthesiology
All India Institute of Medical Sciences, New Delhi

**Jitin Narula**
Associate Consultant
Department of Cardiac Anesthesiology
Max Superspeciality Hospital, Patparganj, New Delhi

**Kulbhushan Saini**
Assistant Professor
Department of Anesthesiology
All India Institute of Medical Sciences, New Delhi

**Minati Choudhury**
Professor
Department of Cardiac Anesthesiology
All India Institute of Medical Sciences, New Delhi

**Milind P Hote**
Professor
Department of CTVS
All India Institute of Medical Sciences, New Delhi

**Neeti Makhija**
Professor
Department of Cardiac Anesthesiology
All India Institute of Medical Sciences, New Delhi

**Parag Gharde**
Professor
Department of Cardiac Anesthesiology
All India Institute of Medical Sciences, New Delhi

**Palletti Rajashekar**
Associate Professor
Department of CTVS
All India Institute of Medical Sciences, New Delhi

**Poonam Malhotra Kapoor**
Professor
Department of Cardiac Anesthesiology
All India Institute of Medical Sciences, New Delhi

**Sandeep Chauhan**
Professor, Department of Cardiac Anesthesiology
All India Institute of Medical Sciences, New Delhi

**Sambhunath Das**
Professor, Department of Cardiac Anesthesiology
All India Institute of Medical Sciences, New Delhi

**Suruchi Hasija**
Associate Professor
Department of Cardiac Anesthesiology
All India Institute of Medical Sciences, New Delhi

**Suruchi Ladha**
Senior Resident, Department of Cardiac Anesthesia
All India Institute of Medical Sciences, New Delhi

**Shiv Kumar Choudhary**
Professor Department of CTVS
All India Institute of Medical Sciences, New Delhi

**Ujjawal K Choudhary**
Professor Department of CTVS
All India Institute of Medical Sciences, New Delhi

**Usha Kiran**
Professor and Head
Department of Cardiac Anesthesiology
All India Institute of Medical Sciences, New Delhi

**Vishwas Malik**
Professor, Department of Cardiac Anesthesiology
All India Institute of Medical Sciences, New Delhi

**V Devagourou**
Professor Department of CTVS
All India Institute of Medical Sciences, New Delhi

I am extremely pleased to witness the book *Textbook of Vascular Anesthesia* by the joint contribution of the faculty of departments of Cardiac Anesthesia and Cardio-Thoracic and Vascular Surgery.

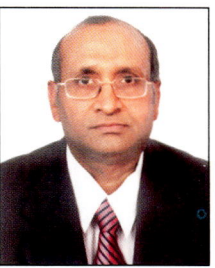

The vascular surgery carries a high risk causing dynamic lability which may result in end organ ischemia, renal deficiency and cerebrovascular complications. Risk of thrombosis and embolism adds to postoperative morbidity. Comorbid conditions increase the perioperative risk. All the preventive measures employed before initiating surgery have been described in this book. A separate chapter is dedicated to the postoperative management.

Aortic dissection is the most common life-threatening disorder affecting aorta with mortality rate rising as high as 1% per hour for several hours and often needs emergent surgery. Such a challenging situation can only be handled with utmost care with low intraoperative morbidity and mortality if the anesthesiologists are well trained in taking care of these patients.

This *Textbook* will prove highly beneficial for all the anesthesiologists, especially those who are undergoing postgraduation in anesthesia, DM, three-years postdoctoral courses and cardiac anesthesia fellowship and vascular surgery fellowship training programs. All senior resident trainees of cardiac anesthesia and all kinds of subspecialties of anesthesia will also be enormously benefited by this book as it is starting from history, anatomy and pathophysiological details of aorta. Management of lesions of ascending aorta, arch and descending aorta, abdominal aorta including chronic diseases and pathology of acute conditions like aortic dissection and aortic rupture are discussed in detail. A special chapter on transesophageal echocardiography for aortic surgery has been included. The information with images reflects the vast variety of knowledge and skills the anesthesiologist requires to practice vascular anesthesia

I am thankful to all the contributors whose great endeavor in collecting latest data for providing comprehensive authoritative text proved worthy for this book. Their own expertise in managing acute and chronic aortic surgery and peripheral–vascular conditions is highly appreciated. Their effort for streamlining protocols for complex aortic and vascular surgery, advanced monitoring and rapid blood transfusion is remarkable. The stated aim of this book is to give clear and concise guidance on the management of anesthesia for peripheral vascular and aortic surgery patients.

I am sure that all the trainees of anesthesiology, postgraduate students, postdoctoral fellows and established cardiovascular anesthesiologists, perfusion technology trainees and vascular surgery trainees will enjoy reading this book.

**Balram Airan** MS, MCh, FIACS
Professor and Head
Department of Cardio-Thoracic and Vascular Surgery
Chief, Cardio-Thoracic Sciences Centre
Dean, All India Institute of Medical Sciences
New Delhi

Our aspiration in writing *Textbook of Vascular Anesthesia* was to assemble the experience of the entire faculty of cardiac anesthesia and cardiovascular surgery gained by working in one superspecialty institute for over thirty years. Understanding and management of aortic and other vascular surgery is the mandatory concern for anesthesiologists. We aim to focus on anesthesia concerns during aortic surgery. A few chapters like anesthesia for carotid artery surgery and peripheral artery surgery are also included. The approach depends more on surgical technique and the organ being affected. Aorta being the main blood vessel carrying blood from the heart to the body, its aneurysms at various sites may be encountered by an anesthesiologist. This aneurysm continues to grow, increasing the risk of rupture and aortic dissection. Techniques for repair of aortic aneurysm and dissection have undergone a dramatic change in last 3 decades. A remarkable addition of biotechnology in the field of anesthesiology and related postoperative care has been added in this book. A separate chapter is included for management of ruptured aortic aneurysm. Readers will find inspiring ideas for handling ruptured or leaking aortic aneurysm.

Transesophageal echocardiography (TEE) has made anaesthesia for aortic surgery safe. Leaving aside the diagnostic value, the adequacy of fluid and inotropes infusions are easily discerned by TEE. The text is dealing elaborately with TEE during perioperative period for patients undergoing aortic surgery.

The perioperative management is highly challenging not just due to high risk profile of the patient but also because of complex surgical procedures they are undergoing. Chronic hypertension is the commonest comorbid condition in patients with vascular disease. It is logical to have an optimal perioperative control of blood pressures. Role of beta-blockers are discussed in detail in the chapter dealing with descending thoracic aortic surgery. Complications prolong the postoperative course, hence all efforts should be made to detect and stabilize the blood pressure and ischemic cardiac disease before aortic surgery. Management of the postoperative complications has been covered in the chapter on postoperative management of vascular surgery. Rapid blood transfusion and technical advances are also discussed.

I firmly believe that *Textbook of Vascular Anesthesia* will be an invaluable asset in learning and teaching the subject. This is the result of dedication and thoughtfulness of contributing authors. The book will provide sustained benefit to the patients.

**Usha Kiran**

# Acknowledgements

I express my extreme gratefulness to all the contributing authors. They all are my colleagues in Cardio-Thoracic Sciences Centre having 10 to 30 years of expertise in providing anesthesia and perioperative care to cardiac and vascular surgery patients. Despite their busy clinical work schedule in operation room and ICU, in research and academics and teaching DM and MCh students, they agreed to support me by contributing various chapters.

I express my heartful thanks to Prof MC Misra, Director, AIIMS, for being kind enough to permit me to write *Textbook of Vascular Anesthesia*.

I am particularly grateful to Prof Balram Airan, Dean, AIIMS, Head, Department of Cardio-Thoracic and Vasular Surgery, and Chief, Cardio-Thoracic Sciences Center; along with the entire faculty of cardiac thoracic surgery for their cooperation.

I would like to take the opportunity to express my gratitude to all the patients who have helped us learn about the disease. This book would not have been possible without the challenges posed by the patients who underwent complex aortic surgeries. They helped us with the opportunity to learn and improve.

The contribution by the nursing and technical staff of cardiothoracic centre is highly appreciated.

Hearty thanks to Mr YN Arjuna (Sr VP, CBS Publishers & Distributors) and the coordinated endeavor of his team by visits from time to time and follow up with extreme patience to get this book published with great enthusiasm.

Special thanks to the senior residents of the department of cardiac anesthesia for their association and support in writing the book.

**Usha Kiran**

# Contents

# CHAPTER 1

# Introduction (Historical Aspects and Background)

Balram Airan, Usha Kiran, Kulbushan

## HISTORICAL BACKGROUND OF VASCULAR ANESTHESIA

This historical background of anesthesia will tell us of our heritage, of how we got to where we are. Little has been written on the history of anesthesia and its subspeciality cardiac/vascular anesthesia. Here is the rememberance of our glorious past. Anesthesia as we know it started in the early to mid 1840s. In 1842, Crawford Long of Jefferson, Georgia, removed a small tumor from a patient under diethyl ether anesthesia.[1] Afterwards, in 1844, Horace Wells a dentist, had used nitrous oxide in his dental practice.

William TG Morton, another dentist in anesthesia's history, successfully etherized a patient at the Massachusetts General Hospital in Boston on October 16, 1846.[2] The news of this event spread worldwide. Morton tried to patent his discovery under the name of Letheon. Oliver Wendell Holmes, dean of Harvard Medical School, only 2 months after Morton's epochal demonstration of surgical anesthesia, suggested the term "anesthesia" to describe the state of sleep induced by ether.

John Snow, from London, was the first physician to devote his energies to anesthetizing patients for surgical operations. In 1853, he administered chloroform to Queen Victoria for the delivery of her son Prince Leopold and successfully used anesthesia to alleviate the pain of childbirth.[3]

Those were the beginnings. By now, the two earliest anesthetic vapors, diethyl ether and chloroform, have been modified hundreds of times. Many congeners have come and gone, but their great-grand children still find daily use.

Afterwards, intravenous drugs have secured an increasingly prominent place in anesthesia. A steadily growing pharmacopoeia of analgesics, hypnotics, neuromuscular blockers, anxiolytics, and cardiovascular drugs now fill the drug cabinets.

As the era of thoracic surgery began the problem was how to ventilate the patient when the chest was open. Some ingenious approaches were explored, such as placing the patient's head in a positive pressure box [Brauer (1904) and Murphy (1905)] or operating within a negative pressure chamber with only the patient's head outside [Sauerbruch (1904)]; for a while, even into the 1940s, positive-pressure ventilation via a tight-fitting mask was used, particularly for children. The solution, however, was endotracheal ventilation. The first elective oral endotracheal intubation for anesthesia was performed by the Scottish surgeon, William Macewan, in 1878. In 1888, the American surgeon, Joseph O'Dwyer, designed metal endotracheal tubes with a conical tip to occlude the larynx and added a bellows device to provide positive-pressure ventilation. This was first used and advocated as the best means of preventing pulmonary collapse during thoracic surgery by the surgeon Rudolph Matas of New Orleans in about 1899.[4]

Advances in vascular surgery spurred the development of vascular anesthesiology. We changed from open drop ether to modern anesthetics and ventilation via tracheal tubes. In 1951, Keown described anesthetic management with hypothermia for the conduct of mitral commissurotomy. This recognized the importance of light anesthesia with minimal cardiac depression, and the benefit of letting the temperature drift down, i.e. of producing mild hypothermia.

In 1953, Gibbon used a heart–lung machine (Fig. 1.1) to allow closure of an atrial septal defect under direct vision.[5] Gibbon's invention, refined and adopted by

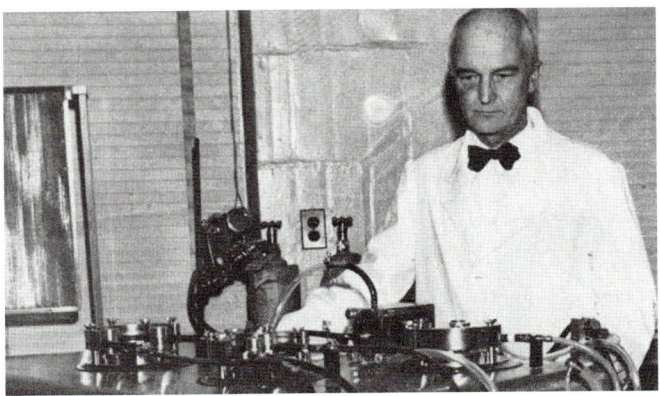

Fig. 1.1: John Gibbon with his heart–lung machine

many, revolutionized cardiac surgery by giving the surgeon a bloodless field and a time limited by how long a hypothermic heart could tolerate no coronary blood flow (about 30 minutes).

In 1967, Barnard performed the first heart transplant.[6] In 1973, surgeons stopped the heart beating (cardioplegia), thereby protecting it, by infusing cold hyperkalemic solutions into the coronary arteries. Myocardial protection techniques with a cold hyperkalemic (high potassium concentration) solution (cardioplegia) facilitated the expansion of cardiac surgery, giving surgeons well over an hour to perform their work.[7]

The development of deep hypothermic circulatory arrest during the 1950s brought potential for cardiac operations not previously possible. DHCA theoretically uses induced hypothermia (nasopharyngeal temperatures less than 24°C) to protect the brain during cessation of flow to the brain, in order to provide bloodless surgical field for visualization of the great vessels.[8] DHCA allows the surgeon to have good visualization for complex cardiac procedures. It can be used also in pulmonary embolectomy and neurovascular surgeries. The theory is to cool the patient, cease blood flow to the brain, and rely on the hypothermic protective effects of decreased cerebral metabolic rate of oxygen ($CMRO_2$). DHCA is used for open heart procedures where the ability to perfuse the brain through the head vessels is not possible with standard proximal aorta cannulation. Repair of the aortic arch, congenital repair involving the aortic arch, repair to the head and neck great vessels, or neurosurgical and pulmonary endarterectomies may require DHCA. Blood gas and electrolyte management is crucial during DHCA and evaluation should be done often. Several options for neurologic monitoring exist. EEG monitoring, BIS monitoring, transcranial Doppler ultrasound, cerebral oximetry and jugular bulb oxygen saturation ($SjVO_2$) have all been used to monitor neurological status during DHCA.

The first patients undergoing cardiac surgery were anesthetized with minimal monitoring, such as a finger on a carotid artery! However, as the surgery became more complex, and particularly after cardiopulmonary bypass was employed, monitoring of hemodynamic variables became an important component of vascular anesthesiology. In 1972, Civetta and Gabel described the use of the pulmonary artery (Swan-Ganz) catheter intra- and postoperatively[9], and in 1973, Lappas *et al.*, demonstrated that pulmonary capillary wedge pressure accurately reflected left atrial pressure intraoperatively, which in turn reflected left heart filling an function.[10]

As the cardiac surgery started, monitoring in cardiac anesthesia practice lacked visualization of the anatomy of the heart. Anatomy is crucially important because many operations propose to repair or palliate anatomic defects such as incompetent valves or ventricular septal defects, and because visualization of malfunctioning areas of the heart can provide clues to explain impaired circulation. Cardiac anesthesiologists and surgeons had no view of the internal anatomy of the heart as complexity of surgery progressed. Transesophageal echocardiography (TEE) changed that. Matsumoto[11] introduced M-mode (one dimensional) transesophageal echocardiography (TEE) in 1980, followed in 1982 by Cahalan's description of 2-dimensional TEE[12], and deBruijn and colleagues report of color-flow Doppler TEE[13] in 1987.

Most recently, TEE allows a 3-dimensional view[14] of structures and even better visualization. TEE has permitted cardiac anesthesiologists to literally look into the heart and become intraoperative cardiac diagnosticians, the intraoperative counterpart of the cardiologists providing the preoperative diagnosis guiding the surgeon to the appropriate procedure. Cardiac anesthesiologists can now inform surgeons in real time, of new intraoperative findings, make new diagnosis, confirm proper repair of the cardiac lesion, and specify needs for further immediate surgical management.

Lowenstein[15] reported the use of high dose morphine for cardiac anesthesia in 1969, and Stanley reported use of high dose fentanyl in 1973, suggesting benefit in patients with valvular and congenital disease.

In the 1980s, Slogoff and Keats showed that increased heart rate endangered the myocardium of patients with coronary artery disease (CAD).[16] Cardiac anesthesiologists then showed that beta-blockers decreased long term mortality after non-cardiac surgery.[17] In 2006, Mangano's group demonstrated that although aprotinin decreased transfusion requirements in patients undergoing open heart surgery, it increased the incidence of kidney failure and death.

Although, we still listen for breath sounds, we still watch color and respiration, and we still feel the pulse, but today we are helped by the most subtle techniques of sensing invisible signals and the most invasive methods with tubes snaking through the heart. Today we have the knowledge of management of anticoagulation, knowledge of cardiac assist devices and pacemakers, and interpretation of measurements obtained from pulmonary artery catheters and of echocardiography images.

## REFERENCES

1. Long CW (1849). "An account of the first use of Sulphuric Ether by Inhalation as an Anaesthetic in Surgical Operations". Southern Medical and Surgical Journal 5:705–13. Retrieved 2010-09-13.

2. Wells, H (1847). A History of the Discovery of the Application of Nitrous Oxide Gas, Ether, and Other Vapors to Surgical Operations. Hartford: J. Gaylord Wells. Retrieved 2010-09-13.

3. EY Euliano, JS Gavenstein, N Gavenstein, D Gavenstein. A short history of anaesthesia. In: Essential Anaesthesia: From Science to Practice, 2nd Cambridge: Cambridge University Press, 2011:1–2.

4. Calverley RK. Anesthesia as a specialty: past, present, future. In: Barash PG, Cullen BF, Stoelting RK, editors. Clinical anesthesia, 3rd ed. Philadelphia: Lippincott-Raven; 1997:3 p3.

5. Gibbon JH Jr. Application of a mechanical heart and lung apparatus to cardiac surgery. Minn Med. 1954; 37:171–85.

6. HesseL EA. History of cardiac surgery and anesthesia. In: Barash PG, Estafanous FG, Reves JG, editors. Cardiac anesthesia principles and clinical practice. 2nd ed. Philadelphia: JB Lippincott Co; 2001. p1–35.

7. Gay WA Jr, Ebert PA. Aorta-to-right pulmonary artery anastomosis causing obstruction of the right pulmonary artery. Management during correction of tetralogy of Fallot. Ann Thorac Surg. 1973; 16:402–10.

8. Drew CE, Anderson 1M. Profound hypothermia in cardiac surgery: report of three cases. Lancet. 1959; 1:748–50.

9. Civetta JM, Gabel JC. Flow directed-pulmonary artery catheterizationin surgical patients: indications and modifications of technic. Ann Surg. 1972; 176:753–6.

10. Lappas D, Lell WA, Gabel JC, Civetta 1M. Lowenstein E. Indirect Measurement of left-atrial pressure in surgical patients-pulmonary capillary wedge and pulmonary-artery diastolic pressures compared with left-atrial pressure. Anesthesiology. 1973; 38:394–7.

11. Matsumoto M, Oka Y, Strom J, Frishman W, Kadish A, Becker RM, Frater RW, Sonnenblick EH. Application of transesophageal echocardiography to continuous intra-operative monitoring of left ventricular performance. Am J Cardiol. 1980; 46:95–105.

12. Cahalan MK, Kremer P, Schiller NB, et al. Intraoperative monitoring with two-dimendional transesophageal echocardiography. Anesthesiology. 1982; 57:A 152.

13. deBruijn NP, Clements FM, Kisslo JA. Intraoperative transesophageal color flow mapping: initial experience. Anesth Analg. 1987; 66:386–90.

14. Kwak J, Andrawes M, Garvin S, D' Ambra MN. 3D trans-esophageal echocardiography: a review of recent literature 2007-2009. Curr Opin Anaesthesiol. 2010; 23:80–8.

15. Raja SN, Lowenstein E. The birth of opioid anesthesia. Anesthesiology. 2004; 100:1013–5.

16. Slogoff S, Keats A. Randomized trial of primary anesthetic agents on outcome of coronary artery bypass operations. Anesthesiology. 1989; 70:179–88.

17. Devereaux PJ, Yang H, Yusuf S, Guyatt G, Leslie K, Villar JC, Xavier D, Chrolavicius S, Greenspan L, Pogue J, Pais P, Liu L, Xu S, Malaga G, Avezum A, Chan M, Montori VM, Jacka M, Choi P. Effects of extended-release metoprolol succinate in patients undergoing non-cardiac surgery (POISE trial): a randomised controlled trial. Lancet. 2008; 371:1839–47.

18. Mangano DT, Tudor IC, Dietzel C. The risk associated with aprotinin in cardiac surgery. N Engl J Med. 2006; 354:353–65.

# CHAPTER 2

# Pathophysiology of Vascular Diseases

Usha Kiran, V Devagourou, B Uma

## PATHOGENESIS OF AORTIC DISEASES

Aorta is the largest artery in the body. Aorta is not simply a passive conduit; its elastic properties make it a dynamic organ responsible for interaction of whole cardiovascular system. The elastic recoil makes it secondary passive pump in addition to serving as conducting vessel. Decreased aortic distensibility which may occur with aging may precipitate left ventricular dysfunction. Knowledge about the anatomy and embryology is mandatory before going into the depth of etiology and pathogenesis of aortic diseases.

## EMBRYOLOGY

Development of aorta is a complex process and starts during the third week of gestation. In the beginning there is formation of endocardial tube. Primitive aorta has ventral and dorsal segments. A sac is formed by fusion of two ventral aortae and midline descending aorta is formed by fusion of dorsal aortae. Between ventral aorta and dorsal aorta, six branchial arch arteries, also called paired aortic arches, develop (Fig. 2.1). Dorsal aorta, in addition gives of several intersegmental arteries. The vessel developed from each arch is given in *Box 2.1*.

### Anatomy

The aorta starts from aortic valve three sinuses, traverses up through the thorax and abdomen giving branches and ends by dividing into iliac arteries (Fig. 2.2). Aortic root and proximal ascending aorta are in pericardial sac. Aorta after its origin ascends and is known as ascending aorta. Its right border is superior vena cava and right atrium. Left border has left atrium and pulmonary vascular trunk (Fig. 2.3). It turns anteriorly and superiorly to the left up to T4 level, passing over main

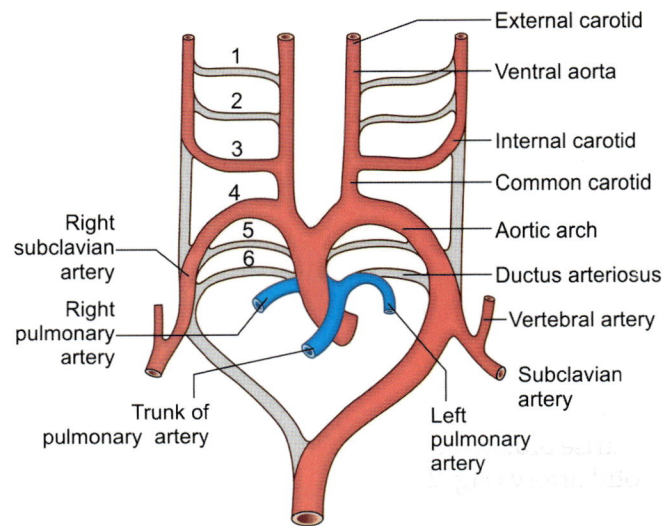

Fig. 2.1: Development of aorta

| Box 2.1 | Development of aorta |
| --- | --- |

- *Ventral aorta* gives rise to ascending aorta and pulmonary trunk
- *Large dorsal aorta* develops into descending aorta
- *First branchial arch*: Contributes to development of external carotid artery and maxillary artery
- *Second branchial arch*: Contributes to development of stapedial artery
- *Third bronchial arch*: Contributes to development of internal carotid artery and is also known as carotid arch
- Arch of aorta develops from *fourth brachial arch*: The left arch contributes to formation of left aortic arch between left common carotid and subclavian arteries. The right fourth arch contributes to formation of proximal right subclavian artery
- The fifth pair does not contribute much
- *Sixth pair*: Left 6th arch contributes by development of main and left pulmonary artery, and ductus arteriosus. The right sixth contributes to development of right pulmonary artery

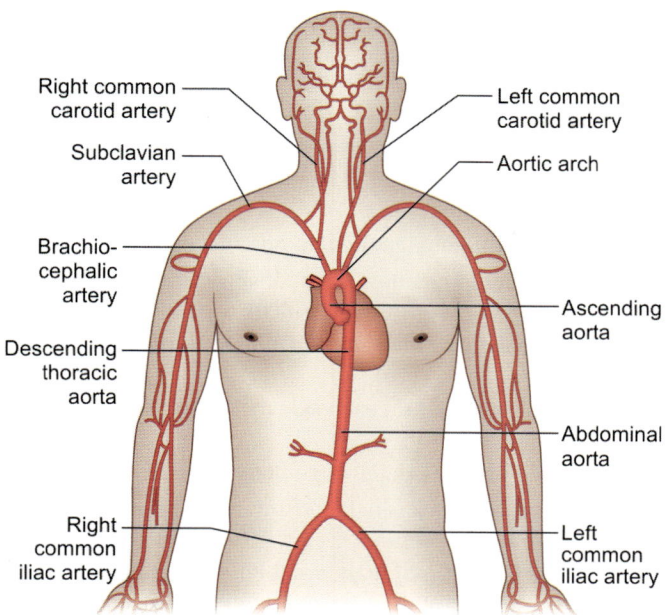

Fig. 2.2: Anatomy of aorta

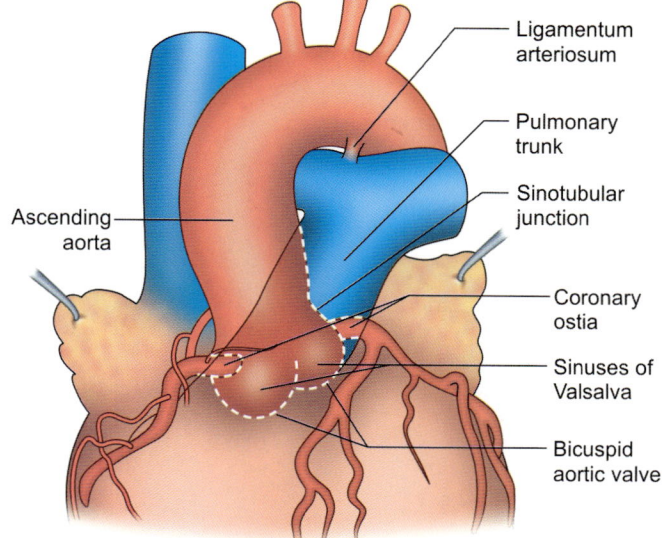

Fig. 2.3: Adjacent structures of aorta as it ascends

pulmonary artery and is known as aortic arch. From there it descends inferiorly to the left of the spine. The part of descending aorta that passes through chest is called thoracic aorta and the part which descends through abdomen is called abdominal aorta. After giving various branches, it ends in iliac arteries at L4 level (Fig. 2.2 )

*Branches of aorta*: The first branches of aorta are left and right coronary arteries. From upper surface of aortic arch arise bracheocephalic trunk, right and left common carotid artery (Fig. 2.4). Left subclavian and aorta starts

descending in front of the spine. The internal diameter at this level is 2.5 cm in adults. Branches arising from thoracic aorta are mentioned in *Box 2.2* and Fig. 2.5. *Aortic isthmus* is that segment of aorta where the distal arch descends down to form descending aorta. The isthmus is an important structure because from here onwards aorta is fixed to the posterior thoracic cage by pleural reflection, intercostal arteries and ligamentum arteriosum. This area is highly vulnerable to traumatic injury when subjected to high sheer force due to blunt trauma.

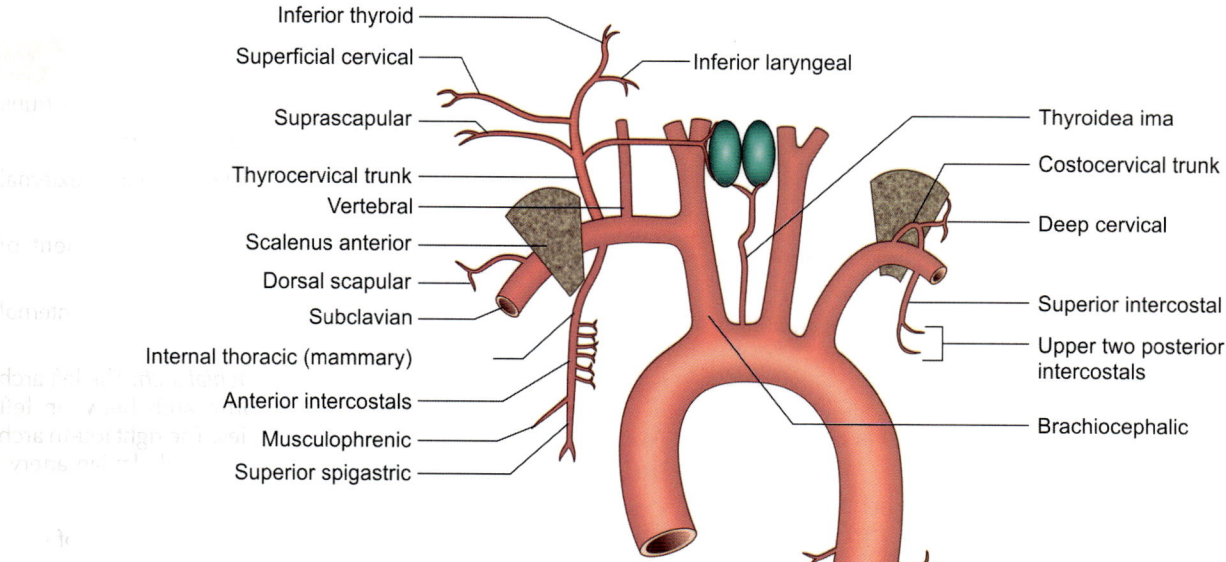

Fig. 2.4: Branches from ascending aorta and arch of aorta

- Nine bilateral posterior intercostals arteries 3rd to 11th intercostals space
- Two subcostal arteries
- Two left bronchial arteries
- Esophageal branches
- Pericardial branches
- Mediastinal branches
- Superior phrenic arteries

- Phrenic (paired) originates just below the diaphragm: Supplying it from below
- Celiac (single) large anterior branch
- Superior mesenteric (single) large anterior branch: Arises just below celiac trunk
- Middle supra-adrenal (paired) to adrenal gland
- Renal (paired) large artery each, arising from the side of the aorta: Supplies corresponding kidney
- Gonadal (paired) ovarian artery in females and testicular artery in males
- Lumbar (paired) four on each side that supply the abdominal wall and spinal cord
- Inferior mesenteric (single) large anterior branch
- Median sacral artery (single) arising from the middle of the aorta at its lowest part
- Common Iliac (paired) branches (bifurcates) to supply blood to the lower limbs and the pelvis, ending the abdominal aorta

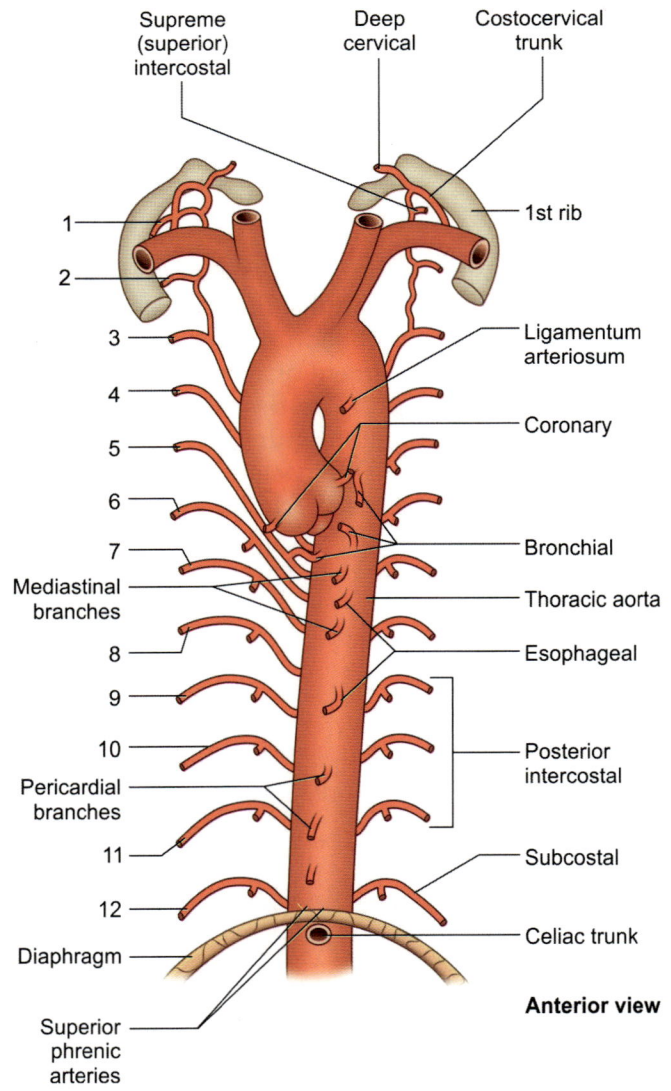

Fig. 2 5: Branches of thoracic aorta

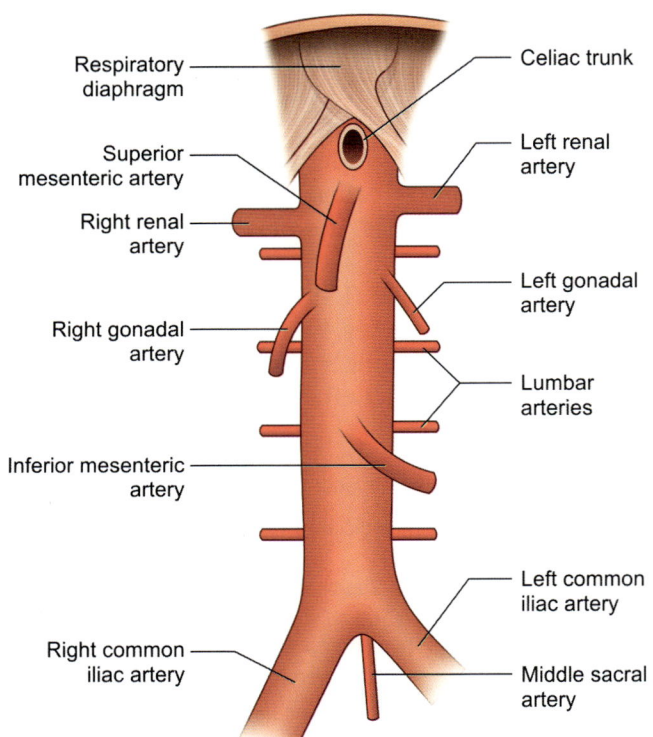

Fig. 2.6: Branches of abdominal aorta

The abdominal aorta supplies blood to much of the abdominal cavity. It begins at T12. Branches of abdominal aorta are mentioned in *Box 2.3* and Fig. 2.6.

## HISTOLOGY

Aorta as well as all arteries are composed of three layers. **Intima** lined by endothelium is the inner lining of the vessel. Endothelium is responsible for control of hemostasis, by acting as a barrier between subendothelial hemorrhagic layer and the blood circulating in the vessel by producing platelet inhibiting prostaglandin I.

Endothelium, due to direct contact with blood is easily traumatized and prone to atherosclerosis. The medial part is known as **media**. This is a thick layer constituting almost 50% of aortic wall thickness. Media is mainly composed of smooth muscle cells. These smooth muscles are binded by collagen and elastin. Media provide tensile strength and elasticity to the vessel. The third and the outermost layer is **adventitia** (Fig. 2.7). It is composed mainly of collagen and vasa vasorum. However, vasa vasorum is absent in infrarenal part of aorta. The blood supply to the intima and media are by diffusion from blood circulating in the lumen while the interstitium is nourished from vasa vasorum. However the infrarenal part of aorta is deficient in vasa vasorum. Probably that explains the increased incidence of aneurysm in infrarenal region.

These three histological layers cannot be distinguished by echocardiography or seen by currently available imaging techniques. However, dissection, diseases or trauma which produces separation of layers can be picked up by imaging techniques like MRI or computerized tomography or angiography.

*Classification of aortic diseases*: Aortic diseases are classified according to:

1. Underlying pathological condition
2. Location of lesion, whether in ascending aorta thoracic aorta or abdominal aorta
3. Depending upon absence or presence of dissection.

Commonest classification used is depending upon amenability to surgery (*Box 2.4*).

| Box 2.4 | Diseases of aorta which are amenable to surgery |
|---|---|

1. **Acute conditions**
   Acute trauma
   Acute aortic dissection
   Impending rupture

2. **Chronic disease of aorta**
   *Aneurysms*:
   *Developmental*: Marfan's syndrome, Ehlers Danlos syndrome
   *Degenerative*: Cystic medial degeneration, atherosclerotic
   *Chronic post-traumatic*: Blunt trauma
   *Inflammatory*:
   ▪ Takayasu's arteritis
   ▪ Kawasaki disease
   ▪ Behcet's disease
   ▪ Giant cell disease
   *Infected*: Bacterial, fungal, spirochetal viral
   *Mechanical*: Poststenotic associated with arteriovenous fistula
   *Anastomotic*: Postarteriotomy
   **False aneurysm**
   **Chronic aortic dissection (dissection more than 14 days old)**
   Type A (Debakey Types I and II) ascending aorta involved
   Type B (Debakey Type III) descending aorta involved
   **Intramural or penetrating atherosclerotic ulcers: Rare condition**

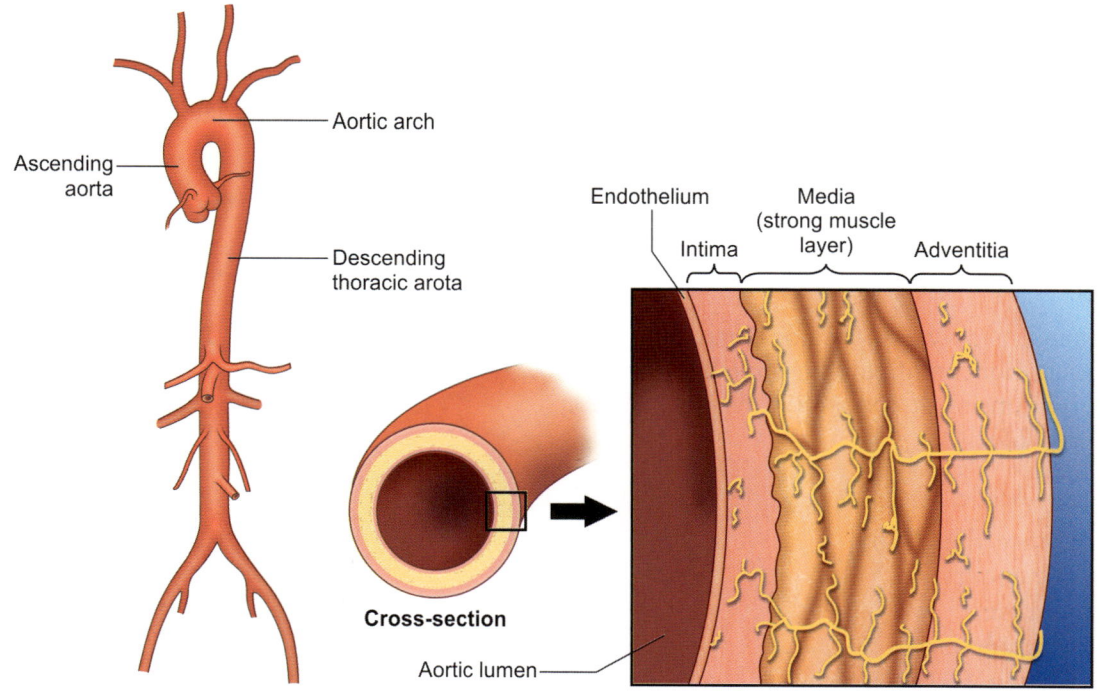

**Fig. 2.7:** Histology of aorta

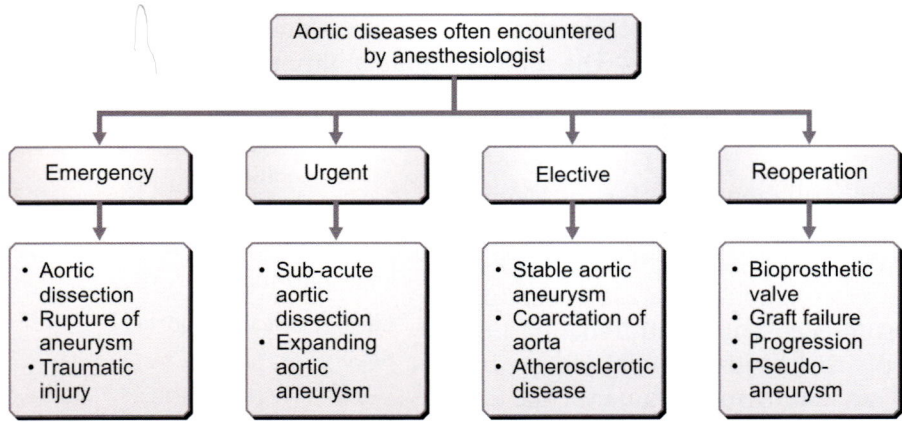

**Fig. 2.8:** Aortic diseases encountered by anesthesiologist

Anesthesiologists encounter most often aneurysm and dissection of aorta presenting for urgent emergent or elective surgery (Fig. 2.8) as mentioned below. Thereby they should be familiar with the extent of disease pathophysiology and etiopathogenesis of aortic aneurysms and aortic dissection in detail.

## PATHOGENESIS OF AORTIC ANEURYSM

### Definitions

*Aneurysm*: Permanent localized aortic dilatation which has at least 50% increase in diameter and include the entire three walls.

*Ectasia*: Aortic dilatation is less than 50% of normal.

*Annuloaortic ectasia*: Isolated dilatation of ascending aorta, aortic root, and aortic valve annulus. Annuloaortic ectasia involves fibrous components of aortic annulus and annulus is primarily enlarged. Dilatation includes the sinuses of valsalva and proximal ascending aorta later. Non-coronary sinus is first to dilate. Association with Marfan's disease and bicuspid aortic valve has been found. This condition frequently leads to aortic regurgitation, acute dissection or combination of both. Annuloaortic ectasia is commonly seen in men during 4 to 6 decade of life.

*Pseudoaneurysm or false aneurysm*: Localized dilatation of aorta that does not contain all the three layers of the vessel wall and consist of connective tissue and clot (Fig. 2.9 and *Box 2.5*).

### Classification of Aortic Aneurysm

*According to location* (Fig. 2.10)
Ascending aortic aneurysm
Aortic arch aneurysm
Descending aortic aneurysm
Thoracoabdominal aortic aneurysm
Abdominal aortic aneurysm

| Box 2.5 | Causes of false aneurysm |
|---|---|

- They arise by intimal rupture or these are caused by contained rupture of aorta
- Penetrating atheroma is also one of the causes
- Partial dehiscence of the suture line at the site of previous aortic prosthetic vascular graft may result in postoperative pseudoaneurysm

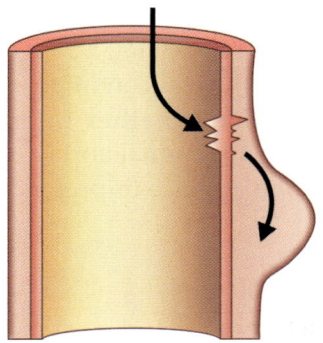

**Fig. 2.9:** False aneurysm

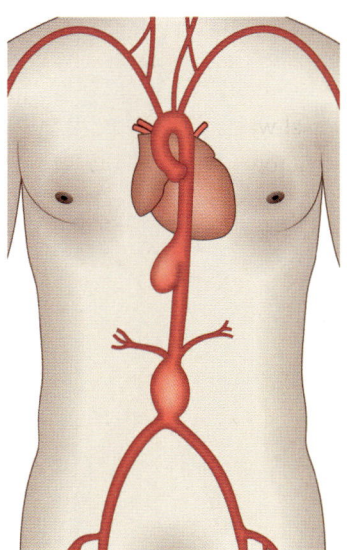

**Fig. 2.10:** According to location

## As per the shape of aortic aneurysm

- Fusiform
- Sacular
- Pseudoaneurysm (Fig. 2.9)

Special focus is being given on aortic aneurysm (Fig. 2.11) and dissections as these are commonly managed by the anesthesiologist in the preanesthesia period and perioperatively during elective or emergent surgery.

## ETIOPATHOGENESIS OF AORTIC ANEURYSM

Pathology of aortic aneurysms is not only multifactorial it is highly complex. Significant genetic and environmental risk factors and numerous co-morbid conditions are associated with aortic diseases. Research studies in the last two decades have aided in understanding the etiology and pathogenesis of aortic aneurysm. Epidemiological risk factors are listed in *Box 2.6*.

Characteristic histological features of aortic aneurysms are destruction of elastic and collagen predominantly in media and adventitia layers (*Box 2.7*). Thinning of vessel wall occurs due to loss of smooth muscle cells.

| Box 2.6 | Risk factors involved in aortic aneurysm |
| --- | --- |

- Male sex
- Cigarette smoking
- Hypertension
- Advanced age
- Atherosclerosis
- Genetic predisposition
- Overweight
- High cholesterol
- Family history of cardiovascular or peripheral vascular disease

| Box 2.7 | Characteristic histological picture of aortic aneurysm |
| --- | --- |

- Destruction of elastic and collagen in media and adventitia
- Thinning of vessel wall due to loss of smooth muscles
- Infiltration of macrophages and leukocytes

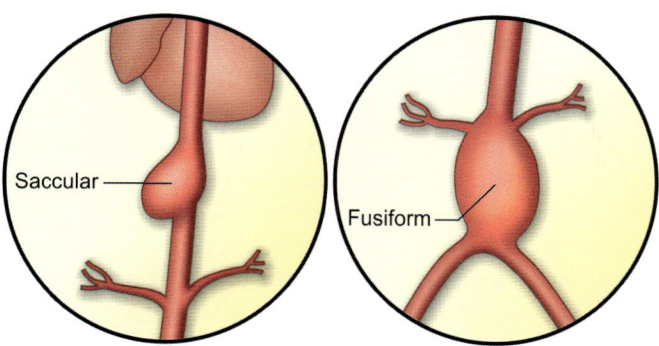

**Fig. 2.11:** Sacular and fusiform aneurysms

Wassef et al (2001) in UK in Natural Biology Research Programme summarized the aortic aneurysm pathogenesis under broad, four headings (*Box 2.8*).

| Box 2.8 | Pathogenic mechanism leading to aortic aneurysm |
| --- | --- |

1. Proteolytic degradation of aortic wall connective tissue
2. Inflammation and immune response
3. Molecular genetics
4. Biochemical wall stress

Figure 2.12 explains various sequences of events. In pathogenesis factors like localized hemodynamic, biochemical wall stress, genetic predisposition and fragmentation of medial layer are involved in formation of aneurysm through a complex mechanism which attracts inflammatory cells in aortic wall and release immulological mediators and chemokines. Metallo proteases cathepsins and serine proteases get induced resulting in medial degeneration and apoptosis ultimately forming aneurysmal dilatation. Continued wall stress eventually result in rupture.

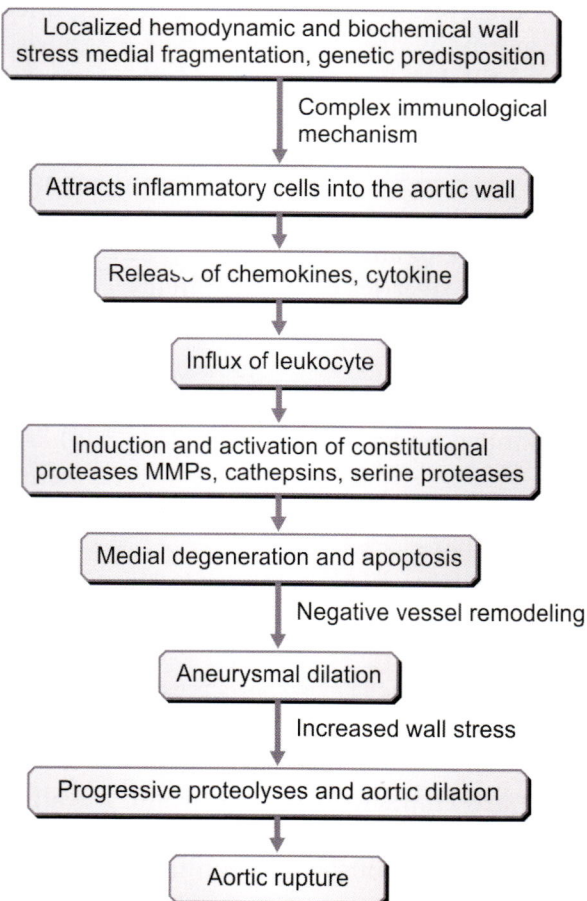

**Fig. 2.12:** Sequence of events in pathogenesis of aortic aneurysm

Little differences have been noticed in aneurysm arising at various sites (*Box 2.9*).

| Box 2.9 | Aneurysm arising at various sites |
|---------|-----------------------------------|
| Ascending aortic aneurysm | Underlying bicuspid valve in 75% of patients |
| Thoracic aortic aneurysm | Predominantly show cystic medial degeneration<br>Fragmentation of elastic lamellae<br>Non-inflammatory loss of media |
| Abdominal aortic aneurysm | Severe intimal atherosclerosis<br>Chronic transmural inflammation<br>Neovascularization<br>Elastic media show destructive remodeling |

Bicuspid aortic valve has been associated with almost 75% of patient being operated for ascending aortic aneurysm. Thoracic aortic aneurysm features more of cystic medial degeneration, fragmentation of elastic lamellae but not much of inflammatory reaction. Abdominal aortic aneurysm in majority remain silent for years as they are asymptomic. They are more in men than women but in women these carry significantly higher morbidity and mortality. Their diagnosis may be missed till they become aged and die of some other causes.[2] Proteolysis plays a predominant role in addition to atherothrombosis. Abnormal production of proteolytic enzymes and elastidase has been demonstrated. Immune mediated changes and deficiency of collagen elastin may also be an etiological factor.[3] Research studies in the last two decades have aided in understanding of etiology and pathogenesis of aortic aneurysm.[4]

*Proteolytic atherothrombosis*: Characteristic pathological features of abdominal and thoracoabdominal aneurysm are mentioned under four headings (*Box 2.10*).

| Box 2.10 | Pathology of aortic aneurysm |
|----------|------------------------------|
| ■ Presence of hemoglobin-rich intraluminal thrombus |
| ■ Medial destruction role of proteases, metalloprotein proteases ( MMP) |
| ■ *Adventitial reaction*: Immunoinflammatory and fibroblastic |
| ■ Genetic susceptibility |

These are characterized by chronic intraluminal thrombus (ILT), medial destruction and are also associated with significant adventitial reaction.

*Intraluminal thrombus*: Hemoglobin rich: It is a laminated structure made up of many layers of fibrin clot. ILT has been shown to play an important role in aneurysmal dilatation whatever is the site of aneurysm. Thinned out arterial wall is evident in association with ILT.[5] Presence of ILT has been found to be participating in aneurysmal dilatation.[6] The luminal layer of ILT is biologically active characterized by red blood cell hemagglutination. This process releases free hemoglobin and fibrin formation by activation of platelets and thrombin and tissue plasminogen activation and plasminogen reaction.[7, 8] It has also been linked with enhanced activity of oxidant enzymes. The hem group liberated as a process of hemoglutination generates free radicals and reduces activity of oxidant chelators.[9] Neutorophils are more numerous in ILT and associated with increased level of MMP2 and MMP9.[10]

## Medial Degeneration

It is a complex process of destruction of aortic media and reduction in smooth muscle density to the extent that elastic lamallae may also be absent. The degradation of elastic fibers is related to release of matrix metalloprotein proteases.[11] Matrix metaloproteinase proteases (MMPs) are derived from macrophages. Neutrophil and aortic smooth cell play a critical role during aneurysm formation. MMP2 and MMP9 both have elastolytic and collagenolytic properties. Elastase is elevated in serum from patients with abdominal aortic aneurysm. It has been documented to play a role in expansion and rupture of aortic aneurysm.[12] The other biomarkers which are useful in diagnosis are serum elastin peptides, amino terminal propeptide of type III, procollagen.[13,14] Recently D dimer and plasmin-antiplasmin has been correlated with aortic diameter and ILT as well as with aneurysm growth in patients with aortic aneurysm.[15]

| Box 2.11 | Response in adventitia |
|----------|------------------------|
| ■ Neoangiogenesis |
| ■ Immunoinflammatory |

Adventitia reacts to centrifugal insult by immune inflammatory response and angiogenic response. (*Box 2.11*) Pathogenic fibrosis of adjacent retroperitoneum and adherence to adjacent structure is commonly seen in association with inflammatory abdominal aortic aneurysm.[16] Neoangiogenesis remain localized in adventitia and outer part of media. Correlation exists between degradation of elastic fibers neoangiogenesis and leukocyte infiltration.[16] Extensive transmural infiltration of macrophages and lymphocytes is the predominant histological feature of aortic wall in aortic aneurysm. Exposed elastin degradation products in the aortic wall are the possible chemotactic attractant to induce infiltration of macrophages. Pro-inflammatory cytokines are also elevated in aortic aneurysmal wall leading to secretion of MMPs.[12] Mast cells have also been shown to contribute to pathogenesis of aortic aneurysm.[17,18] Presence of mast cell has been associated with neoangiogenesis. Mast cells present in the outer media and adventitia of abdominal aortic aneurysm has been correlated with aneurysmal diameter and presence of ILT and high circulatory level of IgE and IgG4.[19,20] Nitric oxide has been known to play its role in aortic aneurysm formation due to its property to alter vessel wall remodeling. NO induces MMP9 which initiate vessel wall degeneration and aneurysm formation[21].

## Biochemical Wall Stress

Infrarenal site is the preferential site for abdominal aortic aneurysm. This is because of a natural decrease of number of elastic layer to almost half in infrarenal aorta as compared to thoracic aorta. Diminished elastin predisposes to aortic dilation. Super added collagen degradation may result in aortic rupture. Increased MMP9 activity is reported in infrarenal aorta as compared to thoracic or abdominal aorta.[22] Increased wall stress is an important factor for accelerating dilation and risk of rupture. Turbulent blood flow results from expansion of flow stream from normal to dilated aorta further leading to aortic expansion. Increased stress has been found at the interface between the less distensible proximal part of abdominal aortic aneurysm and more distensible distal part of abdominal aortic aneurysm which may result in rupture. Beta blockers are recommended to reduce the wall stress as a protection against continued aneurysm dilation and rupture.

## MOLECULAR GENETICS IN AORTIC ANEURYSM

Though thoracic and abdominal aortic aneurysm are not associated with any syndrome, still genetic factors have been shown to play a role in etiology.[23] At least 20% of aneurysm result from inherited disorders like Marfan's syndrome, Ehlers-Danlos syndrome and others.[23] Genome scan for familial aortic aneurysm using sex and family history as covariates suggested genetic heterogeneity linkage with 19q13 chromosome.[24] In monozygotic twins with affected parents, the risk of developing abdomin aortic aneurysm is seven times higher than in monozygotic twins of unaffected parent.

## Aortic Dissection

Acute aortic dissection is the most common life-threatening disorder affecting the aorta.[26] The immediate mortality rate in aortic dissection is as high as 1% per hour over the first several hours, making early diagnosis and treatment critical for survival. When blood from normal aortic channel enters under pressure through an intimal tear it separates the aortic wall, cleaving the medial layer, the lesion is named as aortic dissection. This results in formation of false lumen and may extend proximally to the extent of aortic valve producing aortic regurgitation or distally or both sides.[27] The weakened aortic wall has a tendency to rupture.

*Predisposing factors*: Dissection of ascending aorta is more common, between 50 and 60 years of age. At later ages descending aortic dissections are more frequent. Most often the aortic wall of patient in whom dissection occur shows their pathology report as essentially normal as per their age group.[28-30] Hypertension is present in 75% of individuals with aortic dissection. Genetically triggered disorders affecting the aorta are important and often under recognized as a cause of aortic dissection. Marfan's syndrome, Loeys-Dietz syndrome, vascular Ehlers-Danlos syndrome, bicuspid aortic valve, Turner syndrome are all genetic conditions associated with thoracic aortic.[28-34] Prior cardiac surgery, especially

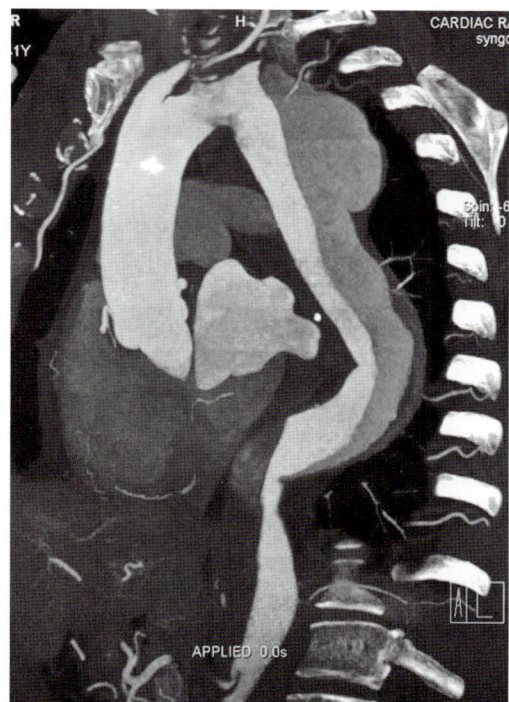

**Fig. 2.13:** CT angiography showing Type B aortic dissection. The image reveals the false lumen with the white arrow head pointing towards the origin or the entry point of the dissection. A small aneurysm is also seen in the proximal descending thoracic aorta

| Box 2.12 | Risk factors for aortic dissection |

- Age
- Hypertension and atherosclerosis
- *Genetically triggered diseases*:
  - Marfan syndrome
  - Bicuspid aortic valve
  - Loeys-Dietz syndrome
  - Turner syndrome
  - Vascular Ehlers-Danlos syndrome
- *Congenital disease*:
  - Coarctation of the aorta
  - Tetralogy of Fallot
- Trauma blunt injury
- Catheter/stent. Intra-aortic balloon pump
- Aortic vascular surgery
- Coronary artery bypass surgery
- *Inflammatory infectious disease*:
  - Syphilis
  - Aortitis
  - Takayasu's arteritis
  - Giant cell arteritis
- Pregnancy

aortic valve replacement and aortic manipulation (including angiography and stenting), are risk factors for aortic dissection (*Box 2.12*).[37] Acute hemodynamic stress such as that encountered with cocaine use[35], pheochromocytoma, and heavy weightlifting has been associated with aortic dissection. Aortic dissection may complicate aortitis[34], most commonly giant cell arteritis.[36] Acute aortic dissection complicating pregnancy is uncommon.[37] It usually occurs during labour and delivery or in the early postpartum period. Although hormonal changes in the aortic wall have been theorized as playing a potential role, an underlying genetic disorder associated with abnormalities of the aortic wall is most likely the underlying cause for aortic dissection complicating pregnancy. Cystic medial degeneration is the pathology underlying many thoracic aortic dissections as well as in aneurysm. Patients with thoracic aortic aneurysms from any cause are at risk for aortic dissection, with absolute size especially > 5 to 6 cm. The details and classification is narrated in Chapter 7.

*False channel*: False channel formed by dissection enlarges as time passes. In many instances, aortic enlargement is usually diffuse. Slowly the aortic wall tends to weaken and tends to become aneurysmal and saccular or fusiform aneurysm may result. Occasionally the false channel may become partially or total thrombosed.

*Penetrating atheromatous ulcer*: These occur often in descending aorta when atherosclerotic lesion involving intima ulcerate and penetrate the internal elastic lamina of aortic wall.[38]

*Intramural hematoma*: This occurs either because of rupture of an atheromatous plaque or spontaneous rupture of vasa vasoram.

*Diffuse atherosclerotic disease*: Mobile or pedunculated atheromas may occur in any part of aorta resulting in recurrent cerebral vascular accidents. Sometimes this condition is amenable to surgery.[39]

## Pathophysiology of Peripheral Vascular Disease

Peripheral vascular disease usually manifest as thrombosis or embolism. Atherosclerosis obliterans is another name given to peripheral vascular disease. This results from atherosclerosis. Atheroma thrombus in the vessel has a core of cholesterol with protein and fibrous intravascular covering. The atheroma may progress to complete occlusion. Athermatous thrombi occur more frequently in the lower extremities than upper extremities usually occluding medium and large arteries. Factors that predispose to thrombosis are sepsis, low cardiac output, aneurysm or aortic dissection.

*Embolism*: These are the most common causes of sudden peripheral ischemia. In 80% of patients emboli are from cardiac origin but can also originate from proximal atheroma or tumor. Atheromas have tendency to lodge at bifurcations, e.g. femoral artery bifurcation or iliac artery bifurcation.

Peripheral vascular disease whether caused by embolism or atheromas may result in loss of limb or loss of life due to flow stagnation resulting in proximal and distal thrombus formation.

## REFERENCES

1. Wassef M, Baxter BT, Chisholm RL, et al. Pathogenesis of abdominal aortic aneurysm; multi disciplinary research program supported by the National Heart, Lung and blood institute. J Vasc Surg 2001; 34:730–8.

2. Michel JB, Ventura JLM, Egido J, et al. Novel aspect of the pathogenesis of aneurysms of the abdominal aorta in humans. Cardiovasc Res. 2011; 90:18–27.

3. Kouchoukos NT, Dougenis D. Surgery of the thoracic aorta. N. Engl J Med 1997; 336:1876–88.

4. Swensson LG, Crawford ES. Aortic dissection and aortic aneurysm surgery clinical observations, experimental, investigation and statistical analyses. Part III Curr Prob. Surg. 1993; 30:1–163.

5. Kazi M, Thyberg J, Religa P, Roy J, Eriksson P, Hedin U et al. Influence of intramural thrombus on structural and cellular composition of abdominal aortic aneurysm wall. J Vase Surg 2003; 38:1283–92.

6. Von Kodolitsch Y, Csosz SK, Koschyk DH, et al. Intraluminal hematoma of aorta: predictor of progression to dissection and rupture. Circulation 2003; 107:1158–63.

7. Vorp DA, Lee PC, Wang DH, et al. Association of intra luminal thrombus in abdominal aortic aneurysm with local hypoxia and wall weakening. J Vas Surg 2001; 34:291–9.

8. Forntaine V, Jacob MP, Houard X, et al. Involvement of the mural thrombus as a site of protease release and activation in human aortic aneurysms. Am J Pathol. 2002; 161:7101–10.

9. McCormick ML, Gavrila D, Weintraub NL. Role of oxidative stress in the pathogenesis of abdominal aortic aneurysm. Arterioscler thromb Vas Biol 2007; 27:461–9.

10. Houard X, Rouzet F, Touat Z, et al. Topology of fibrinolytic system within the mural thrombus of human abdominal aortic aneurysms. J Pathol 2007; 212:20–8.

11. Ailawadi G, Eliason JL, Upchurch GR Jr. Current concepts in pathogenesis of abdominal aortic aneurysm. J Vasc surg 2003; 38:584–8.

12. Touat Z, Ollivier V, Dai J, Huisse MG, Bezeaud A, Sebbag U et al. Renewal of mural thrombus releases plasma markers and is involved in abdominal aneurysm evolution. Am J Pathol 2006; 168:1022–30.

13. Parry DJ, Al Barjas HS, Chappel L, Rashid T, Ariens RA, Scott DJ. Haemostatic And fibrolytic factors in men with a small abdominal aortic aneurysm. Br J Surg 2009; 96:870–7.

14. Wallinder J, Bergqvist D, Henriksson AE. Haemostatic markers in patients with abdominal aortic aneurysm and the impact of aneurysm size. Thromb Res 2009; 124:423–6.

15. Golledge J Muller R Clancy P, McCann M, Norman PE. Evaluation of the diagnostic and prognostic value of D dimer for abdominal aortic aneurysm. Eur Heart J 2011; 32:354–64.

16. Hellmann DB, grand DJ, Freischlag JA. Inflammatory abdominal aortic aneurysm. JAMA 2007; 297:396–400.

17. Sun J, Zhang J, Lindholt JS, Sukhova GK, Liu J, He A, et al. Critical role of mast cell chymase in mouse abdominal aortic aneurysm formation. Circulation 2009; 120:973–82.

18. Tsuruda T, Kato J, Hatakeyama K, Yamashita A, Nakamura K, Ikamura T el al. Adrenomedullin in mast cells of abdominal aortic aneurysm. Cardiovasc Res 2006; 70:158–64.

19. Mayranpaa MI, Trosien JA, Fontaine V, Folkesson M, Kazi M, Eriksson P, et al. Mast cells associate with neovessels in the media and adventitia of abdominal aortic aneurysm, J, Vasc, Surg 2009; 50:388–95.

20. Kasashimas, Zen Y, Kawashima A, Endo M, Matsumoto Y, Kasashima F. A new clinicopathological entity of IgG 4-related inflammatory abdominal aortic aneurysm, J Vas Surg 2009; 49:1264–71.

21. Johanning JM, Armstrong PJ, Franklin DP, et al. Nitric oxide in experimental aneurysm formation. Early events and consequences of nitric oxide inhibition. Ann Vasc Surg 2002; 16:65–72.

22. Ailawadi G, Knipp BS, Lu G, et al. A nonintrinsic regional basis for increased infrareal aortic MMP9 expression and activity. J Vasc. Surg 2003; 37:1059–66.

23. Kuivanieni H, Platsoucas C, Tilson MD. Aortic Aneurysms: An immense disease with a strong genetic component. Circulation. 2008; 117:242–52.

24. Shibamura H, Olson JM, van Vlijimen – Van Keulen C et al. Genome scan for familial abdominal aortic aneurysm using sex and family history as covariates suggests genetic heterogeneity and identifies linkage to chromosome 19 q I3 Circulation 2004; 109:2103–8.

25. Wahlgren CM, Larsson E, Magnusson PK, Hultgren R, Swedenborg J. Genetic and environmental contribution to abdominal aortic aneurysm development in a twin population J Vasc Surg 2010; 51:3–7.

26. Hager PG, Nienaber CA, Isselbacher M, Bruckman D, Kavairta DJ, russman PL, Evangelista a, Fattar R, Suribi SK, Moore AG, Malouf JF, Gulan D, Das SK, Armstrong WF, Eagle KA, International registry of acute Aortic dissection (IRAD). JAMA 2000; 283:897–903.

27. Golledge J, Eagle K A. Acute aortic dissection Lancet 2008; 372:55–66.

28. Larson EW, Edwards WD. Risk factor for Aortic dissection. A Necropsy study of 161 cases Am J Cardioc 1984; 53:849.

29. Shachter N, Perloff JK, Mulder DG. Aortic dissection in Noonan's syndrome, Am J, Cardiol 1984; 54:464–5.

30. Schlatmann TJ, Becker AE. Histological changes in normal aging aorta implication for dissecting aortic aneurysm. Am J Cardiol 1977; 39:13–20.

31. Anabtawi IN, Ellison RG, Yeh TJ, Hall DP. Dissecting aneurysm of aorta associated with turner's syndrome, J. Thorac. Cardio vasc Surg 1964; 47:750–4.

32. Edwards WD, Leaf DS, Edwards JE. Dissecting aortic aneurysm associated with congenital bicuspid aortic valve. Circulation 1978; 57:1022.

33. Prenger K, Pieters F, Cheriex E, Aortic dissection after aortic valve replacement, incidence and consequences of strategy. J Card Surg. 1994; 9:498–9.

34. Roberts WC. The congenitally bicuspid aortic valve. a study of 85 autopsy cases. Am J Cardiol 1970; 26:72–84.

35. Singh A, Khaja A, Alpert MA. Cocaine and aortic dissection. Vasc Med. 2010; 15:127–33.

36. Gornik HL, Creager MA. Aortitis. Circulation. 2008; 117:3039–51.

37. Kinney-Ham L, Nguyen HB, Steele R, Walters EL. Acute Aortic Dissection in Third Trimester Pregnancy without Risk Factors. West J Emerg Med. 2011; 12:571–4.

38. Harris JA, Bis KG, Glover JL, Bendick PJ, Shetty A, Brown OW. Penetrating atherosclerotic ulcers in the Aorta J Vas Surg 1994; 19:98–9.

39. Muehrecke DD, Grimm RA, Nissen SE, Cosghave DM III. Recurrent cerebral vascular accidents are an indication for ascending aortic endarterectomy Am thorac Surg 1996; 61:1516–8.

# CHAPTER 3

# Anesthesia for Ascending Aortic Aneurysm

Neeti Makhija, Jitin Narula

## INTRODUCTION

Thoracic aortic aneurysms are common and are the 17th most common cause of death and 15th most common cause of death after age of 65 years.[1] The aortic aneurysm tends to affect older patients with the mean age for diagnosis in the sixth decade of life. 45% of thoracic aneurysms involve the ascending aorta, 10% the arch, 35% the descending aorta, and 10% the thoraco-abdominal aorta.[2]

The untreated, 5-year rate of survival for patients with thoracic aortic aneurysms ranges from 13 to 39%. As the aorta typically grows slowly at an approximate rate of 0.1 cm/year the disease process is usually gradual, but may however become virulent due to associated complications like aortic rupture, aortic dissection, aortic regurgitation, mycotic infection, tracheobronchial and esophageal compression, right pulmonary artery or right ventricular outflow tract obstruction and systemic embolism from mural thrombus.

Predictors of poor prognosis include large size (greater than 10 cm maximum transverse diameter), presence of symptoms, and associated cardiovascular disease, especially coronary artery disease, myocardial infarction, stroke and renal involvement.

## ANATOMY OF ASCENDING AORTA

The aorta is the largest artery carrying oxygenated blood from the heart to all parts of the body. The aorta begins at the left ventricular—aortic valve junction just to the right of the midline. Thereafter, it initially ascends superiorly and anteriorly, arches to the left and then descends through the thorax and abdomen and bifurcates into two iliac arteries (Fig. 3.1). Segment of

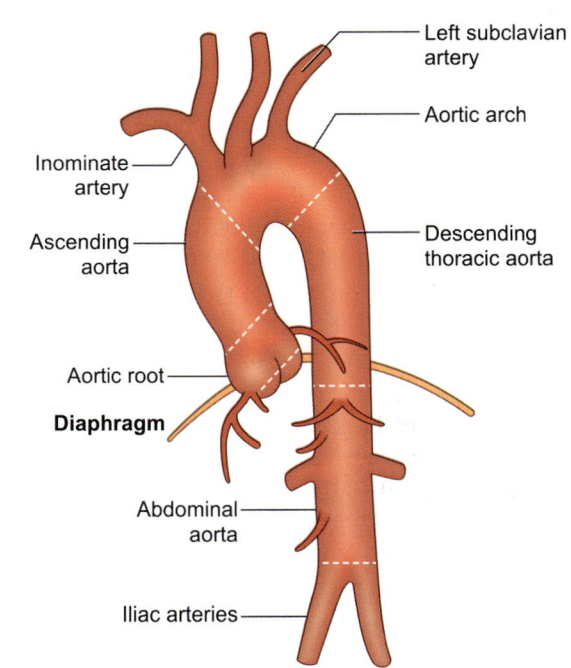

**Fig. 3.1:** Aorta along with its course and division into various segment

aorta from the annulus of the aortic valve up to the origin of innominate artery is called the ascending aorta. The origin of the innominate artery marks the beginning of the aortic arch. The aortic arch is the segment of the aorta between the innominate artery and the left subclavian artery, beyond which is the descending thoracic aorta. The ascending aorta is about 9 cm long in a normal adult and comprises the aortic root and ascending aorta. The aortic root and proximal ascending aorta lie within the pericardial sac. The aortic root includes the aortic valve annulus and the sinuses of Valsalva that terminate at the sinotubular junction (Fig. 3.2). Thus the ascending

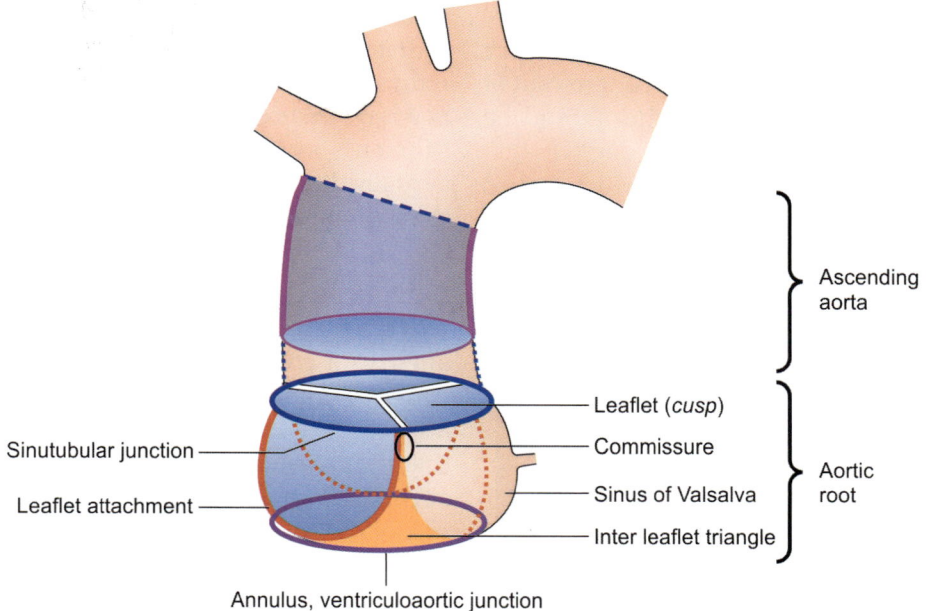

**Fig. 3.2:** Ascending aorta consisting of tubular ascending aorta and the aortic root comprising the aortic valve annulus, the sinuses of Valsalva and terminating at the sinotubular junction

thoracic aortic aneurysm is the aneurysm occurring between the annulus of the aortic valve and the origin of innominate artery.

The size of aorta decreases as the distance increases from the aortic valve. The normal diameter of ascending aorta and descending aorta respectively are <2.1 cm/m² and <1.6 cm/m². The normal diameter is in accordance with age, sex and workload. The size of aorta increases with age.[3] The diameter increases normally by 1–2 mm/ year during childhood and young adulthood. In adulthood, size is related to workload and exercise. With aging, there is loss of compliance and structural changes including increase in collagen content, intimal athero-sclerosis and calcium deposits occurs.[4–6]

*The aortic wall has three layers*: A thin intima or inner layer lined by endothelium, a thick media or middle layer, and a thin adventitia or outermost layer. Aneurysm is defined as localized thoracic aortic dilatation of all three layers of the vessel and having diameter at least 1.5 times normal of that segment. Aneurysms are described morphologically as fusiform or saccular. Fusiform aneurysms are more common, associated with athero-sclerotic or collagen vascular disease, and usually affect a longer segment of the aorta, producing a dilation of the entire circumference of the vessel wall and have a higher operative mortality than saccular aneurysms (Fig. 3.3A). Saccular aneurysms on the other hand are more localized, confined to an isolated segment of the aorta, and produce a localized outpouching of the vessel wall (Fig. 3.3B).

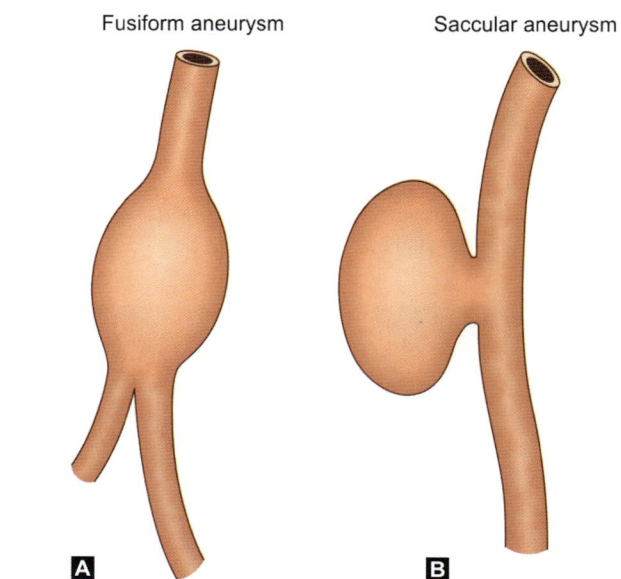

**Figs 3.3 A and B:** (A) Fusiform aneurysm, (B) Saccular aneurysm

Pseudoaneurysm or a false aneurysm is a localized aneurysmal dilation of the aorta that is not surrounded by all the three layers of the aortic wall as compared to the true aneurysm which is a localized dilatation surrounded by all three layers of wall. Pseudoaneurysm is usually a hematoma formed outside the arterial wall as a result of breach in intima or media or leaking hole in the artery. It is thus contained by the adventitia or the surrounding structures of the mediastinum. Pseudoaneurysm is different from arterial dissection, where there is separation of the layers of the wall. Pseudoaneurysm of aorta may develop following trauma, infection or postoperatively at the sites of aortic cannulation, proximal attachment of coronary artery grafts and at suture lines (Fig. 3.4). Pseudoaneurysm of aorta has an inherent risk of rupture and should be operated as early as possible.

Ectasia is localized dilatation of aorta which is less than 150% of normal. Annuloaortic ectasia is defined as an isolated dilatation of proximal ascending aorta, aortic root and aortic valve annulus and is usually associated with severe aortic regurgitation.[7] It may cause thoracic aortic dissection and rupture. It is often associated with Marfan's syndrome and can be a complication of syphilis. It is managed by implanting a composite graft that comprises both a valve and a conduit.

## ETIOPATHOGENESIS WITH RISK FACTORS

Aortic pathology predisposing ascending aortic aneurysm commonly includes cystic medial necrosis, congenital aortic anomalies like bicuspid or unicuspid aortic valve and hypertension. Generalized athero-sclerosis, various infections including mycotic, syphilitic aortitis, trauma and cigarette smoking also increase the risk of thoracic aortic aneurysm (Tables 3.1 and 3.2). At younger ages, cystic medial necrosis is associated with

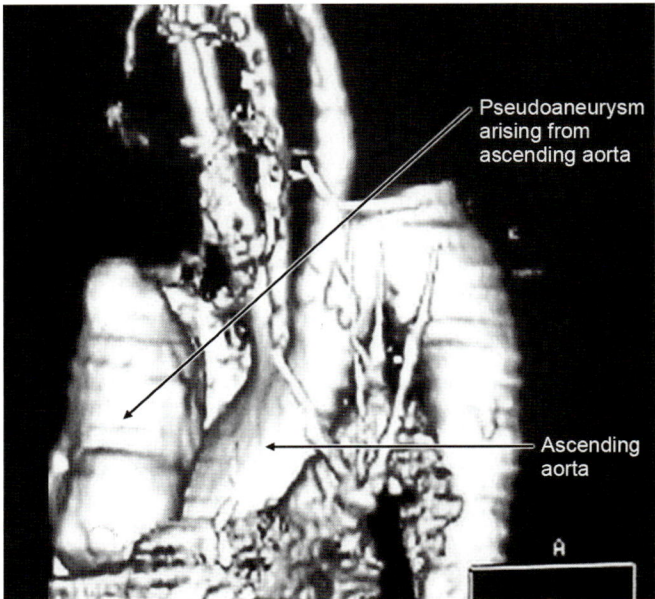

**Fig. 3.4:** A reconstructed computed tomography showing pseudoaneurysm arising from ascending aorta in a postcoronary artery bypass graft patient

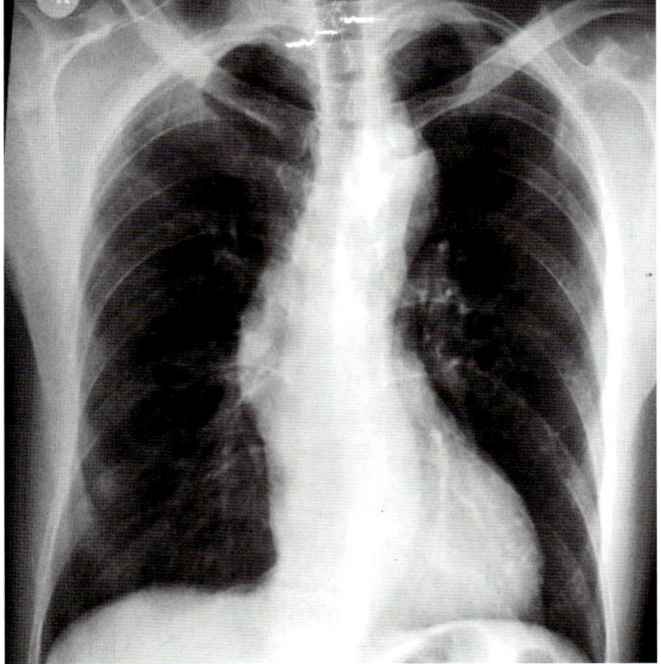

**Fig. 3.5:** X-ray chest posteroanterior view showing ascending aortic aneurysm

| Table 3.1: Etiology of aortic aneurysm | |
|---|---|
| **Congenital** | Cystic medial degeneration<br>· Marfan's syndrome<br>· Ehlers-Danlos syndrome<br>· Loeys-Dietz syndrome (LDS)<br>Bicuspid aortic valve (BAV)<br>Familial thoracic aortic aneurysm syndrome |
| **Hypertension** | |
| **Degenerative** | Atherosclerotic |
| **Post-traumatic** | Acute aortic transection<br>Blunt trauma<br>Penetrating trauma |
| **Inflammatory** | Takayasu's arteritis<br>Behçet's disease<br>Kawasaki disease<br>Giant cell arteritis |
| **Infected** | Bacterial<br>Fungal<br>Spirochetal<br>Viral |
| **Mechanical** | Associated with arteriovenous fistula |
| **Anastomotic** | Post-arteriotomy |
| **Post-stenotic dilation** | Secondary to long-standing aortic stenosis |

| Table 3.2: Risk factors for ascending aortic aneurysms | |
|---|---|
| 1. **Hypertension** | 5. **Chronic obstructive pulmonary disease** |
| 2. **Hypercholesterolemia** | 6. **Male** |
| 3. **Smoking** | 7. **Collagen vascular disease** |
| 4. **Advanced age** | 8. **Family history** |

various connective tissue diseases such as Marfan's syndrome caused by a mutation in the gene for fibrillin-1, Ehlers-Danlos syndrome type IV with a deficiency in type III collagen, Loeys-Dietz syndrome (LDS) due to mutations in transforming growth factor β-receptor genes (*TGFβR1* and *TGFβR2*) and familial/thoracic aortic aneurysm and dissection.[8]

Cystic medial degeneration involves fragmentation and degeneration of elastic fibers in medial layer of aorta. Also, there is abnormal synthesis of fibrillin, a glycoprotein which is component of aortic elastic fibres. Thus as the basophilic amorphous material accumulates, it imparts a cystic appearance to the media. There occurs smooth muscle cell loss.[9]

Marfan's is genetic disorder with defect in chromosome 15, affecting fibrillin synthesis.[10] On histological examination there is cystic medial degeneration, disruption of elastic fibres and fibrosis of media. Majority of patients with Marfan's syndrome have aortic dilatation with resultant aortic regurgitation. The Marfan's syndrome not only affects the cardiovascular system but also causes ocular, pulmonary, musculoskeletal, and central nervous system involvement.

There is growing evidence that many patients with bicuspid aortic valve (BAV) or aortic coarctation have disorders of vascular connective tissue as well, involving loss of elastic tissue.[11] The aortic expansion rate is higher in patients with BAV resulting in dilatation of the aortic root or ascending aorta, even in the absence of hemodynamically significant aortic valve stenosis or regurgitation.[11] Furthermore, the first-degree relatives of patients with thoracic aortic dilatation are also at increased risk and should be evaluated for manifestations of connective tissue disorders.

Atherosclerosis leads to narrowing of the arteries by the gradual formation of intimal plaques inside the arterial walls. Later on, there occurs secondary degeneration of the underlying media. It typically occurs in the elderly. It involves the abdominal aorta more commonly, followed by the descending and ascending aorta respectively, and thus presenting most commonly as thoracoabdominal aortic aneurysm.[12] The aneurysms are typically irregular, fusiform or saccular in contrast to uniform dilatation of cystic medial degeneration.[13] Aging results in changes in collagen and elastin, which lead to weakening of the aortic wall and aneurysmal dilation. Hypertension not only contributes to the formation but also accelerates the expansion of already existing aneurysms.

Aneurysm formation can also occur from medial destruction by inflammatory process. Aneurysm of ascending aorta may be caused by systemic vasculitis, as in giant cell or granulomatous arthritis, often associated with rheumatic disease.[14] Mycotic aneurysm due to primary bacterial infections of ascending aorta, are rare. They most commonly develop after the valvular endocarditis, or infection of aortic jet lesion.[15] Syphilis was a common cause of aneurysm of ascending aorta before the advent of modern antibiotic.

## CLINICAL PRESENTATION

Thoracic aortic aneurysms mostly are asymptomatic. Up to a half of patients with aortic lesions remain asymptomatic and are frequently discovered as an incidental finding. Possible explanations for the lack of symptoms might include distracting injuries in the patient with trauma, a chronic disease process or other masking coexisting disease processes.

Aortic lesions often present with a constellation of symptoms suggesting the ongoing events. These symptoms are a result of expansion, dissection, bony erosion or rupture of the aorta. Severe anterior chest or back pain is the most common presenting symptom. Pain may occur directly from aortic expansion or from involvement of nearby structures. Pain may extend into the neck, shoulders, or abdomen. The intensity of pain may not correlate with the size of the lesion.

Dilation of the aortic valve annulus, aortic root, and ascending aorta leads to the passive stretching of aortic valve leaflets and displacement of commissures causing central aortic regurgitation (AR). As a result of aortic regurgitation, congestive heart failure may develop. A large thoracic aortic lesion can impinge upon and damage the trachea or main-stem bronchus, leading to tracheomalacia and respiratory distress. The intrathoracic "mass effect" from a large thoracic aortic aneurysm can compress local structures to cause hoarseness (recurrent laryngeal nerve), dyspnea (trachea, mainstem bronchus, pulmonary artery), central venous hypertension (superior vena cava syndrome), and/or dysphagia/hematemesis (esophageal compression or erosion). Horner's syndrome may occur as a result of stellate ganglion compression. Expansion of ascending aortic aneurysm can result in dissection and/or rupture which is a surgical emergency and is often accompanied with acute pain with or without hypotension. Refractory hypotension may also result from rupture of the ascending aortic aneurysm into the pericardial cavity leading to cardiac tamponade as ascending aortic aneurysms rupture three fourth of the times into the pericardium.

Atherosclerotic aneurysm with mural thrombus may additionally present with stroke (embolism into carotid artery), mesenteric ischemia, renal insufficiency and/or limb ischemia.

In case of annuloaortic ectasia there may be worsening of aortic regurgitation. A diastolic murmer can be auscultated on the right of sternum. The presence of acute or subacute symptoms with associated chest pain is more common in annuloaortic ectasia patients compared with those of primary aortic regurgitation.

## INVESTIGATIONS

In case of dilatation of the ascending aorta >4.0 cm, evaluation of a possible connective tissue disease should be performed by a multidisciplinary team (cardiologist, geneticist, and ophthalmologist). Patient and family history should be investigated; physical examination should be undertaken, diagnostic investigations carried out; and eventually DNA testing should be done. Electrocardiographic findings may be normal or there may be changes consistent with left ventricular hypertrophy (increased QRS voltage) and strain showing ST-segment depression and T wave inversion. There may be ECG changes due to myocardial ischemia/infarction or pericarditis. Many patients with asymptomatic aneurysm may get detected on routine chest radiograph. Radiological findings may include loss of aortic contour, mediastinal widening, enlarged aortic knob, aortic calcifications and displacement of trachea and esophagus. Ascending aortic aneurysm may have a convex contour on right side of superior mediastinum, which is often difficult to distinguish from mediastinal tumor (Fig. 3.5). Loss of retrosternal airspace is often present on lateral chest radiograph.[16]

Transthoracic echocardiography (TTE) although not able to evaluate the entire length of aorta is a useful bedside first line investigation in patients with suspicion of aortic disease. In patients with shock TTE can screen for aortic dissection. TTE is helpful in examination of the aortic valve, quantification of aortic regurgitation and for identification of pericardial temponade or wall motion abnormalities.[17] Often an unsuspected dilated aortic root or ascending aortic aneurysm may be detected for the first time by echocardiography for assessment of aortic valve regurgitation. The diameter of the ascending aorta should be measured at 4 levels: The level of the annulus, the aortic sinuses, the sinotubular junction, and the proximal ascending aorta (Fig. 3.6). Transthoracic echocardiography can provide a reasonable examination of the thoracic aorta, although the acoustic windows are limited by the lungs and imaging of the proximal ascending aorta may be difficult to be visualized by TTE. Transesophageal echocardiography (TEE) helps in rapid detection of any dissection flap, intramural hematoma or intraluminal thrombus. However, distal ascending aorta and proximal arch

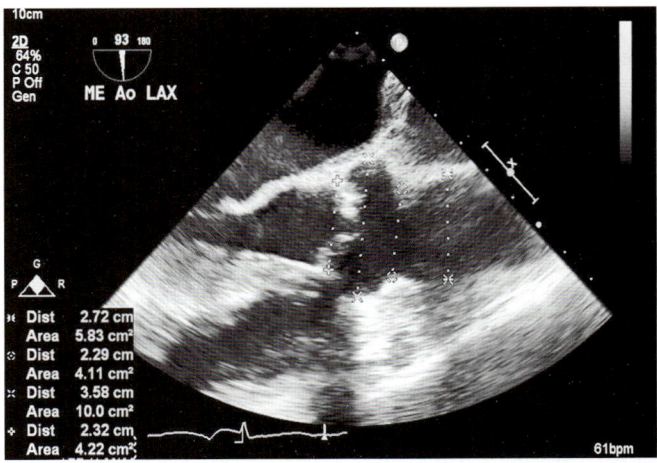

**Fig. 3.6:** TEE image of ascending aortic aneurysm showing measurement of aortic annulus, the aortic root the sinotubular junction, and the proximal ascending aorta

cannot be accurately imaged by TEE. The combined use of TTE and TEE may overcome these limitations. Both TTE and TEE with color interrogation are bedside echocardiographic techniques, used as first priority, for patients with suspected aortic syndromes who are unfit for transportation.[17] A detailed TEE evaluation of aorta for aneurysm is given in Chapter 12.

Computed tomographic angiography (CTA) images the thoracic aorta during the arterial phase of an intravenous radiocontrast agent injection. Arterial phase imaging coincides with arterial contrast opacification. It defines vascular anatomy and surrounding non-vascular structures (Fig. 3.7). A reconstructed 3D CT can show the entire ascending aorta, arch and descending thoracic aorta anatomy along with coronaries (Fig. 3.8). Aneurysm leak is detected as extravascular contrast extravasation. The delayed venous phase imaging helps

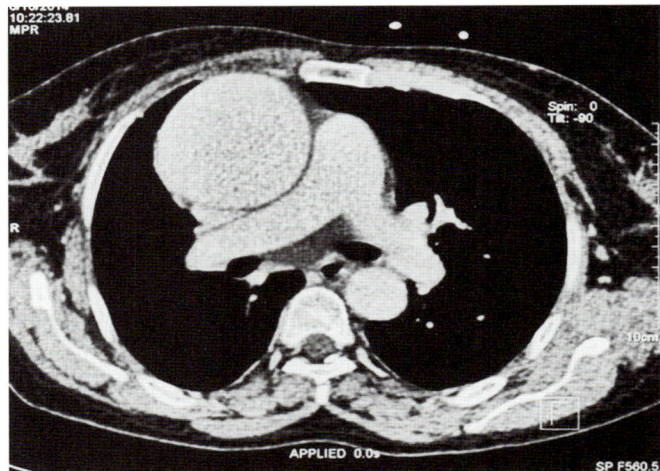

**Fig. 3.7:** Axial CT image showing aneurysm of ascending aorta compressing the superior vena cava between it and right pulmonary artery

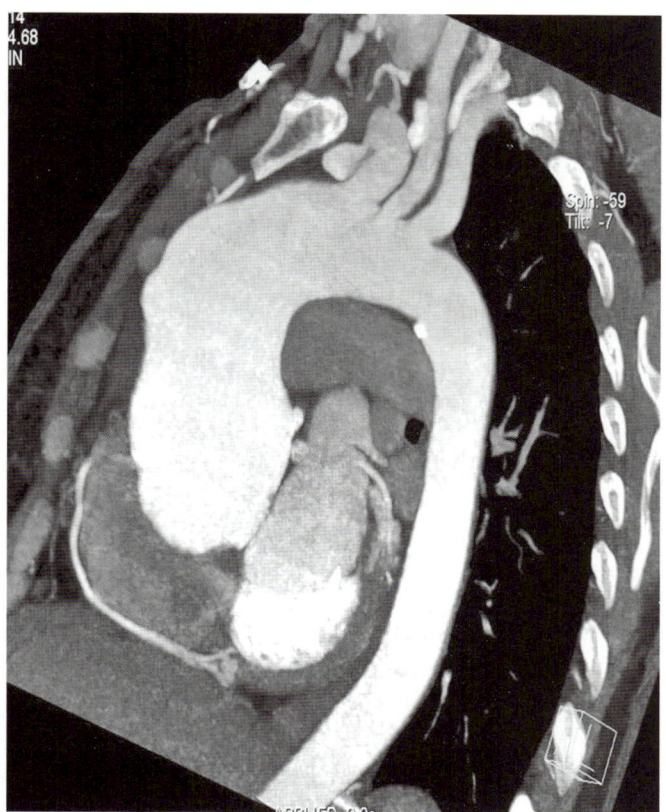

**Fig. 3.8:** Sagittal oblique CT showing entire ascending aorta, arch and descending thoracic aorta anatomy along with coronaries

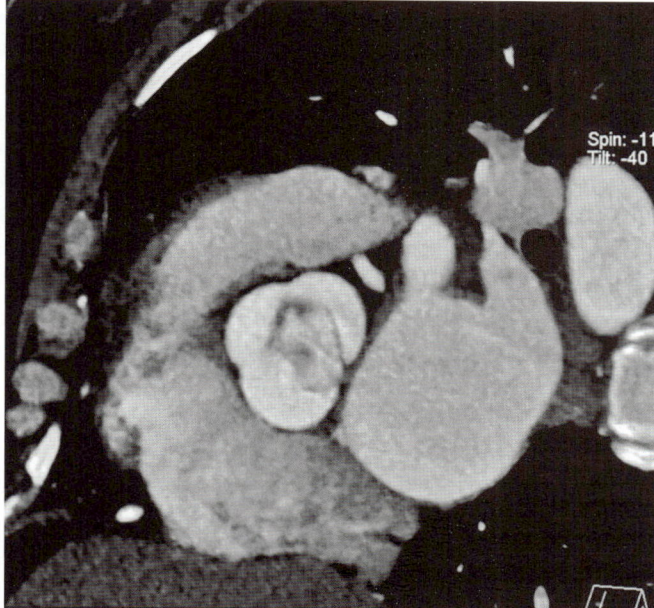

**Fig. 3.9:** Gated CT showing fusion, nodularity in leaflets with functionally bicuspid aortic valve

in evaluation of solid organs for mass lesions or for detection of endoleaks in patients with stent grafts by using 3D reconstruction. Gated CT can detect aortic valve abnormality (Fig. 3.9). This imaging modality has multiple advantages such as high resolution, wide availability, rapid acquisition, imaging in patients with metallic implants, and generation of volumetric aortic images for stent design. However, as CTA requires administration of iodinated contrast agents, it carries a risk for contrast nephropathy, that can be attenuated by ruling out any baseline renal dysfunction, ensuring a good hydration status of the patient before dye injection, administration of acetylcysteine and sodium bicarbonate.[18] Also, a dose of 10 to 25 mSv radiation is a concern in patients subjected to serial cardiovascular imaging.[19]

Magnetic resonance angiography is complementary imaging modality for thoracic aorta. Contrast-enhanced magnetic resonance angiography with gadolinium, has shortened the examination time, images the entire aorta in fine detail and has emerged as preferred MR modality for aortic diseases. Although the spatial resolution of magnetic resonance angiography is slightly inferior to CTA, it does allow for degrees of tissue and fluid characterization. The disadvantages of magnetic resonance angiography include its limited availability, lack of imaging in patients with metallic implants, imaging difficulty in the setting of continuous hemodynamic monitoring, and the time required for image acquisition. MRI is thus less suitable for unstable patients than CT.

Its advantages are the avoidance of ionizing radiation and the lack of renal toxicity associated with iodinated contrast used in CT.[20] MRA had been preferred in patients with renal failure as compared to CT, but with recent discovery of nephrogenic systemic fibrosis in patients with renal dysfunction who received gadolinium, non-enhanced MRA is now considered ideal[21].

Aortography was once an important modality for preoperative evaluation of aortic aneurysm but with the advent of CT and MRI its role has declined. Aortography, not only defines the anatomy of aortic aneurysm and arch vessels but also detects the presence of aortic regurgitation, dilatation of sinuses of Valsalva and displacement of coronary ostia. As a part of the preoperative evaluation in a patient undergoing surgery for aortic disease, coronary angiography is indicated in patients who have any evidence of coronary artery disease or in patients above the age of 40 years. Ascending aortography and left ventriculography may be performed in combination with coronary arteriography.[22] Duplex imaging of carotids is limited to patients more than 65 years of age to rule out any unaddressed severe carotid disease which is a significant risk factor for perioperative stroke.

Intraoperatively epiaortic ultrasonographic imaging of the ascending and descending thoracic aorta is useful for detecting atherosclerosis. Presence of severe atherosclerosis, including mobile or pedunculated atheroma, may necessitate alterations in surgical technique to avoid embolization of atheromatous debris to the brain and other organs during cardiac and thoracic aortic operations. Epiaortic imaging is more accurate than palpating the aorta and, in comparative studies, more accurate than TEE for detecting atheromatous disease in the ascending aorta.[23]

There are no laboratory findings specifically found with asymptomatic aortic aneurysms. Aortic dissections or ruptures will decrease hemoglobin. Dissections may cause elevated cardiac enzymes from coronary artery occlusion, may increase blood urea nitrogen and creatinine from renal artery involvement, and may lead to metabolic acidosis from low cardiac output or ischemic bowel. Fibrinogen may decrease in patients experiencing associated disseminated intravascular coagulation. D-dimer is 100% sensitive (but not specific) for aortic dissection, but D-dimer detects the dissection only after it has occurred.

## MANAGEMENT OF PATIENTS WITH AORTIC DILATATION

When ascending aorta dilates beyond 4.0 cm; evaluation by a multidisciplinary team including cardiologist, geneticist and ophthalmologist is required. Patient history for the presenting illness, family history, examination and investigations are carried out. Evaluation for possible connective tissue disease is carried out. DNA testing is done. TTE is performed for the evaluation of aortic valve, quantification of aortic regurgitation and for assessment of diameter of ascending aorta at the level of annulus, aortic sinuses, sinotubular junction and proximal ascending aorta. MRA and CTA should be performed for evaluation of the entire aorta. History for various risk factors leading to development of aneurysm like hypertension, cigarette smoking and hypercholesterolemia should also be sought and appropriate preventive measures taken. A strict control of arterial blood pressure to less than 120/80 mmHg should be maintained. Physical activity should be restricted and patients should not indulge in competitive and isometric sports. Yearly follow up of aortic diameters with TTE, CTA and MRA should be done. As LDS has a malignant course MRI of thoracic and cervical vessels should be done frequently.[24]

### When to Operate?

Aortic dissection and rupture are associated with high mortality. So to prevent dissection of aorta, surgery should be performed timely. According to the law of Laplace, increase in the transverse aortic diameter leads to an increase in wall stress. So as aorta enlarges to specific dimensions, there occurs an increased risk of rupture or dissection. In the ascending aorta an abrupt hinge-point is typically seen at 6 cm[24]. At 6 cm, the engineering characteristics of the aorta deteriorates markedly. Also, loss of aortic elasticity has been associated with increased risk of dissection.[25] As aorta loses its elasticity and becomes a rigid tube; the force of systolic contraction can no longer be dissipated in expanding the aorta. Aortic dilatation in addition is frequently associated with thrombus along the aneurysmal wall and thus poses the risk of embolization and systemic sequelae.

Surgical repair aims to replace the aneurysmal segment with a tube graft to prevent further complications. As symptoms occur in about 5% of patients and often herald the onset of rupture or dissection, they require urgent surgical intervention. Symptomatic thoracic aortic aneurysm regardless of size is thus a primary indication for repair (ACC/AHA Class I recommendation; level of evidence C).[26]

In asymptomatic patients indications for surgical intervention depend on maximum diameter, the size of the patient, rate of growth, presence of connective tissue disorder or bicuspid aortic valve and whether patient is planning pregnancy. In accordance with 2006 ACC, 2007 ESC guidelines for valvular heart disease, the ACC/AHA guidelines for adult congenital heart disease and recent 2010 ACC Foundation/AHA guidelines, indications for prophylactic surgery of dilated ascending aorta includes.[26–29]

1. An aneurysm with diameter of aortic root or ascending aorta ≥ 5.5 cm or if the rate of expansion is >0.5 cm/year.
2. In the presence of bicuspid aortic valve the threshold for ascending aorta repair decreases to 5.0 cm.
3. Marfan's or familial thoracic aortic aneurysm with diameter of ascending aorta ≥5.0 cm.
4. Severe aortic regurgitation in patients with ascending aortic aneurysm is often a primary indication.
5. An aorta which is twice the diameter of normal segment.
6. In patients with a family history of type A aortic dissection, the aortic root should be replaced earlier at a diameter of >5 cm.
7. Aortoannular ectasia with aortic root aneurysm.
8. Refractory pain.

9. In patients undergoing aortic valve replacement with aortic diameter of 4.5 cm, as the incidence of aortic dissection is high after valve replacement. Therefore, concomitant repair of the aortic root or replacement of the ascending aorta is indicated if the diameter of aorta is >4.5 cm

10. It is reasonable to consider prophylactic replacement of the aortic root and ascending aorta in a woman with Marfan's syndrome who is planning a pregnancy and who has an aortic root or ascending aortic diameter larger than 4.0 cm.

11. If the maximal cross-sectional area of the aortic root or ascending aorta (in square centimeters) divided by the patient's height (in meters) exceeds a ratio of 10, then surgical repair is a reasonable option (ACC/AHA Class IIa recommendation; level of evidence C).[26] The rationale behind indexing the aortic dimensions to body size is that shorter adults dissect and rupture their aortas at smaller diameters. Therefore, lower thresholds are considered for short statured individuals.

12. For patients with LDS or confirmed *TGFβR1* or *TGFβR2* mutation, it is reasonable to undergo aortic repair earlier when the aorta diameter exceeds 4.5 cm as these patients have an accelerated and malignant course.

13. Pseudoaneurysms should always be repaired as early as possible as these increase in size progressively, erode into adjacent structures and are prone to rupture.

*Cannulation options for CPB*: The aneurysm's location, extent, presence or absence or dissection/rupture determine the operative strategy and related perioperative complications. Ascending aortic lesions are repaired through a median sternotomy under full cardiopulmonary bypass, instituted by cannulation of ascending aorta and right atrium, without the requirement for one-lung ventilation (OLV) under mild to moderate hypothermia. If the entire ascending aorta is involved and there is no space for placement of aortic cannula and aortic cross clamp proximal to the origin of right subclavian artery, then an alternative arterial access is sought for institution of cardiopulmonary bypass. Femoral and axillary arteries are the alternative sites for cannulation. The femoral artery cannulation provides a retrograde flow from the femoral artery toward the great vessels and has the advantage of rapid and percutaneous cannulation.[30] The femoral artery cannulation has the disadvantage of retrograde showering of descending

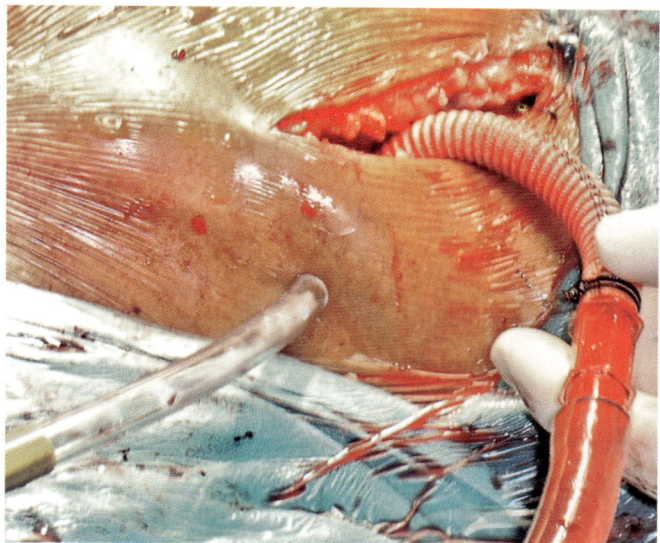

**Fig. 3.10:** Axillary atery being perfused with a side graft sewn to the artery at one end and connected to the arterial cannula at the other end

aortic debris into the cerebral circulation.[31] Cannulation of the right axillary or subclavian artery is an alternative approach, allowing perfusion into the innominate artery and then into the aorta in an antegrade manner. Alternately axillary cannulation also allows for antegrade cerebral perfusion. Left subclavian/axillary artery cannulation is not preferred as it does not share circulation with left carotid artery. The axillary artery cannulation has been associated with improvement in neurological outcomes as manipulation of atherosclerotic aorta can be avoided. The axillary artery itself is seldom involved in atherosclerosis.[32-34] The axillary artery cannulation should be avoided in subclavian stenosis as it can result in right arm overperfusion and edema. Axillary artery cannulation can be direct but is preferably perfused with a side graft sewn to the artery (Fig. 3.10). The side graft avoids the problem of insufficient flow during CPB because of narrow vessel. Venous cannulation usually is obtained via the right atrium. The application of aortic cross clamp interrupts coronary circulation and necessitates cardioplegic cardiac arrest.

In case the disease process extends into the arch and descending thoracic aorta, surgery is managed under deep hypothermic circulatory arrest, and is described in chapter on arch and descending thoracic aorta. In patients with aneurysm rupture, intramural hematoma or false lumen thrombus, aortic dissection variable cannulation and perfusion techniques are required which are discussed in appropriate chapters.

## Surgical Procedures

The type of surgical repair whether repair, replacement or re-implantation is required depends on aortic valve function and the aneurysm extent based on re-evaluation on intraoperative TEE. If the aortic valve and aortic root are normal, a simple tube graft can be used to replace the ascending aorta. If the aortic valve is diseased but the sinuses of Valsalva are normal, an aortic valve replacement combined with a tube graft for the ascending aorta without need for re-implantation of the coronary arteries can be performed. In this procedure a rim of aortic root containing right and left coronary ostia are left behind. The procedure is known as 'Wheat procedure' (Figs 3.11A to F, ACC/AHA class 1 recommendation; level of evidence C).[26] If disease involves both the aortic valve and the aortic root along with ascending aorta, the patient requires aortic root replacement and a composite valve-graft conduit is indicated (Bentall's procedure, Figs 3.12A to C, ACC/AHA Class I recommendation; level of evidence C).[26] Aortic root replacement typically requires Cabrol

technique in which anastomosis of right and the left coronary arteries to 8–10 mm prosthetic tube graft is done, which is anastomosed to the aortic root on the other end (aortocoronary bypass grafting, Fig. 3.13).

Various valve sparing procedures for aortic root aneurysms are described in case the valve cusps whether tricuspid or bicuspid are intact without calcifications, thickening or fenestrations and the aortic root is involved. There are basically two technique of valve sparing aortic root replacement namely the Yacoub technique and the David technique.[35,36] In both these techniques the sinus of Valsalva is first resected out leaving a rim of 3–4 mm of tissue on sides of all commissures, and along the line of attachment of cusps. The coronary ostiae are left in place. The aortic root is then replaced by vascular graft. The aortic valve is then reimplanted into the vascular graft (David technique)[35] or is remodeled into the vascular graft (Yacoub technique)[36] (Figs 3.14 and 3.15). Whenever aortic root is replaced coronary re-implantation is required.

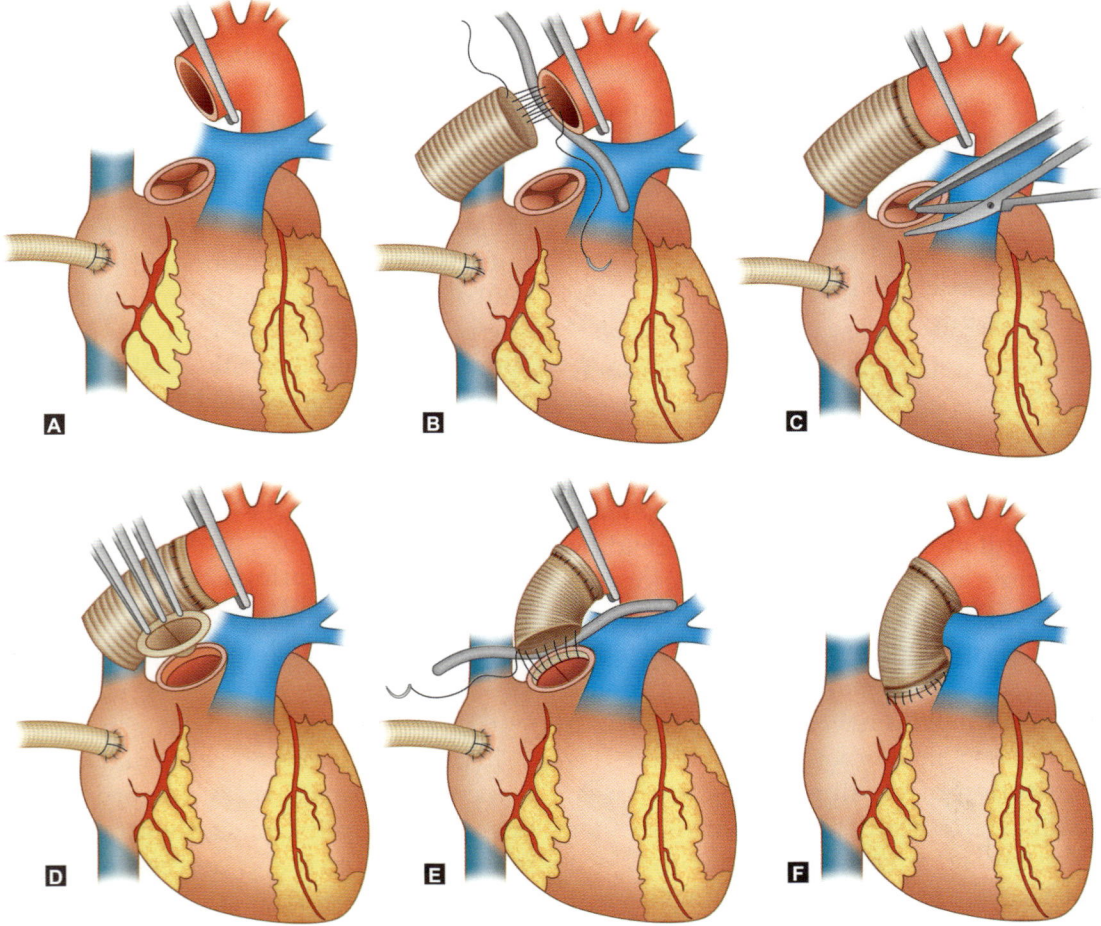

**Figs 3.11A to F:** A, B and F show replacement of ascending aorta with prosthetic tube graft when aortic valve and root are normal in ascending aortic aneurysm. C, D and E show replacement of aortic valve also when aortic valve is diseased in addition to ascending aortic aneurysm. A small rim of the native aortic root containing the right and left coronary ostia is left behind

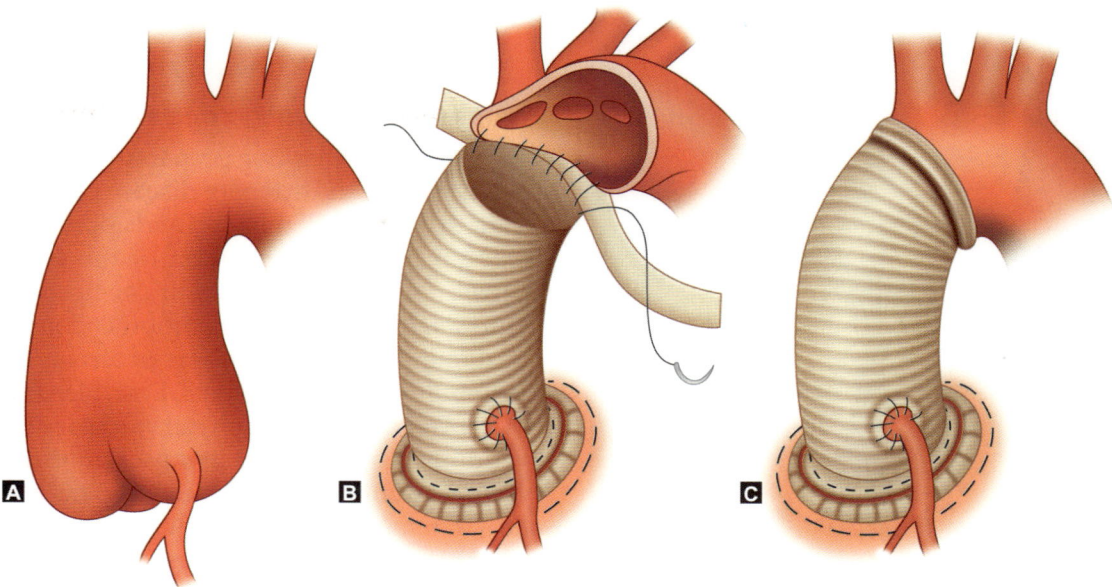

**Figs 3.12A to C:** Replacement of the entire aortic root with composite valved conduit where both aortic valve and aortic root along with all ascending aorta are involved in aneurysm. The underside of aortic arch is also seen incorporated within the graft. In addition right and left coronary arteries are reimplanted into the graft

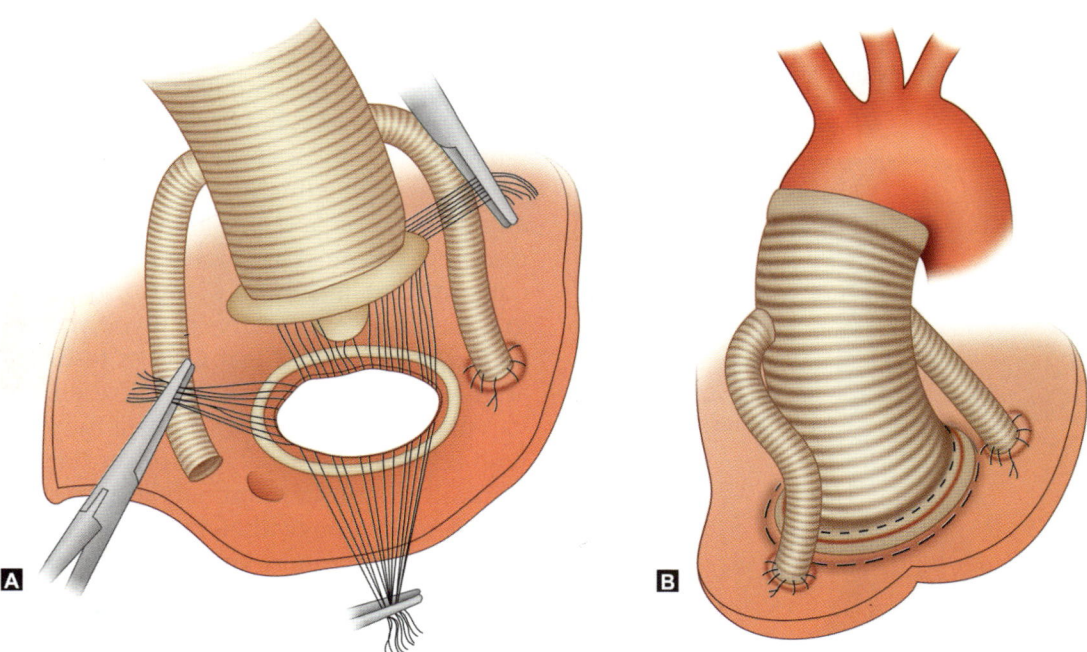

**Figs 3.13A and B:** Replacement of the entire root with composite valved conduit for ascending aortic aneurysm involving aortic valve and aortic root. The procedure is combined with end to end anastomosis of both coronary arteries to 8–10 mm prosthetic tube graft that is anastomosed to the aortic root

Ascending aortic aneurysm may extend into the proximal aortic arch and may require a partial arch replacement (hemiarch technique) in which a tubular graft is interposed between the ascending aorta or aortic root and the underside of the aortic arch (ACC/AHA class II a recommendation; level of evidence B).[26] Ascending aorta with hemiarch reconstruction is performed by an open technique using DHCA with or without antegrade/retrograde cerebral perfusion to make distal anastomosis feasible without crossclamping the aorta. Repair of ascending aorta along with whole of arch and DTA is beyond the scope of this chapter and is given in the relevant chapters.

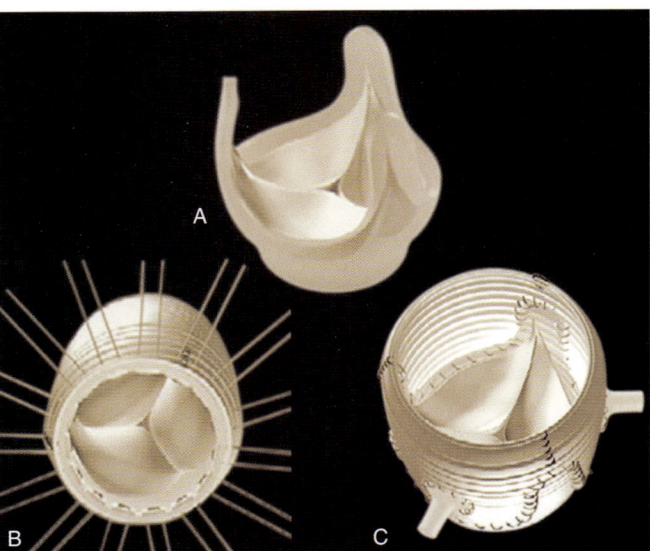

**Figs 3.14A to C:** A valve sparing reimplantation (David) procedure. (A) The aortic root is resected first leaving only the crown-like attachments of the aortic valve cusps with 3–4 mm of surrounding tissue and the coronary ostiae in place. (B) The vascular graft is put over the aortic valve and secured below the aortic valve attachment with several U-stitches. (C) Then, the basal aortic valve attachment and the commissures are sewn into the graft with three continuous sutures. As the vascular graft has been left tubular, no pseudosinuses are created. Finally, the coronary ostiae are reimplanted into the graft[35]

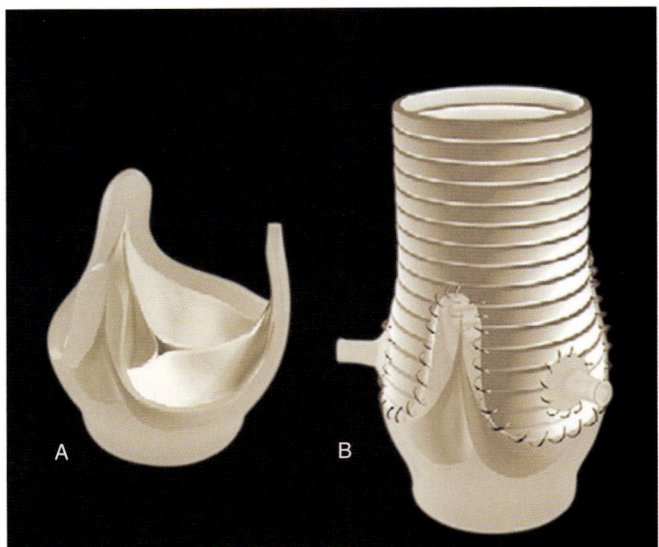

**Figs 3.15A and B:** A valve sparing remodeling (Yacoub) procedure. (A) The aortic root is resected first leaving only the crown-like attachments of the aortic valve cusps with 3–4 mm of surrounding tissue and the coronary ostiae in place. (B) The vascular graft is incised at its base in such a way that the incisions match the height of the commissures—the graft now looks as if it has three "tongues". Then, the basal aortic valve attachment and the commissures are sewn into the graft and between the "tongues" with three continuous sutures. The three "tongues" of the vascular graft act as pseudosinuses. Finally, the coronary ostiae are reimplanted into the graft[36]

## ANESTHETIC MANAGEMENT

### A. Pre-anesthetic Management

#### Preoperative Evaluation and Preparation

The goal of preoperative preparation is evaluation and understanding the extent of disease process, the type of repair that would be required and appropriate measures to be taken for optimization of the patient prior to surgery. Also the assessment for need of any other concomitant surgical intervention is done. A thorough questioning for the symptoms of airway compression, cardiopulmonary status, renal, liver, bleeding diasthesis, cerebrovascular and peripheral vascular disease is done. In addition to general and airway examination, a detailed systemic examination is done. Preoperative X-ray chest and CT scans should be evaluated to rule out airway involvement. As major causes of perioperative morbidity and mortality after aortic surgeries result from myocardial infarction, respiratory failure, renal failure, and stroke, a thorough preoperative assessment of the functions of these organ systems becomes necessary.

#### Cardiac Function

As there is a high incidence of coronary artery disease in the elderly, particularly those with degenerative aneurysms, assessment of cardiac function is imperative when elective aortic surgery is contemplated, especially for those with a history of myocardial infarction or angina pectoris and those older than 50 years. Those planned for elective aneurysm repair and having concomitant ischemic symptoms or electrocardiographic changes indicative of myocardial ischemia must be further evaluated using stress testing and coronary angiography when indicated. Presence of associated valvular heart disease warrants a thorough evaluation with echocardiography and/or cardiac catheterization. Clinically, important coronary lesions should be treated with percutaneous catheter interventional techniques or bypass grafting, and valvular heart disease by valve repair or replacement either before or at the time of the aortic surgery.

#### Pulmonary Function

Predictors of poor respiratory outcome include long standing history of smoking and presence of chronic obstructive pulmonary disease. Pulmonary function tests including spirometric tests and arterial blood gas analysis should be performed in these patients. Cessation of smoking, short course antibiotic therapy and inhaled bronchodilators should be administered preoperatively in patients with reversible restrictive disease or excessive sputum production.

## Renal Function

Preoperative renal dysfunction is the single most important predictor of acute renal failure after surgery on thoracic aorta. Even though preoperative blood urea nitrogen and serum creatinine are routinely measured, they are associated with a low predictive value for postoperative renal dysfunction. Preoperative maintenance of adequate hydration, avoidance of nephrotoxic drugs including iodinated contrast, and avoidance of hypotension, low cardiac output, and hypovolemia in the perioperative period are important mechanisms for reducing the prevalence of this complication.

## Neurologic Function

In patients with a history of stroke, transient ischemic attack, or other risk factors for cerebrovascular disease, duplex imaging of the carotid arteries and/or angiography of the brachiocephalic and intracranial arteries, should be performed preoperatively when indicated to minimize the risk of stroke.

Laboratory investigations like complete blood count, serum electrolytes, blood urea nitrogen, creatinine, coagulation indices and blood type and cross match should be performed. Availability of blood and blood products are ensured.

The risk factors such as hypertension, cigarette smoking, and hypercholesterolemia should be aggressively managed. Moderate restriction of physical activity should be advised. Patients should avoid exertion at maximal capacity and specifically should not engage in competitive, contact, or isometric sports.

## Discussion with Patient

The ascending aortic aneurysm repair is complex and involves considerable morbidity and mortality. At times decision about the arch repair is taken intraoperatively which further increases the complexity of the procedure. Although our surgical colleagues do discuss with the patient, but major issues associated with the anesthesia and postoperative care should be discussed with patient, and the attendants. Discussion should include the possible risks of major cardiac events, major neurological complications, transfusion reactions as well as risks of massive transfusion, respiratory failure requiring prolonged ventilation and the risk of death.

## Planning

Planning should include discussion with the surgeon about the surgical plan including sites of invasive arterial pressure monitoring, need of cerebral protection strategies as to the depth of hypothermia, cerebral perfusion strategies and adjunct medications.

## Premedication

Preoperative hemodynamic optimization is essential in patients who present for elective repair of aortic lesions. Oral antihypertensive agents may include beta-blockers, calcium channel blockers, diuretics, and ACE inhibitors. Simultaneous blood pressure and heart rate control can be achieved using calcium channel and beta-blocking agents. Besides ACEIs, it is essential to continue all preoperative vasoactive medications until the morning of surgery, as rebound tachycardia or hypertension from medication withdrawal in such patients may be disastrous. Additionally anxiolysis using benzodiazepines assists in controlling hypertension and tachycardia and, therefore, minimize aortic wall tension. In addition, at our center patients undergoing elective surgery are premedicated with injection morphine sulphate 0.1 mg/kg and injection promethazine 0.5 mg/kg administered 45 minutes prior to induction of anesthesia.

## B. Intraoperative Management

### Intraoperative Goals

Control of both blood pressure and ejection velocity are the mainstays of hemodynamic optimization of the patient with an aortic lesion (Table 3.3). Increased blood pressure and ejection velocity are capable of causing an aneurysm rupture or extending an already existing dissection. Simultaneous control of both blood pressure and ejection velocity is best obtained with a combination of beta-blockers and vasodilators.

### Pre-induction Preparation

Preparations must be made for rapid and massive transfusion and preferably two large bore (14-gauge or 16-gauge) intravenous catheters should be placed in bilateral upper-extremity. All necessary vasopressors, vasodilatory agents; and at least six units of typed and cross-matched blood should be available in the operating room as the patient is wheeled in. External defibrillator paddles may additionally be applied. Rapid infuser sets and fluid warmers should be made available for use in surgery for aortic aneurysm.

For surgeries involving only the ascending aorta radial arterial catheter may be inserted into the left or right radial artery. If arterial cannulation of the right

| Table 3.3: Hemodynamic goals in patients undergoing aortic surgery | |
|---|---|
| MAP | 70–90 mmHg |
| HR | 60–80/min |
| CI | 2–2.5 L/min/m² |

axillary, subclavian, or innominate artery is planned for CPB and ACP, bilateral radial arterial catheters often are required to measure cerebral and systemic perfusion pressures.

Epidural catheters often are used after confirming normal coagulation status in patients undergoing elective procedures. Caution must be exercised as inadvertent vascular or subarachnoid placement of the catheter may delay the procedure. A test dose with 3 ml of 2% lidocaine with 1:2,00,000 epinephrine is essential to confirm correct placement of the catheter. Neuraxial anesthetic techniques are not recommended in patients at risk for neuraxial hematoma as in the setting of concomitant thienopyridine antiplatelet therapy, low-molecular weight heparins, and clinically significant anticoagulation (ACC/AHA Class III recommendation; level of evidence C).[37] Anticoagulation status must be similarly reviewed at the time of removal of the catheter in the postoperative period.

### Induction and Maintenance of Anesthesia

Essential preinduction monitoring includes a 5-lead electrocardiogram, invasive arterial blood pressure and pulse oximetry. There is no single anesthetic technique recommended for induction in aortic surgery. The main deciding factor in choosing any anesthesia plan for induction is hemodynamic control. The induction of general anesthesia requires beat to beat hemodynamic monitoring, with anticipation of changes because of anesthetic depth; and profile of drugs used for induction and tracheal intubation. For elective procedures, an opioid based induction technique using fentanyl (15–25 µg/kg) or sufentanil (1–3 µg/kg) can be used to minimize hemodynamic disturbances. The authors commonly use a balanced anesthesia technique using sleep dose of thiopentone (3–5 mg/kg), fentanyl 2–5 µg/kg, midazolam 0.01–0.02 µg/kg with oxygen-air and isoflurane 0.5–2% for induction of anesthesia. Tracheal intubation may be facilitated using rapidly acting dose of rocuronium (0.9 mg/kg) or vecuronium bromide 0.1 mg/kg. Utmost care should be taken to avoid tachycardia and hypertension during laryngoscopy and intubation as these can lead to rupture of aneurysm. The addition of beta-blockade, xylocaine or vasodilator therapy before laryngoscopy helps to attenuate this undesirable response. On the other, and combination of anesthetic agents and antihypertensive agents have the potential to cause a precipitous fall of blood pressure especially in a patient with poor left ventricular function and hypovolemia. As discussed previously, aortic lesions may cause both tracheal and bronchial compression and caution should be exercised in tube placement. After induction, monitoring of end-tidal carbon dioxide is started. General anesthesia maintenance is typically with a balanced technique and deepening the anesthetic depth with a supplemental narcotic dose to improve hemodynamic stability. An intermediate-acting, nondepolarizing neuromuscular blocker such as vecuronium (0.1 mg/kg), or cisatracurium (0.5 mg/kg) can be used for maintenance of muscle relaxation. Amnesia can be accomplished with intermittent boluses of short acting benzodiazepines like midazolam and/or inhalational agents. Appropriate prophylactic antibiotic therapy should be completed at least 30 minutes before skin incision to achieve adequate bactericidal tissue levels. It is to be noted that anesthetic requirement decreases during hypothermia and any over dosage can lead to vasodilatation and hypothermia in the post CPB period. In the authors experience usually a total doses of fentanyl 20–25 µg/kg and midazolam 5–10 mg are typically required.

After the induction of general anesthesia, additional venous accesses and other monitoring lines are placed for monitoring right atrial pressure, which include triple lumen central venous catheter or a pulmonary artery catheter, transesophageal echocardiography (TEE) probe and any other additional arterial line if required in accordance with the surgical plan. A large bore venous sheath of 8F is also inserted into the right internal jugular vein or femoral vein for rapid volume administration. Both rectal and nasopharyngeal temperature probe are required for monitoring the absolute temperature of the periphery and core, as well changes during deliberate hypothermia and subsequent rewarming. Neurological monitoring in the form of processed EEG monitors as bispectral index (BIS) or patient state index (PSI) can prevent unnecessary anesthetic drug administration especially in the post CPB period and can improve outcomes.[38] Cerebral oximetry using near-infrared spectroscopy (NIRS) monitoring is especially required where involvement of arch is a possibility and antegrade cerebral perfusion may be required, as high risk of neurological sequelae is associated with aortic surgery. In one of the case reported by the authors, use of NIRS has been found to be beneficial for detection of cerebral ischemia by superior vena cava obstruction in a patient with ascending aortic aneurysm during left internal artery harvesting.[39]

Intraoperative TEE can image the thoracic aorta from the aortic valve to the distal ascending aorta and from the distal aortic arch to the proximal abdominal aorta. The intervening zone including the distal ascending aorta and proximal aortic arch is known as the "blind spot" of TEE as it cannot be reliably imaged by TEE because of the intervening trachea and left main stem bronchus obstructing the acoustic window. Intra-operative TEE can be used to make or confirm the diagnosis; and can evaluate the aortic valve structure and function to guide the surgical intervention (reimplantation, repair or replacement) for which the measurement of diameters of the aortic annulus, aortic root, ascending aorta, and aortic arch is essential. In case of emergency where patient has not preoperatively been assessed by CT/MRI, the intraoperative TEE can help locate a possible dissection site, and identify the true/false lumen. In addition, it can help assess the adequacy of perfusion during cardiopulmonary bypass (CPB), myocardial performance, signs of ischemia, valve status, and post-repair aortic integrity. Details of trans-esophageal echocardiographic assessment in aortic diseases are given in Chapter 12.

In a patient undergoing elective surgery for ascending aortic aneurysm, (Fig. 3.16) hemodynamics needs to be maintained not only during induction but also throughout the surgical procedure. The heart rate and blood pressure both need to be controlled. The blood pressure should be kept within normal range with the help of rapidly acting vasodilators and β-blockers (Table 3.4).

| Table 3.4: Drugs for rapid control of blood pressure | |
|---|---|
| *Drug* | *Dosage* |
| SNP | 0.5–2.5 g/kg/min |
| NTG | 0.5–4 g/kg/min |
| Fenolodopam | 0.05–0.1 g/kg/min |
| Nicardipine | 2–15 mg/h |
| Metoprolol | 2.5–5 mg up to 15–20 mg |
| Labetalol | 0.25 mg/kg followed by 0.5–2 mg/min |
| Esmolol | 0.5 mg/kg followed by 50–300 g/kg/min |

SNP: Sodium nitroprusside, NTG: Nitroglycerine

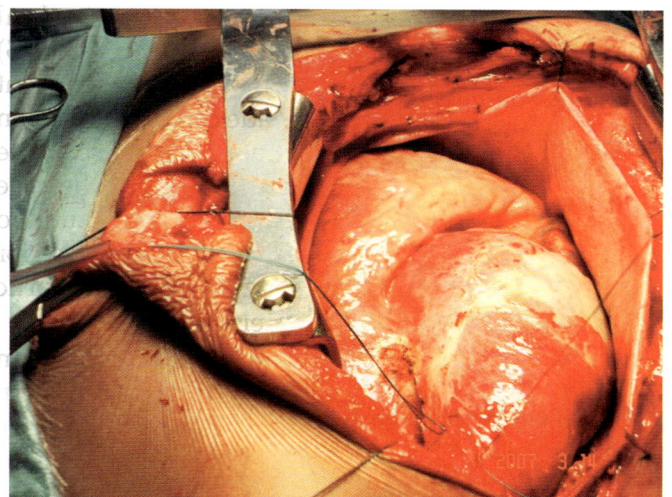

Fig. 3.16: Preoperative view of ascending aortic aneurysm

The other group of patients with ascending aortic aneurysms where aneurysm complicates into aortic dissection or rupture with hemopericardium (cardiac temponade), severe aortic regurgitation or myocardial ischemic due to coronary artery involvement may present with compromised hemodynamics for emergency repair. In such a situation, it becomes a challenge for the anesthesiologist to rapidly secure airway, maintain ventilation, circulation and quickly obtain arterial and central venous assess, and the surgeon simultaneously prepares to institute CPB. The details of management of dissection and rupture are described in separate chapters in this book.

In addition, monitoring of hourly urine output, intermittent arterial blood gases, electrolytes, blood glucose levels and activated coagulation time (ACT) is done. A baseline activated coagulation time (ACT) is measured prior to CPB and post-hepainization with 400 U/kg of heparin. An ACT of above 480 seconds is maintained during cardiopulmonary bypass. During CPB, ACT is monitored every 30 minutes and post CPB after reversal of heparin with protamine sulphate.

### The Conduct of Cardiopulmonary Bypass

The CPB is conducted using membrane oxygenation and mild to moderate hypothermia. On the onset of CPB, packed red blood cells are added and during re-warming phase conventional ultrafiltration is performed to maintain a hematocrit of 30%. Myocardial protection is achieved by using cold blood cardioplegia solution. Cerebral protection is provided by ACP if in case arch is involved. Perfusion pressure is maintained between 50–70 mm Hg.

### Weaning from Cardiopulmonary Bypass

Patient should be adequately re-warmed to a naso-pharyngeal temperature of 35–36°C, ensuring that the gradient of temperature between the bath and the patient is always less than 10°C to avoid cerebral injury from warm blood directed towards cerebral circulation. Ventricular fibrillation may occur if the clamp is released at a very low temperature or if there is associated myo-cardial dysfunction. Hemofilter must be used to regulate the intraoperative fluid balance and achieve a target hematocrit of 30% at the time of weaning from cardio-pulmonary bypass. Inotropic support may be required in patients with associated preoperative myocardial dysfunction or poor myocardial preservation. Volume and sodium bicarbonate injection should be administered as the limb perfusion is restored after the removal of the femoral arterial cannula. Anticoagulation with heparin is antagonized with protamine sulphate in the dose of 1.3 mg/100 U of heparin. An additional dose of protamine may have to be administered to ensure an ACT close to pre-heparinization levels or between 110 and 150 seconds.TEE is performed to ensure normal aortic valve function, cardiac functions and adequacy of repair of aorta. In the post CPB period, it important to prevent any hypertension with the use of vasodilators and beta blockers to prevent any disruption of aortic suture lines. Also, maintenance of normal arterial blood gases, electrolytes, blood glucose, hematocrit and prevention of temperature drift are all very important.

## Strategies of Blood Conservation

As there is a potential for significant bleeding in aortic surgery, implementation of strategies to decrease bleeding and transfusion in these procedures is essential. These include a timely preoperative recognition of patients with high risk of bleeding and performing all possible blood conservative measures. Patients with advanced age, preoperative anemia, congenital and acquired coagulation disorders, preoperative anti-platelet and antithrombotic therapy, complex and redo surgery, small sized individuals, emergency surgical procedure, prolonged CPB duration and multiple comorbidies are the patients likely to bleed.[40] Also the aortic surgery itself is associated with altered hemostasis and risk of bleeding due to platelet dysfunction, disruption of coagulation cascade, CPB with associated hypothermia, inflammation, fibrinolysis and systemic anticoagulation. Appropriate measures like timely cessation of anticoagulants and anti-platelet medications should be taken. Blood conservation strategies like pre-operative autologous donation, intraoperative auto-logous collection of blood prior to CPB in case patient is stable and has an adequate hematocrit (acute normo-volemic hemodilution) can reduce the homologous blood transfusion. Intraoperatively use of cell-saver circuit can help to recoup the blood from the operative field in case of profuse bleeding which can later on be transfused. Also, the blood remaining in the extra-corporeal circuit after cessation of CPB can be processed using ultrafiltration and re-infused. In addition, the use of antifibrinolytic therapy, the biologic glue, activated factor VII, and avoidance of perioperative hypertension can help to decrease bleeding. At the end of CPB, adequate reversal of the effects of heparin is important. An additional dose of 25–50 mg of protamine has to be administered after transfusion of heparinized blood of cell saver. Post CPB, after ensuring adequate surgical hemostasis, in case of persistent bleeding, platelet concentrates and fresh frozen plasma may be transfused.

The use of point of care tests if available can help in the judicious use of these blood products.

Various antifibrinolytic agents like lysine analogs and aprotinin have been used to mitigate the effect of fibrinolysis that occurs during CPB and thus decreases the perioperative bleeding. Aprotinin, a serine protease inhibitor was the commonly used antifibrinolytic agent until 2007 when it was withdrawn from the market following blood conservation using antifibrinolytics in a randomized trial (BART) study, where it was found to have increased all-cause mortality.[41] Presently lysine analogs epsilon aminocaproic acid (EACA) or tranexamic acid (TXA) are commonly used antifibrinolytics in reducing perioperative bleeding. In a study conducted by the authors, both EACA and TXA were found to be equally effective in reducing the perioperative blood loss and transfusion requirement in patients undergoing thoracic aortic surgery.[42] The use of antifibrinolytic agents is avoided in patients with renal disease.

## C. Postoperative Management

In most cases, the general anesthesia continues for several hours after admission to the intensive care unit (ICU) to permit a controlled anesthetic emergence. Fast tracking and early anesthetic emergence is preferable for early assessment of neurological function in the absence of any intraoperative complications. Epidural catheter if inserted, should be used with extreme caution in the postoperative phase administering only a dilute solution of local anesthetic and narcotic in order to minimize sympathectomy associated postoperative hypotension, and to minimize motor blockade to allow serial neuro-logic assessment of lower extremity function.

Antibiotic prophylaxis is continued for 48 hours after surgery to minimize surgical infection risk.

Common postoperative complications have been listed in Table 3.5. Postoperative management should be targeted towards prevention of these complications. Adequate analgesia is essential to ensure adequate patient comfort, prevent hypertension/myocardial ischemia resulting from tachycardia and sympathetic stimulation secondary to pain. Precise control of blood

| Table 3.5: Postoperative complications | |
|---|---|
| · Hypothermia | · Myocardial ischemia |
| · Bleeding | · Embolism |
| · Anemia | · Stroke, agitation and confusion |
| · Hypertension/hypotension | · Renal failure |
| · Hyperglycemia | · Prolonged ventilation |
| · Acid base/electrolyte disturbances | · Prolonged (>6 hrs) inotropic support |

pressure with the use of appropriate vasodilators and inotropes is essential. Use of forced air warmers should be continued in the postoperative period to prevent hypothermia. Blood glucose monitoring is essential to prevent hyperglycemia which is associated with an, wound infection, adverse neurologic outcomes and increased ICU morbidity and mortality. Serial chest radiographs should be done to rule out any pleural/ pericardial effusion or collection, pulmonary edema, pneumothorax and confirmation of endotracheal tube and central venous cannula position.

Besides the routine hemodynamic monitoring, patients should be evaluated regularly for adequacy of ventilation, using arterial blood gas analysis and assessment of various ventilatory parameters. Urine output, chest tube drainage, collection of blood in mediastinum, and peripheral pulses should be monitored on an hourly basis. For control of postoperative bleeding, it is essential to avoid hypertension, maintain ACT, administration of blood products as per point of care testing using thromboelastography or sonoclot, ensure normothermia, as well as administration of antifibrinolytics like EACA and TXA. Recombinant Factor VIIa (90 µg/kg) repeated after 2 hrs may be tried for refractory medical bleeding. Gauze packing of mediastinum followed by removal after 12–24 hours in anticipation of pressure effect from inserted gauzes can also be attempted in cases of refractory microvascular ooze.

## Key Notes

1. Ascending aortic aneurysm is often associated with connective tissue disorders and congenital heart disease.

2. Repair of ascending aortic aneurysm is not as simple as it appears. In spite of preoperative diagnostic investigations, important intraoperative decision making is often required.

3. A thorough understanding of the anatomy is essential for understanding the complexities of aortic repair.

4. Transesophageal echocardiography is an important intraoperative tool in the hands of anesthesiologists, that helps in important decision making, as to feasibility and type of repair or replacement of the aortic valve or ascending aorta.

5. A possibility should always be borne in mind for the likely involvement of arch and the additional complexity in the perfusion system especially the cerebral protection. An anesthesiologist should be prepared for the additional monitoring as well as other complexities associated with the management.

6. Management of hemodynamics is very important and the necessary arrangement should be kept ready at all times during conduct of surgery.

7. The surgery for ascending aortic aneurysm has a potential to bleed. So blood and blood products should be in hand and important blood conservation techniques should be adopted.

## REFERENCES

1. Lazar HL, McDonnell M, Chipkin SR, Furnary AP, Engelman RM, Sadhu AR, Bridges CR, Haan CK, Svedjeholm R, Taegtmeyer H, Shemin RJ; Society of Thoracic Surgeons Blood Glucose Guideline Task Force. The Society of Thoracic Surgeons practice guideline series: Blood glucose management during adult cardiac surgery. AnnThorac Surg. 2009 Feb; 87(2):663–9.

2. Bickerstaff LK, Pairolero PC, Hollier LH, Melton LJ, Van Peenen HJ, Cherry KJ, Joyce JW, Lie JT. Thoracic aortic aneurysms: a population-based study. Surgery, 1982 Dec; 92(6):1103–8.

3. Roman MJ, Devereux RB, Kramer-Fox R, O'Loughlin J. Two-dimensional echocardiographic aortic root dimensions in normal children and adults. Am J Cardiol. 1989 Sep 1; 64(8):507–12.

4. Erbel R, Alfonso F, Boileau C, Dirsch O, Eber B, Haverich A, Rakowski H, Struyven J, Radegran K, Sechtem U, Taylor J, Zollikofer C, Klein WW, Mulder B, Providencia LA. Task Force on Aortic Dissection, European Society of Cardiology. Diagnosis and management of aortic dissection. Eur Heart J. 2001 Sep; 22(18):1642–81.

5. Aronberg DJ, Glazer HS, Madsen K, Sagel SS. Normal thoracic aortic diameters by computed tomography. J Comput Assist Tomogr. 1984 Apr; 8(2):247–50.

6. Hager A, Kaemmerer H, Rapp-Bernhardt U, Blücher S, Rapp K, Bernhardt TM, Galanski M, Hess J. Diameters of the thoracic aorta throughout life as measured with helical computed tomography. J Thorac Cardiovasc Surg. 2002 Jun; 123(6):1060–6.

7. Coselli JS, Crawford ES. Composite valve-graft replacement of aortic root using separate Dacron tube for coronary artery reattachment. Ann Thorac Surg. 1989 Apr; 47(4):558–65.

8. Albornoz G, Coady MA, Roberts M, Davies RR, Tranquilli M, Rizzo JA, Elefteriades JA. Familial thoracic aortic aneurysms and dissections-incidence, modes of inheritance, and phenotypic patterns. Ann Thorac Surg. 2006 Oct; 82(4):1400–5.

9. Fuster V, Halperin JL. Aortic dissection: a medical perspective. J Card Surg. 1994 Nov; 9(6):713–28.

10. Dietz HC, Cutting GR, Pyeritz RE, Maslen CL, Sakai LY, Corson GM, Puffenberger EG, Hamosh A, Nanthakumar EJ, Curristin SM, et al. Marfan syndrome caused by a recurrent de novo missense mutation in the fibrillin gene. Nature. 1991 Jul; 352(6333):337–9.

11. Tadros TM, Klein MD, Shapira OM. Ascending aortic dilatation associated with bicuspid aortic valve: pathophysiology, molecular biology, and clinical implications. Circulation. 2009 Feb 17; 119(6):880–90.

12. Agmon Y, Khandheria BK, Meissner I, Schwartz GL, Sicks JD, Fought AJ, O'Fallon WM, Wiebers DO, Tajik AJ. Is aortic dilatation an atherosclerosis-related process? Clinical, laboratory, and transesophageal echocardiographic correlates of thoracic aortic dimensions in the population with implications for thoracic aortic aneurysm formation. J Am Coll Cardiol. 2003 Sep 17; 42(6):1076–83.

13. Galloway AC, Colvin SB, LaMendola CL, Hurwitz JB, Baumann FG, Harris LJ, Culliford AT, Grossi EA, Spencer FC. Ten-year operative experience with 165 aneurysms of the ascending aorta and aortic arch. Circulation. 1989 Sep; 80:249–56.

14. Salisbury RS, Hazleman BL. Successful treatment of dissecting aortic aneurysm due to giant cell arteritis. Ann Rheum Dis. 1981 Oct; 40(5):507–8.

15. Feigl D, Feigl A, Edwards JE. Mycotic aneurysms of the aortic root. A pathologic study of 20 cases. Chest. 1986 Oct; 90(4):553–7.

16. Guthaner DF. The plain chest film in assessing aneurysms and dissecting hematomas of the ascending aorta. In: Taveras JN, Ferruci JT, eds. Radiology diagnosis-imaging-intervention. Philadelphia: JB Lippincott, 1994:1.

17. Nienaber CA, Kische S, Skriabina V, Ince H. Noninvasive imaging approaches to evaluate the patient with known or suspected aortic disease. Circ Cardiovasc Imaging. 2009 Nov; 2(6):499–506.

18. Brown JR, Block CA, Malenka DJ, O'Connor GT, Schoolwerth AC, Thompson CA. Sodium bicarbonate plus N-acetylcysteine prophylaxis: a meta-analysis. JACC Cardiovasc Interv. 2009 Nov; 2(11):1116–24.

19. Einstein AJ, Henzlova MJ, Rajagopalan S. Estimating risk of cancer associated with radiation exposure from 64-slice computed tomography coronary angiography. JAMA. 2007 Jul 18; 298(3):317–23.

20. Halvorsen RA. Which study when? Iodinated contrast-enhanced CT versus gadolinium-enhanced MR imaging. Radiology. 2008 Oct; 249(1):9–15.

21. Kuo PH, Kanal E, Abu-Alfa AK, Cowper SE. Gadolinium-based MR contrast agents and nephrogenic systemic fibrosis. Radiology. 2007 Mar; 242(3):647–9.

22. Israel DH, Sharma SK, Ambrose JA, Ergin MA, Griepp RR. Cardiac catheterization and selective coronary angiography in ascending aortic aneurysm or dissection. Cathet Cardiovasc Diagn. 1994 Jul; 32(3):232–7.

23. Wilson MJ, Boyd SY, Lisagor PG, Rubal BJ, Cohen DJ. Ascending aortic atheroma assessed intraoperatively by epiaortic and transesophageal echocardiography. Ann Thorac Surg. 2000 Jul; 70(1):25–30.

24. Cozijnsen L, Braam RL, Waalewijn RA, Schepens MA, Loeys BL, van Oosterhout MF, Barge-Schaapveld DQ, Mulder BJ. What is new in dilatation of the ascending aorta? Review of current literature and practical advice for the cardiologist. Circulation. 2011 Mar 1; 123(8):924–8.

25. Nollen GJ, Groenink M, Tijssen JG, Van Der Wall EE, Mulder BJ. Aortic stiffness and diameter predict progressive aortic dilatation in patients with Marfan syndrome. Eur Heart J. 2004 Jul; 25(13):1146–52.

26. Hiratzka LF, Bakris GL, Beckman JA, Bersin RM, Carr VF, Casey DE Jr, Eagle KA, Hermann LK, Isselbacher EM, Kazerooni EA, Kouchoukos NT, Lytle BW, Milewicz DM, Reich DL, Sen S, Shinn JA, Svensson LG, Williams DM; ACCF/AHA/AATS/ACR/ASA/SCA/SCAI/SIR/STS/ SVM guidelines for the diagnosis and management of patients with Thoracic Aortic Disease: a report of the American College of Cardiology Foundation/American Heart Association Task Force on Practice Guidelines, American Association for Thoracic Surgery, American College of Radiology, American Stroke Association, Society of Cardiovascular Anesthesiologists, Society for Cardiovascular Angiography and Interventions, Society of Interventional Radiology, Society of Thoracic Surgeons, and Society for Vascular Medicine. Circulation. 2010 Apr 6; 121(13):e266–369.

27. American College of Cardiology; American Heart Association Task Force on Practice Guidelines (Writing Committee to revise the 1998 guidelines for the management of patients with valvular heart disease); Society of Cardiovascular Anesthesiologists, Bonow RO, Carabello BA, Chatterjee K, de Leon AC Jr, Faxon DP, Freed MD, Gaasch WH, Lytle BW, Nishimura RA, O'Gara PT, O'Rourke RA, Otto CM, Shah PM, Shanewise JS, Smith SC Jr, Jacobs AK, Adams CD, Anderson JL, Antman EM, Fuster V, Halperin JL, Hiratzka LF, Hunt SA, Lytle BW, Nishimura R, Page RL, Riegel B. ACC/AHA 2006 guidelines for the management of patients with valvular heart disease: a report of the American College of Cardiology/American Heart Association Task Force on Practice Guidelines (writing Committee to Revise the 1998 guidelines for the management of patients with valvular heart disease) developed in collaboration with the Society of Cardiovascular Anesthesiologists endorsed by the Society for Cardiovascular Angiography and Interventions and the Society of Thoracic Surgeons. J Am Coll Cardiol. 2006 Aug 1; 48(3):e1–148.

28. Vahanian A, Baumgartner H, Bax J, Butchart E, Dion R, Filippatos G, Flachskampf F, Hall R, Iung B, Kasprzak J, Nataf P, Tornos P, Torracca L, Wenink A; Task Force on the Management of Valvular Hearth Disease of the European Society of Cardiology; ESC Committee for Practice Guidelines. Guidelines on the management of valvular heart disease: The Task Force on the Management of Valvular Heart Disease of the European Society of Cardiology. Eur Heart J. 2007 Jan; 28(2):230–68.

29. Warnes CA, Williams RG, Bashore TM, Child JS, Connolly HM, Dearani JA, del Nido P, Fasules JW, Graham TP Jr, Hijazi ZM, Hunt SA, King ME, Landzberg MJ, Miner PD, Radford MJ, Walsh EP, Webb GD. ACC/AHA 2008 Guidelines for the Management of Adults with Congenital Heart Disease: a report of the American College of Cardiology/American Heart Association Task Force on Practice Guidelines (writing committee to develop guidelines on the management of adults with congenital heart disease). Circulation. 2008 Dec 2; 118(23):e714–833.

30. Shimazaki Y, Watanabe T, Takahashi T, Minowa T, Inui K, Uchida T, Koshika M, Takeda F. Minimized mortality and neurological complications in surgery for chronic arch aneurysm: axillary artery cannulation, selective cerebral perfusion, and replacement of the ascending and total arch aorta. J Card Surg. 2004 Jul-Aug; 19(4):338–42.

31. Fusco DS, Shaw RK, Tranquilli M, Kopf GS, Elefteriades JA. Femoral cannulation is safe for type A dissection repair. Ann Thorac Surg. 2004 Oct; 78(4):1285–9.

32. Reuthebuch O, Schurr U, Hellermann J, Prêtre R, Künzli A, Lachat M, Turina MI.Advantages of subclavian artery perfusion for repair of acute type A dissection. Eur J Cardiothorac Surg. 2004 Sep; 26(3):592–8.

33. Moizumi Y, Motoyoshi N, Sakuma K, Yoshida S. Axillary artery cannulation improves operative results for acute type A aortic dissection. Ann Thorac Surg. 2005 Jul; 80(1):77–83.

34. Pasic M, Schubel J, Bauer M, Yankah C, Kuppe H, Weng YG, Hetzer R. Cannulation of the right axillary artery for surgery of acute type A aortic dissection. Eur J Cardiothorac Surg. 2003 Aug; 24(2):231–5.

35. David TE, Armstrong S, Manlhiot C, McCrindle BW, Feindel CM. Long-term results of aortic root repair using the reimplantation technique. J Thorac Cardiovasc Surg. 2013 Mar; 145(3 Suppl):S22–5.

36. Yacoub MH, Fagan A, Stassano P, Radley-Smith R. Results of valve conserving operations for aortic regurgitation. Circulation 1983; 68:III-321–4.

37. Horlocker TT, Wedel DJ, Rowlingson JC, Enneking FK, Kopp SL, Benzon HT, Brown DL, Heit JA, Mulroy MF, Rosenquist RW, Tryba M, Yuan CS. Regional anesthesia in the patient receiving antithrombotic or thrombolytic therapy: American Society of Regional Anesthesia and Pain Medicine Evidence-Based Guidelines (Third Edition). Reg Anesth Pain Med. 2010 Jan-Feb; 35(1):64–101.

38. Edmonds HL Jr. Advances in neuromonitoring for cardiothoracic and vascular surgery. J Cardiothorac Vasc Anesth. 2001 Apr; 15(2):241–50.

39. Makhija N, Vasdev S, Jagia P. Use of near-infrared spectroscopy for detection of cerebral ischemia by superior vena cava obstruction in a patient with an ascending aortic aneurysm during left internal mammary artery harvesting. J Cardiothorac Vasc Anesth. 2012 Oct; 26(5): e62–3.

40. Society of Thoracic Surgeons Blood Conservation Guideline Task Force, Ferraris VA, Ferraris SP, Saha SP, Hessel EA 2nd, Haan CK, Royston BD, Bridges CR, Higgins RS, Despotis G, Brown JR; Society of Cardiovascular Anesthesiologists Special Task Force on Blood Transfusion, Spiess BD, Shore-Lesserson L, Stafford-Smith M, Mazer CD, Bennett-Guerrero E, Hill SE, Body S. Perioperative blood transfusion and blood conservation in cardiac surgery: the Society of Thoracic Surgeons and The Society of Cardiovascular Anesthesiologists clinical practice guideline. Ann Thorac Surg. 2007 May; 83(5 Suppl):S27–86.

41. Makhija N, Sarupria A, Choudhary S' Das S, Lakshmy R, Kiran U. Comparison of epsilon aminocaproic acid and tranexamic Acid in thoracic aortic surgery: clinical efficacy and safety. J Cardiothorac Vasc Anesth. 2013 Dec; 27(6):1201–7.

**Acknowledgment**

I hereby acknowledge Dr Priya Jagia, Additional Professor, Department of Interventional Cardiac Radiology for the contribution of CT images.

# CHAPTER 4

# Anesthesia for Arch of Aorta Diseases

Parag Gharde, Shiv Kumar Choudhary

## ANESTHESIA FOR AORTIC ARCH SURGERY

### Introduction

Aortic arch aneurysm incidence in isolation is very rare. It is often involved as an extension of the disease from the adjacent aortic segment. Though rare compared to other aortic aneurysm, it demands careful planning regarding aortic cannulation site selection and cerebral protection strategies and monitoring during an open surgical procedure.

## AORTIC ARCH ANATOMY AND ITS VARIANTS

Aortic arch is a segment of thoracic aorta, which lies transversely between the distal ascending aorta and the proximal descending thoracic aorta. The arch can be divided into a proximal segment from where the innominate artery originates and a distal segment that gives rise to the left common carotid and left subclavian artery. The arch is widest in its proximal portion and gradually narrows towards the distal segment. The narrowest portion of the thoracic aorta is in fact the isthmus, which lies between the distal segment of the aortic arch (i.e. distal to the left subclavian artery) and the ductus arteriosus.

Three vessels arise from the arch and are commonly referred to as arch vessels (Fig. 4.1).

The first in line is the *innominate artery* or the brachiocephalic artery that further branches into the right subclavian artery and the right common carotid artery. The next arch vessel is the left common carotid artery, which branches into left internal and external carotid artery. The last of the arch artery is the left subclavian artery. This normal branching pattern of the arch vessels is seen in nearly 70% of individuals. Bovine

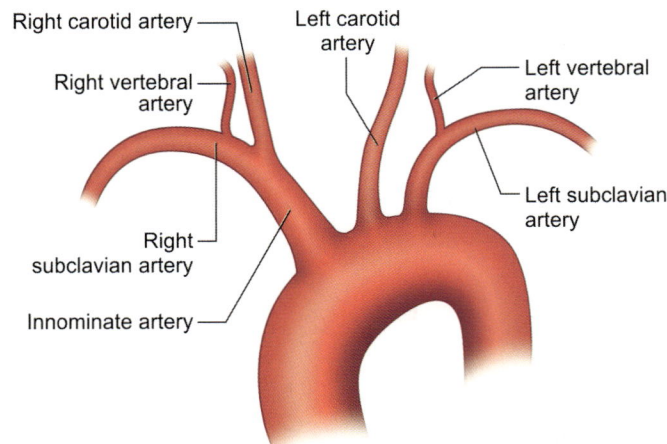

**Fig. 4.1:** A normal aortic arch branching pattern. Three arch vessels having separate origin first is the innominate artey. Second is the left common carotid artery. The last arch vessel is the left subclavian artery

trunk is the commonest variant of arch vessels, seen in approximately 20% of individuals. Bovine trunk comprises of only two arch vessels. The innominate and the left common carotid artery have a common origin, while the left subclavian artery originates as a separate vessel (Fig. 4.2 ).

In another variant, the left common carotid originates from the innominate artery (Fig. 4.3 ). Some[1] consider these variant of arch branching pattern as a misnomer, since in a true bovine arch a single vessel originates from the arch (as seen in cattle). This large brachiocephalic trunk gives rise to the innominate artery, left common carotid artery and the left subclavian artery (Fig. 4.4). There are clinical implications of bovine trunk (including misnomers) during the arch surgery. Perfusion through cannulation of the right axillary, or innominate artery

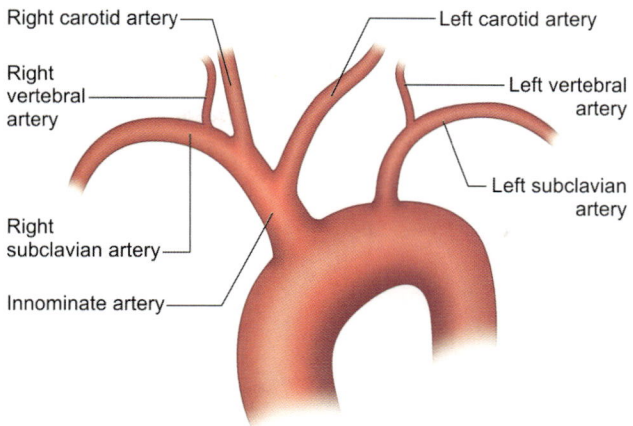

Fig. 4.2: A variant of bovine arch, not a true bovine arch. The innominate and the left common carotid have a common origin, while the left subclavian artery originates separately

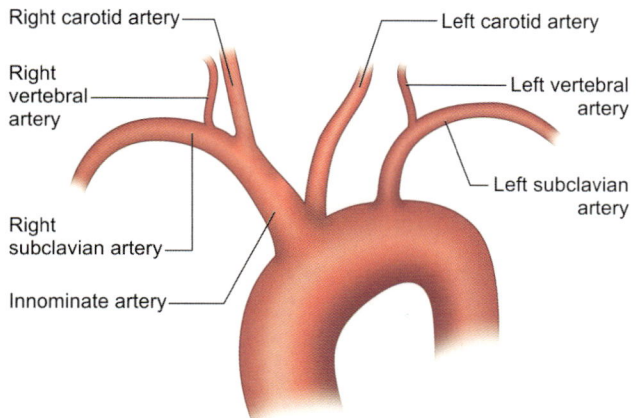

Fig. 4.3: The first branch of the arch is the innominate artery which bifurcates into right brachiocephalic and the left common carotid artery. The left subclavian artery again has a separate origin

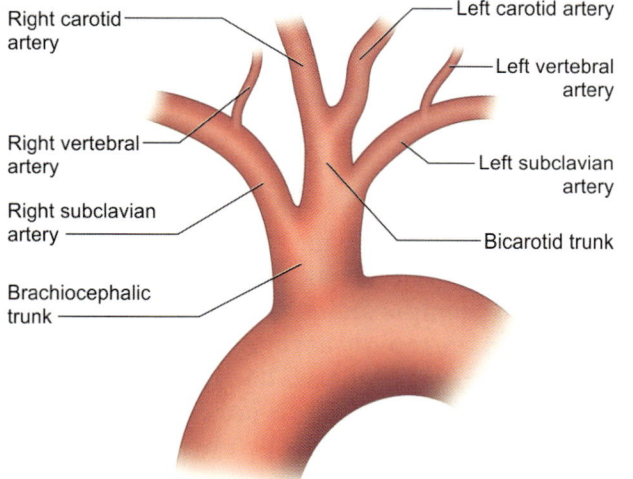

Fig. 4.4: This is an image of a true bovine arch as in the cattle. There is a single arch vessel, which post its origin trifurcates into right subclavian artery, the bi-carotid trunk and the left subclavian artery

or the right common carotid artery, will result in bilateral cerebral circulation. Thus, this may not necessitate separate cannulation of left common carotid for its perfusion or its separate anastomosis to the arch graft.

A study from United Kingdom[2] involving 861 patients selected randomly from the population underwent CT scan analysis of their aortic arch pattern. The result shows a bovine pattern in 20% of studied subjects. A 4-vessel arch with the left vertebral artery take off from the arch was the next common variant in 6%. Four-vessel arch with an aberrant right subclavian artery was seen in 0.5%, while a right-sided arch was seen in only 0.2% cases.

The aberrant right subclavian artery will result in compressive symptoms depending upon the course it follows. In about 80% of cases it originates from the descending thoracic aorta (DTA), coursing behind the esophagus, resulting in symptoms of reflux or difficulty in food intake. The clinical implication of an aberrant right subclavian artery is most significant. If an aberrant right subclavian artery originating from DTA is used for pressure monitoring, it will not reflect cerebral perfusion pressure (as in case of its normal origin from the innominate artery), when innominate/right carotid artery is used for CPB inflow during arch surgery. In such a case, a side pressure measurement from the aortic cannula can be used as a surrogate for cerebral perfusion pressure. The author though doesn't rely on the pressure monitoring as a surrogate for cerebral perfusion but follow the trend of near infrared spectroscopy. Knowledge of this variation will be critical for cerebral protection strategy. The axillary/subclavian artery is an attractive choice for arterial cannulation during CPB, as it also caters for unilateral antegrade cerebral perfusion. If the right axillary artery has been used for initiation of CPB before sternotomy, a separate cannulation of right or left common carotid or both is required for antegrade cerebral perfusion. Alternatively, the right common carotid artery can be used for the initiation of CPB and this will also provide cerebral protection during lower body systemic circulatory arrest, once the arch is opened for repair. Thus, detailed anatomical verification of the arch vessel is of great clinical significance during arch surgery, as anatomical variation can have impact on cerebral perfusion strategy and initiation of CPB.

## Clinical Features

Patients are usually asymptomatic with slow growing aneurysm. Symptom development in arch aneurysm is due to compressive effect on the surrounding structures. The aortic arch shares close relationship with trachea, left main bronchus and esophagus (Fig. 4.5).

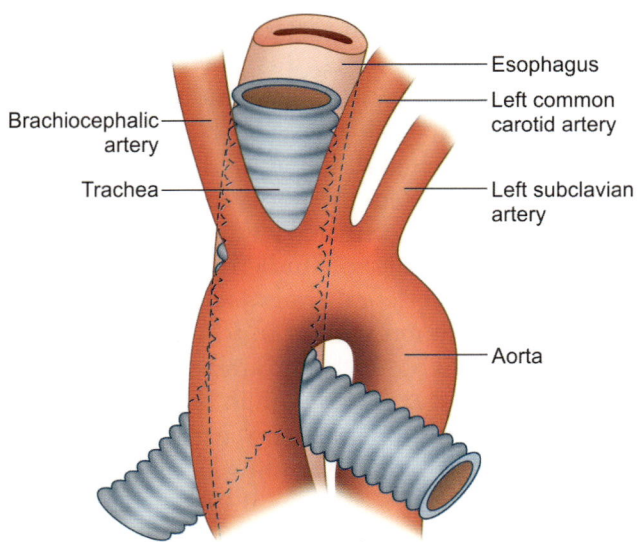

**Fig 4.5:** Structures surrounding arch of aorta

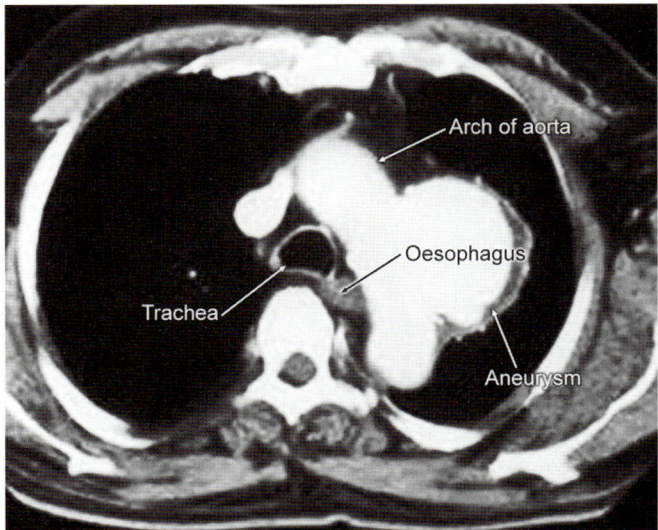

**Fig. 4.6:** Note the relation of arch of aorta with trachea. The image shows a saccular aneurysm along the greater curvature of the aortic area with thrombus in the sac

The primary complaint most commonly is of retrosternal pain in case of a rapidly enlarging aneurysm or if the aneurysm has already attained a significant size. Compression of left recurrent laryngeal nerve will result in complaint of hoarseness of voice. Difficulty in swallowing will reflect esophageal compression. Tracheal compression or left bronchus obstruction may elicit a complaint of difficulty in breathing or feeling of choking. History of hemoptysis due to aortopulmonary fistula development may bring the patient to the hospital for evaluation.

Stroke or transient ischemic attacks may occur due to thrombus embolization that can form as a result of sluggish circulation in the aneurysmal portion of the aorta.

During preliminary examination of the patient, history taking should also involve leading question of any family history of aortic disease, aortic dissection and sudden death. A positive history on this front will have significant implication on management, with pressing need for early intervention or frequent close follow-up if the aneurysm is small.

## Evaluation

Imaging is crucial, not only to reach an accurate diagnosis but also to follow-up patients with aortic disease. Ultrasonography is an attractive choice for the initial assessment. Once the diagnosis has been reached, the patient can then be subjected to the advanced imaging. Transthoracic ultrasonography scores over transesophageal ultrasonography in terms of being non-invasive with better ability to visualize the arch vessels. Multislice CTA and MRA have now almost replaced digital subtraction angiography for preoperative assessment and post-procedural follow-up. CTA is the preferred diagnostic tool for aortic aneurysm.

It is also the first choice for aortic emergencies, as it is faster than MRA and less operator dependent compared to transesophageal ultrasonography.

**Imaging modalities for aortic arch aneurysm**

- Chest X-ray
- Transthoracic echocardiography
- Multi-slice computed tomography angiography (CTA)
- Magnetic resonance imaging angiography (MRA)

**Key information from imaging**

- Morphology
- Maximum aortic dimension
- Extension
- Involvement of aortic branches
- Relationship with adjacent structure (compression effect)
- Presence of thrombus

## Aneurysm Growth and its Significance

Thoracic aortic aneurysm on an average has slow growth rate, taking years before posing clinical symptoms or complications. The descending thoracic aorta grows more rapidly as compared to the ascending aorta—0.30 cm/year versus 0.10 cm/year respectively. Rapid growth of an aneurysm is rather unusual and may occur in presence of uncontrolled hypertension, infection of aneurysm or post-dissection of the aneurysm. Also, a faster growth rate is seen as the aneurysm becomes bigger. Despite the fact that the descending thoracic aorta grows faster than the ascending aorta, the ascending aortic aneurysm shows a staggering rise in the incidence of dissection and rupture to the tune of 34% once it assumes the size of 6.0 cm. The descending thoracic aorta aneurysm shows such a behavior when the size reaches 7.0 cm in diameter. This differential risk behavior is not fully understood, but may be related to the difference in the level of stress these arteries are exposed to, due to their relative position from the heart.

Isolated aortic arch aneurysm incidence is low when compared to ascending and descending thoracic aortic aneurysm. Most often the aortic arch is involved as an extension either from the distal ascending aorta or proximal descending thoracic aortic disease (Fig. 4.7).

Due to paucity of available data on isolated aortic arch aneurysm no specific criteria or growth map can be formulated regarding the ideal time for intervention. The decision is most often taken based on the size of aorta, proximal or distal to the arch. The data from previous studies have shown sudden increase in the incidence of rupture, dissection and death, once the ascending aorta aneurysm size exceeds 6.0 cm and descending thoracic aorta aneurysm 7.0 cm. These dimensions are often referred to as 'hinge points' (Fig. 4.8), beyond which there is sudden escalation in incidence of complications. Therefore, it is wiser to intervene before this size is reached and hence have become the basis of the recommendation for intervention. Intervention can be planned based on symptom development and size of the aneurysm. Thoracic aneurysm of size ≥5.5 cm is an indication for intervention. Those with connective tissue disorder or having family history of dissection, rupture or sudden cardiac death, an early intervention at 5 cm is undertaken.

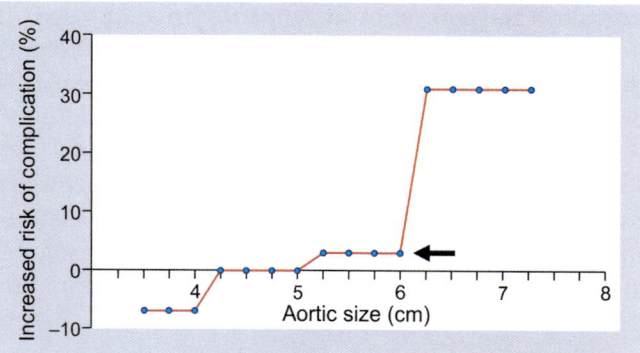

**Fig. 4.8:** This graph depicts the relationship between the size of the ascending aortic aneurysm (plotted on X-axis) and the incidence of complications-rupture or dissection (plotted on Y-axis). The bold arrow points the 'hinge point' at 6 cm aneurysm size from where there is sudden escalation in the incidence of complications

## MANAGEMENT OF ARCH ANEURYSM

There is paucity of data on the natural history of isolated aortic arch aneurysm and this is reflected in the decision making as well, since any kind of intervention (surgical or endovascular) is associated with the risk of stoke and

**Recommendations for aortic arch aneurysms 2010 AHA Guidelines[4]**

*Class IIa*

1. For thoracic aortic aneurysms also involving the proximal aortic arch, partial arch replacement together with ascending aorta repair using right subclavian/axillary artery inflow and hypothermic circulatory arrest is reasonable. (*LOE: B*)

2. Replacement of the entire aortic arch is reasonable for acute dissection when the arch is aneurysmal or there is extensive aortic arch destruction and leakage. (*LOE: B*)

3. Replacement of the entire aortic arch is reasonable for aneurysms of the entire arch, for chronic dissection when the arch is enlarged, and for distal arch aneurysms that also involve the proximal descending thoracic aorta, usually with the elephant trunk procedure. (*LOE: B*)

4. For patients with low operative risk in whom an isolated degenerative or atherosclerotic aneurysm of the aortic arch is present, operative treatment is reasonable for asymptomatic patients when the diameter of the arch exceeds 5.5 cm. (*LOE: B*)

5. For patients with isolated aortic arch aneurysms less than 4.0 cm in diameter, it is reasonable to reimage using computed tomographic imaging or magnetic resonance imaging, at 12-month intervals, to detect enlargement of the aneurysm. (*LOE: C*)

6. For patients with isolated aortic arch aneurysms 4.0 cm or greater in diameter, it is reasonable to reimage using computed tomographic imaging or magnetic resonance imaging, at 6-month intervals, to detect enlargement of the aneurysm. (*LOE: C*)

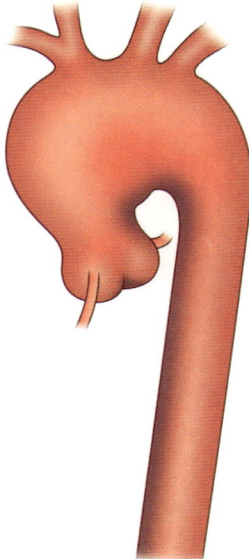

**Fig. 4.7:** Aneurysm of arch of aorta extending to ascending and proximal descending aorta

mortality. Surgery should be contemplated when the maximum diameter of the arch aneurysm is ≥5.5 cm or those who present with sign of compressive features.[3]

## Medical Management

A small aneurysm detected accidentally on medical investigation require tight control of blood pressure as it will decrease the shear stress on the diseased segment and retard the progressive dilatation of the aneurysmal segment. Beta-blocking agents are commonly initiated to achieve this. History of smoking is quite common in aortic aneurysm. Smoking also accelerates aneurysm expansion and therefore its cessation is advocated.[5]

## Closed Repair

If the aneurysm is large and patient is symptomatic then an intervention is warranted. The choice of intervention has to be made between an open repair and a closed endovascular stent repair (thoracic endovascular aortic repair—TEVAR). The choice is mostly governed by presence of severe comorbidity and life expectancy. TEVAR for an isolated arch aneurysm often requires surgical revascularization of arch vessels (hybrid approach), so as to provide healthy landing zone for the stent, which may cover the arch branches. The landing zone classification is based on its relationship with the arch vessels (Figs 4.9A to C). Landing zone-0 is proximal to the innominate artery, landing zone-1 is between the innominate artery and the left common carotid artery, while the zone-3 is distal to the left subclavian artery. Aortic arch aneurysm stenting requiring stent positioning in the landing zone-0 and 1 will require a de-branching procedure. A debranching procedure involves branched graft to arch vessel from the ascending aorta. This procedure requires median sternotomy. Patients at increased surgical risk may undergo carotid-to-carotid grafting if the landing zone is in zone 1. These surgical procedures require close neurological monitoring to avoid neurological complications. Revascularization of the left subclavian artery may be required if limb ischemia complication develops after stenting. Prophylactic revascularization is warranted in post-coronary artery bypass grafting with patent left internal mammary artery graft or in patient where significant portion of descending thoracic aorta of going to be covered by stent along with left subclavian artery origin, especially if it gives rise to dominant vertebral artery.

## Open Repair

Surgical repair is the first choice for patients not plagued by severe comorbidities and have good life expectancy, especially when long-term results of stent grafting is still lacking. A well-planned approach is key to the outcome. The right axillary artery is invariably the first choice for arterial cannulation, as it provides antegrade cerebral blood supply during the arch repair. Femoral artery cannulation is often required when the surgical time is expected to be long, to provide blood supply to lower body and spinal cord. When dealing with aortic arch and descending thoracic aortic aneurysm an integrated approach of open arch replacement and

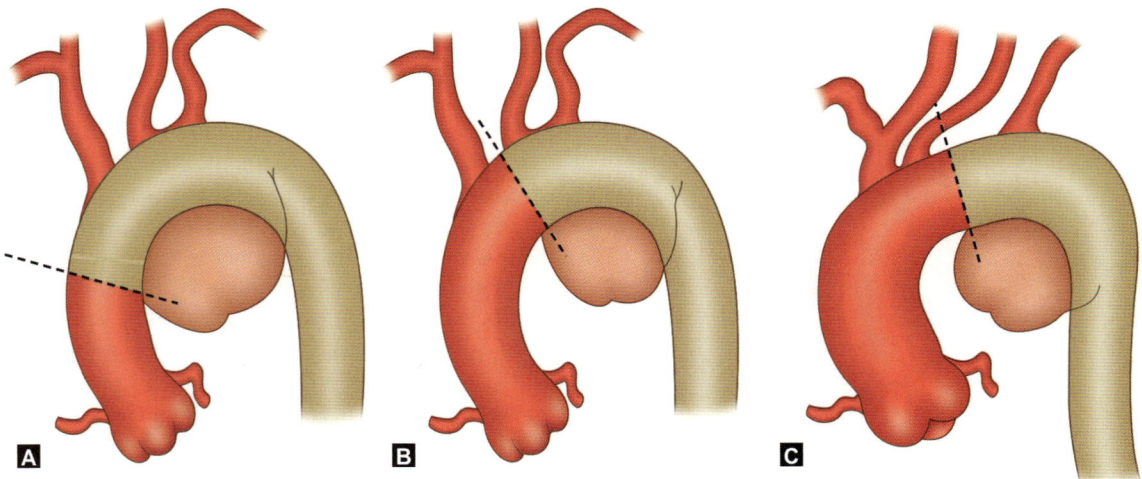

**Figs 4.9A to C:** Stent deployment requires a healthy aorta ~2.0 cm proximally and distally for firm anchorage which will prevent stent migration. The dotted line demarcates the classification of proximal landing zone as described by Ishimaru. (A) Shows presence of an aneurysm on the undersurface/lesser curvature of the aortic arch. Covering this whole portion with a stentgraft will result in obliteration of all the 3 arch branches. This picture is an example of landing zone-0 deployment, while the (B and C) represent landing zone 1 and 2 respectively

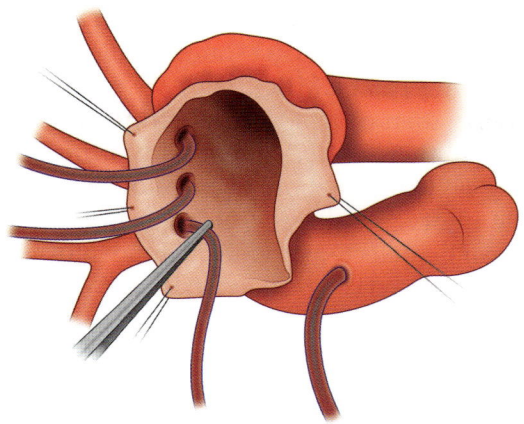

**Fig. 4.10:** Cerebral protection by selective antigrade cerebral perfusion. Note that all the three arch vessels are being perfused

frozen elephant trunk (stent grafting of the descending aorta) as a single-stage procedure sounds like a good proposition, but is highly expensive when compared to the traditional elephant trunk.

## CEREBRAL PROTECTION DURING OPEN ARCH REPAIR

Cerebral protection is one of the core issues of aortic arch surgery. The worst nightmare for an aortic intervention team is neurological injury, stroke and paraplegia. After all the hard work and efforts put in by the team members, postoperative neurological deficiency is heartbreaking. For this very reason great emphasis is laid on cannulation strategy. A careful planning for cerebral protection method to be employed becomes very crucial before the patient is taken up into an operating room (OR). A well thought out plan makes team members aware of their respective roles rather than waiting for the next cue from the surgeon. On most occasions a good protocolled approach bears good results in the end. Neurological complication was found to be associated with high mortality, through the pioneering work by DeBakey *et. al* in 1957.[6]

The brain is just like any other organ in the body. Preservation and protection is purely based on meeting the oxygen demand and supply ratio. Keeping this in mind various methods have evolved for cerebral preservation and each center, from where these protocols emerged, are quite vocal of their own strategy. The DeBakey et al[6] group was the first to come up with selective antegrade cerebral perfusion (ACP) technique in 1957. Griepp et al[7] group introduced deep hypothermic circulatory arrest (DHCA), while Ueda et al[8] introduced retrograde cerebral perfusion.

Each strategy has its own advantages and disadvantages. The author's opinion is to follow the physiology of nature, which has provided cerebral perfusion through carotid arteries. Therefore at the author's center, selective ACP technique is followed. There may be situations where this strategy cannot be followed, as in the case of dissection extending into both the carotid arteries. Therefore, it is best to select a strategy or combine two strategies based upon the prevailing circumstances to provide best cerebral protection possible.

## 1. DHCA

Brain requires constant supply of glucose and oxygen for its metabolic needs, which at rest is about seven times the rest of the body. This demand is met by blood flow to the brain. Cerebral blood flow autoregulation maintains the balance between demand and supply over a wide range of mean perfusion pressure (50–130 mm Hg). This limit is not a fixed number and there will be an upward shift in this in presence of long standing hypertension, advanced age and diabetes. This altered autoregulation predisposes the patient to the risk of hypoperfusion if the mean perfusion pressure falls below the lower limit. Beyond these autoregulatory limits the cerebral flow is proportional to perfusion pressure.

Apart from the above-mentioned conditions, autoregulatory function is transiently lost during long periods of non-pulsatile CPB, pH-stat management of the acid–base balance and during the cooling phase for DHCA. Impairment of autoregulation uncouples the relationship between metabolic demand and supply. A new coupling relationship is established between supply and perfusion pressure. Cerebral cooling decreases the cellular metabolic demand on one hand and impairs the autoregulatory function on the other hand. This result in an environment of extra blood flow above the metabolic needs, a condition termed as "luxury perfusion". The flipside of luxury perfusion state is that it increases the macro and micro-embolic load to the brain due to greater proportion of the pump flow reaching the brain during CPB.[9,10]

Temperature coefficient $Q_{10}$ reflects upon the relationship between cerebral metabolic rate for oxygen ($CMRO_2$) and temperature. There is 50% reduction in $CMRO_2$ for every 10° decrease in temperature. This relationship is valid within the temperature range of 38°C to 14°C.[11]

$$Q_{10} = \frac{CMRO_2 \text{ at } x°C}{CMRO_2 \text{ at } (x°C - 10)}$$

*This study performed on eight dogs concluded the following:*

Between 37°C and 27°C, the $Q_{10}$ was 2.23, but between 27°C and 14°C the $Q_{10}$ doubled to 4.53.

During cooling, the EEG developed burst suppression at or below 22°C. With further cooling, the periods of suppression increased but the burst activity continued in seven of eight dogs even at 14°C.

A study on the effect of norepinephrine on basal $CMRO_2$ during hypothermia in rats by Nemoto et al[12] resulted into an important finding:

Addition of Norepinephrine can nullify the isoelectric EEG effect of thiopentone and hypothermia. Norepinephrine is commonly added to the cardiopulmonary reservoir during CPB to maintain perfusion pressure. This addition may therefore be detrimental in patients who are to undergo DHCA.

McCullogh et al[13] demonstrated that at 15°C the human $CMRO_2$ decreased by 17% of the baseline and at 20°C was 24% of baseline value. This study found $Q_{10}$ in adult humans as 2.3, which was similar to $Q_{10}$ reported from experimental study in canines while cooling from 37 to 27°C.

A leftward shift of the oxyhemoglobin dissociation curve in the erythrocytes is seen with hypothermia, along with decrease in $PaCO_2$, increase in pH and decrease in intracellular concentration of 2, 3-diphosphoglycerate. This shift makes the oxygen bond with hemoglobin stronger and thus there is difficulty in its release at the cellular level. This results in higher values of oxygen saturation for a given $PaO_2$.

DHCA has evolved over the years along with our understanding of physiology involved. However, quite a few shortcomings of this strategy still remain to be tackled.

### Advantages of DHCA

1. Clear visualization of the operative field with no clutter of perfusion cannula and clamps.
2. The method is simple, easy and can be replicated anywhere and does not need any additional perfusion equipment.
3. Avoidance of clamping or cannulation for perfusion reduces the risk for brain embolism.

### Disadvantages of DHCA

1. DHCA offers cerebral protection but has time constraints. The reported range of safe circulatory arrest time is between 30–40 minutes.[3,4,10] Thereafter, incidence of stroke and mortality increases if DHCA alone is used for cerebral protection. There are others* who have indicated safe circulatory anesthesia duration as 25 minutes with DHCA as standalone cerebral protective strategy.
2. Clotting complications.
3. Reperfusion injury.
4. Slow cooling and rewarming prolongs the duration of CPB time with detrimental effect on endothelial, cardiac, cardiac, pulmonary and renal function.

It is to be clearly understood that different areas in brain have different $CMRO_2$ rates and therefore those regions with greater $CMRO_2$ rates are more vulnerable to ischemia than others. Hippocampus[15] is one such region of higher $CMRO_2$ rates and is the centre for acquiring new information. Because of its sensitivity to ischemic injury, subtle sign of brain injury following DHCA can be detected by deficits in memory function during neuropsychological evaluation.[16]

Despite being in clinical use for decades, some significant grey areas still remain with DHCA. The most important issue is the question of safe duration. Due to conflicting reports from various studies, it is best to limit the circulation arrest period to less than 30 minutes. The safe duration of arrest depends on uniform cerebral cooling. Use of pharmacological adjuncts to further suppress $CMRO_2$ is still controversial. The rate of rewarming will also determine the incidence of cerebral injury. Therefore, the duration of the arrest alone is not the only determinant of neurological injury but the conduct of DHCA as a whole has an important bearing.

### Controversies in DHCA strategy

- The degree of hemodilution
- Cooling and warming rates
- pH strategies

The major limiting factors of DHCA are prolonged CPB time resulting in significant coagulopathy and inflammatory reaction.

With all these controversies, it is apt to say that DHCA is not an ideal strategy for cerebral protection. Thus, alternative means and methods are being looked into and many centers are departing from this traditional method of cerebral protection.

All said and done, this will not be the last swan song for DHCA. There are clinical situations when there are no alternative means but DHCA to provide for cerebral protection.

## The Technique of Performing DHCA

Neuromonitoring in form of Bispectral index or near infrared spectroscopy (NIRS) sensors is applied to the forehead after proper cleaning of the skin, to improve contact and decrease impedance. After induction of anesthesia methylprednisolone 30 mg/kg is administered to the patient.

The cooling blanket is set at 4°C for topical cooling during the preparatory phase of the operation. The patient is actively cooled to nasopharyngeal temperature of 18°C over a period no less than 30 minutes during CPB.

Some cool till the burst suppression ratio of 100 is achieved or use a pharmacological agent, like thiopentone (5–10 mg/kg), to achieve burst suppression. Others rely on NIRS, which shows steady rise in cerebral saturation as cellular metabolism is suppressed with hypothermia. Others[17] cool the patient guided by mixed venous oxygen saturation from the SVC drainage cannula. Once the value is above 95%, which suggests adequate suppression of cerebral metabolism, DHCA is initiated.

To prevent passive rewarming from the ambient temperature of the operating room, the head is covered with ice packs, with adequate care taken to avoid direct contact with pinna and eyes.

Before initiating DHCA and opening the arch, the patient is placed in Trendelenburg position. Once the surgical anastomosis is over, CPB is reinitiated with very gradual rewarming over minimum 30 minutes duration. A short period of retrograde cerebral perfusion can be performed to remove any air or debris trapped in the vessel when the arch is opened. This maneuver will help in deairing the graft as well.

## 2. RETROGRADE CEREBRAL PERFUSION

An innovative idea from Mills and Ochsner[10] gave birth to retrograde cerebral perfusion, which was first used in a patient of massive arterial air embolism during CPB. But it was Ueda et al[8] ten years after Mills et al in 1990 who described its first use in thoracic aortic surgery as cerebral protection strategy.

Ueda described the use of RCP as an adjunct to HCA in a series of eight adult patients undergoing aortic arch replacement. There was only one incidence of temporary neurological dysfunction. This historic report from Ueda *et al.* opened up a new avenue for aortic surgeons who were highly dissatisfied with the incidence of neurological events, especially in complex aortic arch repair, which required extension of DHCA period. RCP is an attractive adjunct to the surgeons as in addition to providing oxygenation and metabolic needs it flushed out gaseous as well as particulate embolic debris, thus having additional protective benefit.[19] At the author's center, RCP is very rarely used, as cerebral perfusion is mostly through ACP (Fig. 4.11).

## 3. ANTEGRADE CEREBRAL PERFUSION (ACP)— UNILATERAL OR BILATERAL

Whether the ACP has to be via unilateral or bilateral carotid artery cannulation is generally linked to the completeness of circle of Willis. Every surgeon has their own philosophy regarding the importance of circle of Willis, and some follow the path of what is natural, and

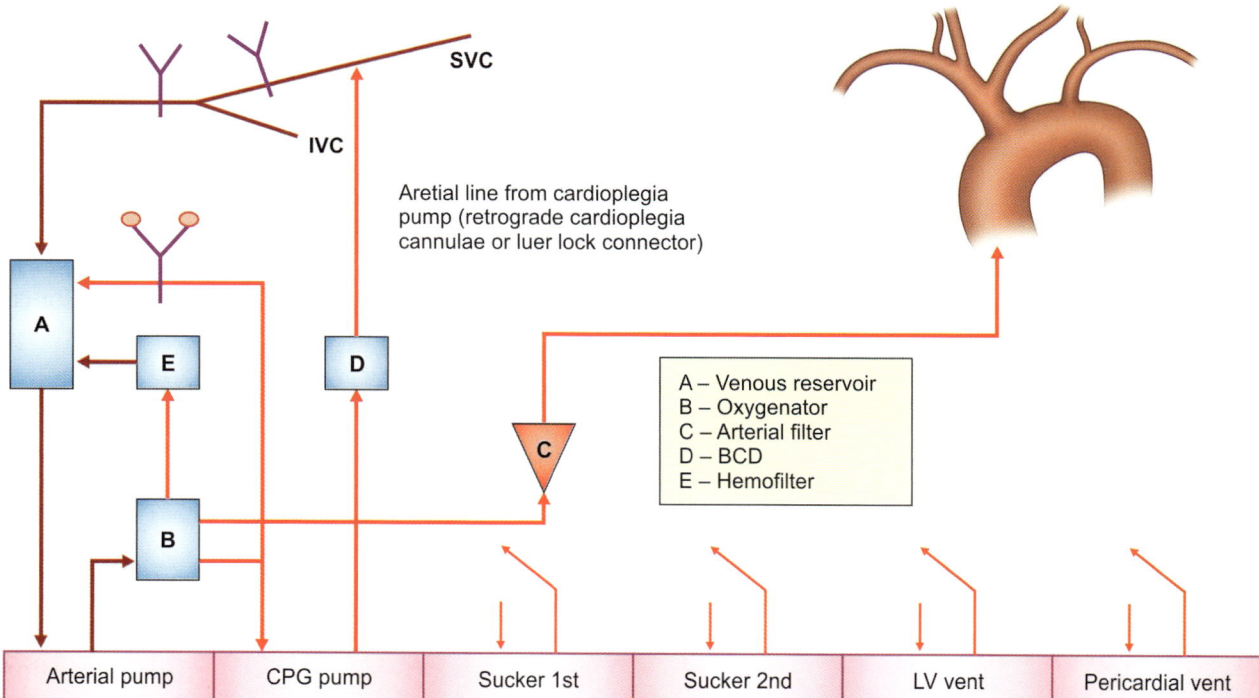

A – Venous reservoir
B – Oxygenator
C – Arterial filter
D – BCD
E – Hemofilter

**Fig. 4.11.** Retrograde cerebral perfusion is achieved by either connecting the superior vena caval cannula to the arterial pump or to the cardioplegia pump of the cardiopulmonary machine (as shown in position D). (*Courtesy*: Mr Yogesh Solanki)

cannulate both the carotids even in presence of complete circle of Willis. But this practice carries its own risk, especially in older population where atherosclerotic disease of the arch vessels is also common, and may in fact increase the incidence of embolic stroke. Others, who call themselves wiser, base their decision on preoperative evaluation of the circle of Willis by cranial computed tomography angiography. Urbanski *et al*[20] confronted the reliance of selection of cerebral perfusion based on circle of Willis. They demonstrated that in cases where the circle of Willis was incomplete cross perfusion did occur through secondary collateral vessels, during unilateral cerebral perfusion. There is a possibility that other collateral systems exists, which may not yet have gained attention (the extra-cranial collateral circulation), which is angiographically invisible, and may dilate to provide cerebral perfusion.

The perfusion via right innominate artery, axillary artery or carotid artery carries the advantage of cerebral supply via the right carotid artery and the right vertebral artery, while the left common carotid artery perfusion lacks the support from the left vertebral artery which originates from the left subclavian artery (Figs 4.12A to D).

The author opines that the decision for unilateral or bilateral cerebral perfusion should not be based on the anatomical status of the circle of Willis but based on function status. To assess the latter, help of neuro-monitoring tool like near infrared spectroscopy should be taken.

Malvindi et al[21], performed a detailed analysis of 17 studies with combined study sample of 3, 548, of these 83.1% (2, 949/3, 548) received bilateral ACP and only 16.9% (599/3, 548) received unilateral ACP. The important conclusion that came from this study analysis was that bilateral ACP is favoured when the aortic arch repair time exceeds 45 minutes to 50 minutes.

Antegrade cerebral perfusion has traditionally been performed with deep hypothermia.[22,23] Recently a few centers have made departure from this tradition to perform ACP with mild to moderate hypothermia, thereby avoiding the ills associated with deep hypothermia.[24]

### Technique of Performing ACP

The conduct of cardiopulmonary bypass during aortic arch surgery has to be well planned in advance, to prevent morbidity and mortality due to ischemic injury. Over the years various aortic sites have been cannulated for arterial flow during CPB, and each group claims and propagates their own strategy as the best. Since there can be multitude of scenarios which can dictate the selection of CPB strategy, the concept of one shoe fits all has to be discouraged. Therefore, the CPB conduct should be planned with an open mind, taking into consideration the pros and cons of each cannulation strategy.

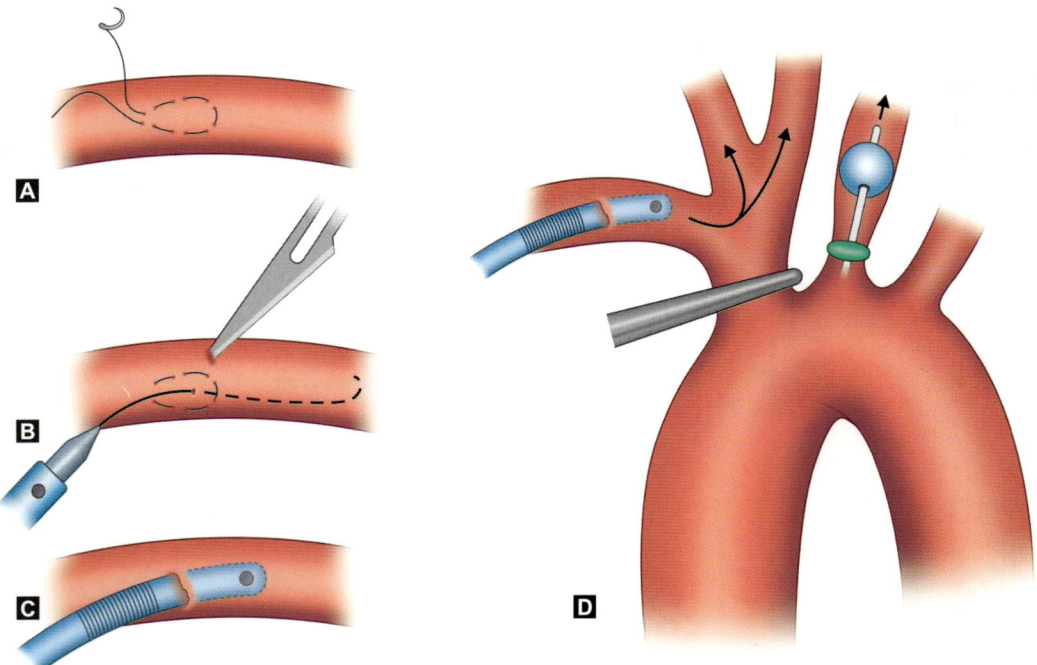

**Figs 4.12A to D:** ACP by subclavian artery cannulation. (A to C) Shows surgical introduction of straight tip cannula into the artery. (D) Shows the base of innominate artery clamped, with the cannula in the subclavian artery, providing antegrade cerebral perfusion. Also note that a separate balloon tipped cannula has been introduced into the left common carotid artery as well

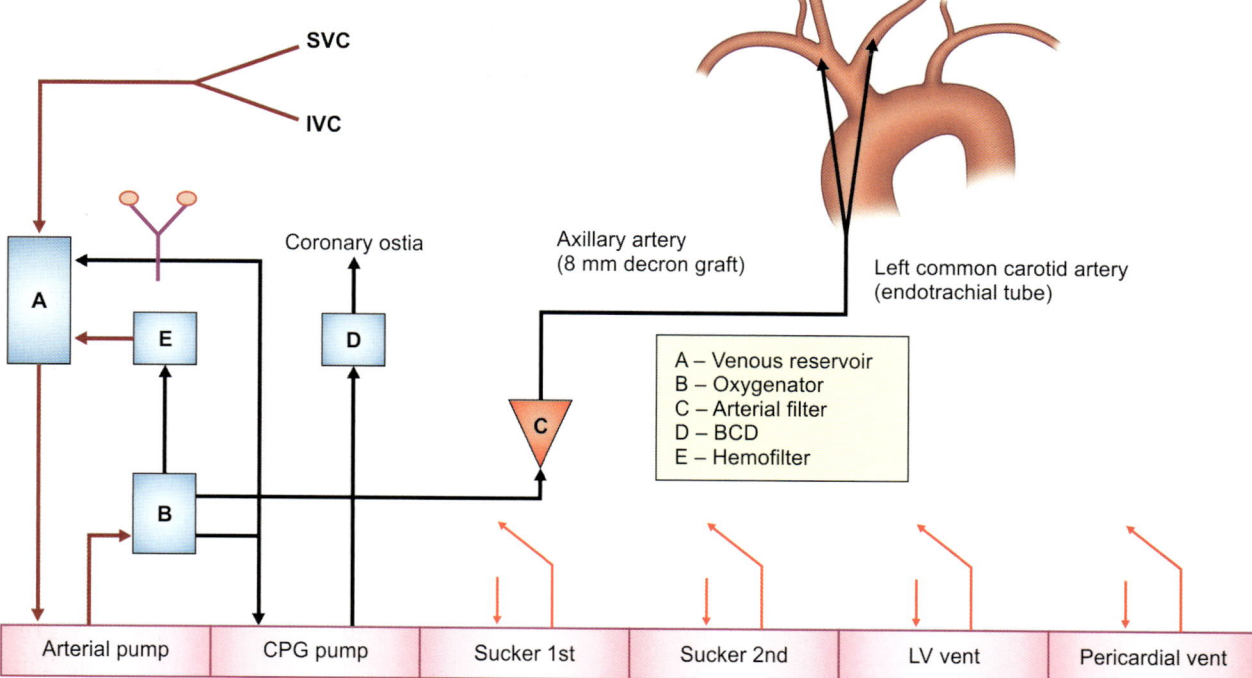

**SVC**

**IVC**

Coronary ostia

Axillary artery
(8 mm decron graft)

Left common carotid artery
(endotrachial tube)

A – Venous reservoir
B – Oxygenator
C – Arterial filter
D – BCD
E – Hemofilter

A

E

D

C

B

| Arterial pump | CPG pump | Sucker 1st | Sucker 2nd | LV vent | Pericardial vent |

**Fig. 4.13:** Antegrade cerebral perfusion can be achieved either through direct cannulation of the carotids once the arch is opened or axillary/innominate artery cannulation with separate cannulation of the left common carotid artery if the need arises. (*Courtesy*: Mr Yogesh Solanki)

The femoral artery (FA) cannulation has been a popular choice in patients undergoing aortic surgery for the following conditions:

Type-A dissection, dissection extending into the arch vessels, significantly dilated ascending aorta aneurysm abutting the sternum, or arch aneurysm. With this technique, DHCA is required for cerebral protection, before the aortic cross clamp is placed over the proximal DTA to repair the arch. If the arch repair is complex, then it should be supported with some source (ACP or RCP) to provide cerebral perfusion. Selective ACP can be performed by special arch vessel cannula or by endotracheal tube. FA may not be an ideal choice, especially if the FA is small in size, as in females, which will limit the size of cannula used. In such conditions bilateral FA cannulation can be done to circumvent this issue. But due to retrograde nature of the flow with FA cannulation, cerebral embolization of atheromatous debris or thrombus or retrograde extension of the dissection flap may fail this strategy.

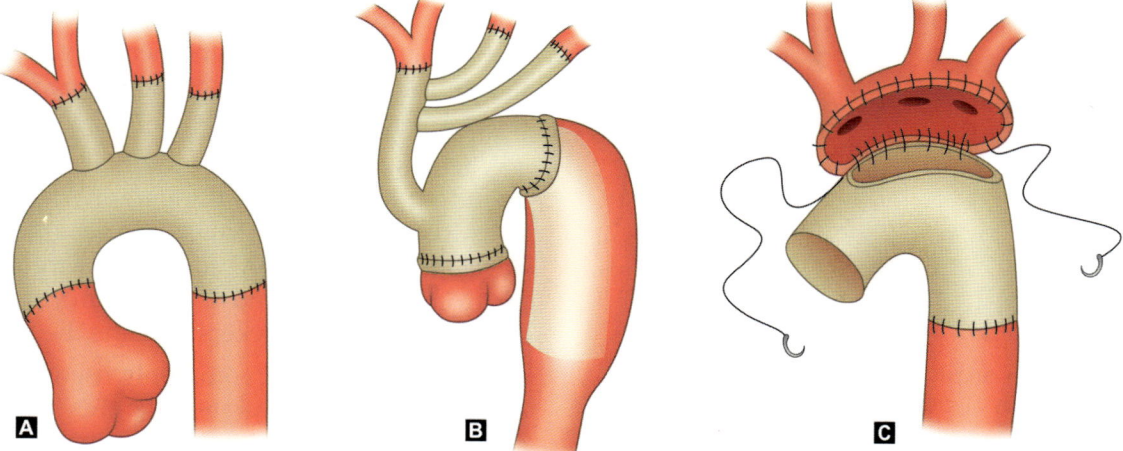

**A**

**B**

**C**

**Figs 4.14A to C:** Open aortic arch replacement. The following figures shows different methods by which the arch is replaced. (B) Shows debranching of the arch vessel with ascending aorta (supracoronary) replacement, note that a length of free graft has been left in the descending thoracic aorta which will be used for stent grafting to cover the aneurysmal aorta, (C) is the classical Carrels patch technique where an island of arch with the arch vessel is reimplanted on to the graft

Axillary artery cannulation is an attractive alternative as it can be used for selective ACP by placing a vascular clamp proximal to the bifurcation of the innominate artery when the sternum is opened, with lower body circulatory arrest. Villard et al[25] in 1976 first described axillary artery cannulation in a case of Type-A dissection. The axillary artery is usually free from atherosclerotic disease and dissection, and therefore, it is a good option for initiation of CPB, and can also provide ACP. Axillary artery cannulation is associated with potential danger of brachial plexus injury, limb ischaemia, axillary artery injury/dissection and neurological complication if the vertebral artery is covered/crossed by the cannula itself.[26,27] Because of the reasons sited above, many surgeons use an 8 mm graft, anastomosed end to side to axillary artery, allowing blood flow to the limb as well (Fig. 4.15).[28] Decannulation is simply performed by transecting the graft and over sewing. One of the other drawback, though not a significant one, is that axillary artery cannulation will require a separate incision. Thus, few have ventured out to directly cannulate the innominate artery through the same sternotomy incision using 22-French or 24-French

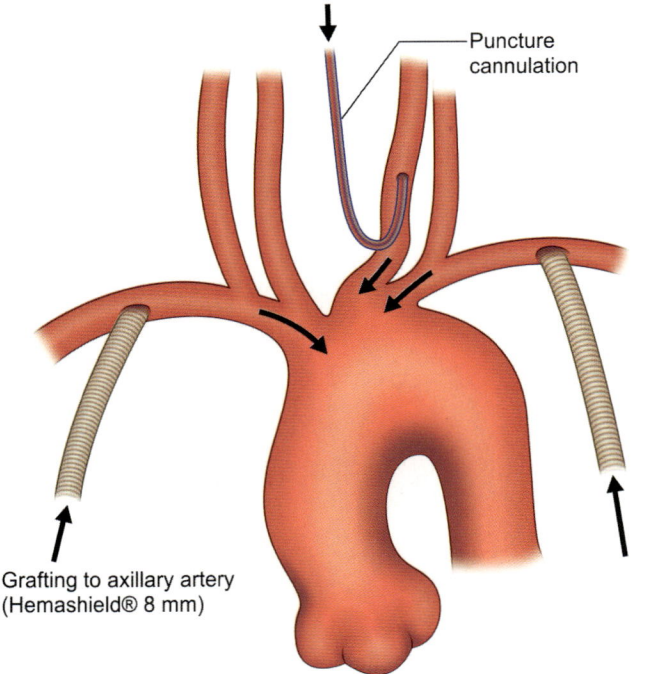

Puncture cannulation

Grafting to axillary artery (Hemashield® 8 mm)

**Fig 4.15:** End to side anastomosis of 8 mm graft to the right subclavian artery is an alternative to direct cannulation and is associated with less incidence of artery injury. If the NIRS values on left side show significant fall during test clamping of left common carotid artery then selective perfusion of left common carotid artery is also warranted. Also note that left subclavian artery use for ACP completely fails if used as stand alone method because only left vertebral artery originates from it

wire-reinforced flexible cannula, which is introduced with the tip pointing towards the aortic arch. Once the arch procedure is to be initiated, the cannula tip is redirected towards the head for selective antegrade cerebral perfusion with clamp proximal to the cannula. Redirecting the angled cannula may cause intimal damage and dissection. Therefore, use of a straight tip cannula can circumvent this potential problem. The Stanford group was the first to report innominate artery cannulation during arch surgery for unilateral cerebral perfusion.[29] Innominate artery cannulation may not be an ideal site in presence of dissection extension into the innominate artery or in patients with large ascending aortic aneurysm abutting or eroding into the sternum, where sternotomy after initiation of partial CPB will be a safer strategy. In such a case, FA cannulation and initiation of partial CPB or carotid artery cannulation via a side graft can be performed. There are potential dangers of cerebral embolism; therefore in the preoperative workup, these vessels should be evaluated by Duplex Ultrasound and CT angiography.[30]

## NEUROPROTECTIVE DRUGS

The total energy utilized by a neuron is divided into 60% for electrophysiological activity and 40% for maintenance of neuronal and glial integrity. Hypothermia reduces energy consumption for both, while anesthetics decrease energy consumption for neuronal electrical activity. Therefore, it can be assumed that adding barbiturates to hypothermia will enhance the neurological protective effect.[31] Experimental studies have shown that decreasing temperature had variable effect on $CMRO_2$. This led to shifting of focus on pharmacological agents who would further decrease $CMRO_2$ as attained by hypothermia and thus improve the neurological outcome and this may perhaps stretch the safe duration of DHCA.

Various pharmacological agents have been tried including barbiturates (thiopentone), lignocaine, and steroids, and mannitol. Now recent interest has developed with NMDA receptor antagonists (ketamine, dextromethorphan and magnesium), statins, alpha-2 agonists and beta-blockers to name the few.

Presently, the most commonly used neuroprotective agents include barbiturates, steroids and Mannitol. A postal survey on practice of use of pharmacological agents as cerebral protectants during DHCA was performed on members of Association of Cardiothoracic Anesthetics. 60% responded to the survey and 80% of them administered some pharmacological agent for neuroprotection. Most commonly used agent was thiopentone (59%) but of them only 35% believed that there is sufficient evidence in support. 48% respondents used steroids but only 16% used it because they felt there was some evidence in support of its use.[32]

Thiopentone among all other barbiturates finds mention in most of the earlier studies and textbooks as a preferred agent for neurological protection. The proposed mechanism behind the neurological benefits of thiopentone includes decrease in $CMRO_2$, suppression of seizure activity, decrease in the release of excitatory amino acids and calcium influx during ischemia and decrease in cerebral blood flow, which benefits by decreasing the embolic load. Thiopentone was earlier given at a high dose (30–50 mg/kg) which resulted in significant cardiac depression, warranting infusion of inotropic agents, delayed awakening, prolonged intubation time, and length of ICU and hospital stay.

Studies that failed to show benefits of thiopentone may have been because of periods of hemodynamic instability due to large doses of thiopentone. The timing of administering thiopentone is also very crucial. If administered before the onset of CPB, then it decreases CBF due to cerebral vasoconstriction and hence may not allow uniform cooling of brain. It should be administered just before the initiation of DHCA.

Etomidate, like barbiturates produces EEG burst suppression and reduces $CMRO_2$. At doses of 0.4–0.5 mg/kg it does not produce hemodynamic instability. This is where etomidate significantly scores over thiopentone, but at the cost of adrenocortical suppression. It may also impair renal function due to propylene glycol.[33]

Steroids are also popular as neuroprotective agents. Methylprednisolone (30 mg/kg) is commonly administered after anesthesia induction. The neuroprotective effect is probably due to inhibition of lipid peroxidation. Both glucocorticoids-dexamethasone and methyl-prednisolone result in hyperglycemia, which in presence of ischemia increases neuronal injury. Apart from this, steroids induce immunosuppression and increase the risk of perioperative infection. A recent study from Germany on intraoperative use of neuroprotective drugs in patients undergoing surgery for type-A aortic dissection concluded that use of Mannitol may be associated with decreased mortality but routine use of steroids requires more investigation.[34] The cosseli group use 1 gm methylprednisolone prior to anesthesia in all patients when the anticipated circulatory arrest time is more than 30 minutes and is continued in the first 48 hours postoperatively (125 mg every 6 hours for 24 hours and then 125 mg every 12 hours for the next 24 hours). In patients whom the circulatory anesthesia time is <30 minutes, the postoperative doses of methylprednisolone are omitted.

## Anesthesia Management for Open Repair

Before taking up the patient with arch aneurysm to the OR, it is pertinent to go through all the investigative reports. This will help in proper planning in advance. As the aortic arch shares close relation with trachea and left main bronchus, there may be deviation or compression of these structures. Preoperative CT angiography will give this information and if present, a wire reinforced endotracheal tube for tracheal intubation will be best suited for the purpose. If there is a history of hemoptysis due to the aneurysm, then it is better to go for lung isolation technique. As there may be left bronchus deviation, the ideal choice will be a right sided double lumen tube, as a left sided tube may be difficult to negotiate into the deviated left main bronchus. Any hoarseness of voice should alert the anesthesiologist of the possibility of laryngeal nerve compression by the

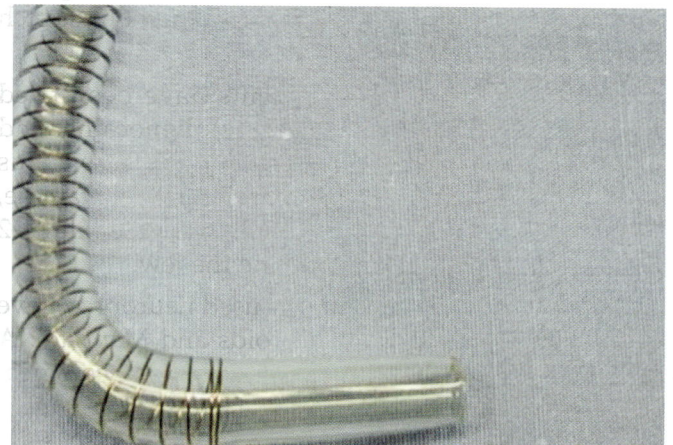

**Fig. 4.16:** A wire reinforced angle cannula commonly used for innominate artery or subclavian artery perfusion

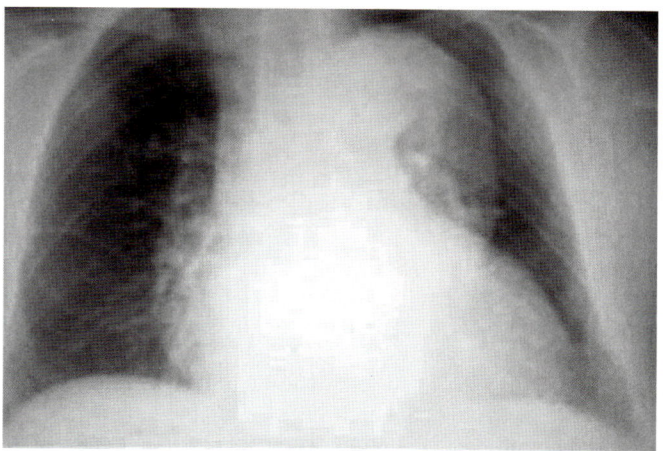

**Fig. 4.17:** Chest X-ray shows aortic arch enlargement

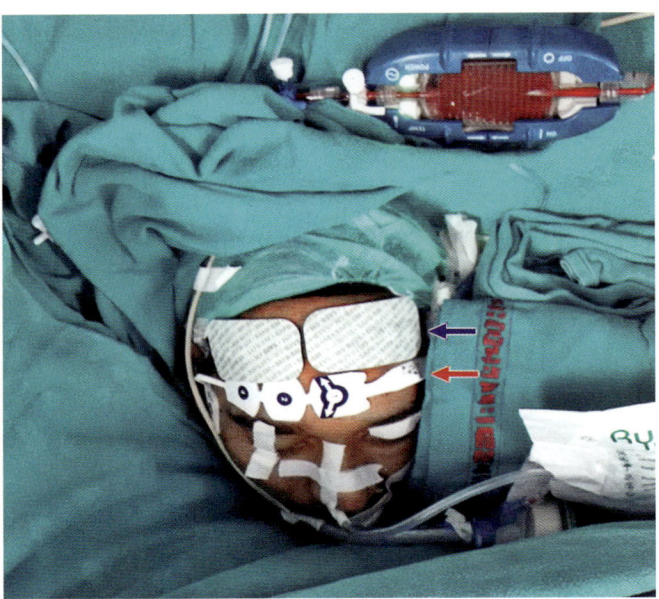

**Fig. 4.18:** Neurological monitoring is an integral part of arch aneurysm repair. The red arrow points towards the bispectral index sensor, while the blue arrow points towards the NIRS sensor

expanding arch aneurysm. A preoperative documentation of vocal cord palsy by indirect laryngoscopy would be ideal.

A history of difficulty in deglutition should be taken to rule out esophageal compression. If the history is positive and the CT angiography shows esophageal compression then one needs to be very careful while inserting transesophageal echocardiographic probe. A

pediatric TEE probe can be an ideal substitute to adult probe in such a case. The author opines that TEE probe should not be inserted in patients with aorto-esophageal fistula. Reports of blood investigation should be looked into, especially hemoglobin, total leukocyte count, platelet count, urea, creatinine, and C-reactive protein. If the patient is diabetic, a good glycemic control should be strived for by adjusting the drug dosages adequately, or best convert them to insulin. Proper glucose control will prevent significant fluctuations in sugar levels intraoperatively. Adequate blood and blood products should be arranged before hand, especially if DHCA has been planned, as coagulopathy is common with prolonged CPB and hypothermia.

Once the patient is in the operating theatre 5 lead electrocardiogram is applied. Two NIRS sensors (Fig. 4.19) are applied over the forehead after proper cleaning, and a baseline value is recorded on room air, which acts as a reference value. The need for selective ACP from the left carotid is determined based on how the NIRS behaves after selective ACP from the right common carotid artery, or innominate artery or the axillary artery. A test clamp of left common carotid artery is done. If the left side NIRS value shows a 20–30% decline over the baseline, it suggests the need for perfusion through the left common carotid artery. A large bore intravenous line is placed under local infiltration. As a protocol, a 20 G catheter is inserted in right radial artery for pressure monitoring. Since right subclavian artery is used for initiation of bypass and also acts as source for antegrade

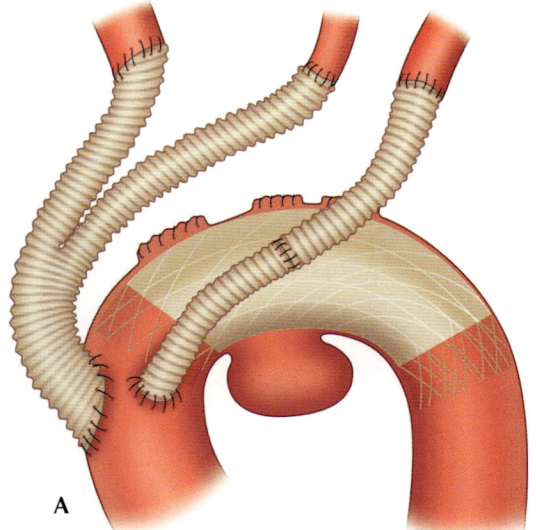

A

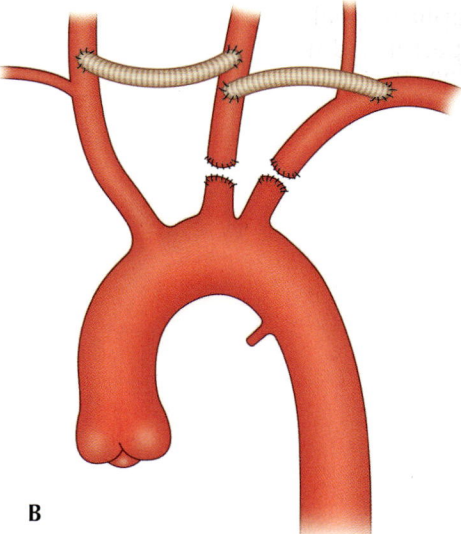

B

**Figs 4.19A and B:** An aneurysm of aortic arch and descending thoracic aorta (A) is amenable to endovascular repair but requires a de-branching procedure of the arch vessel. A branched graft is anastamosed to the proximal aorta with slight lateral location so as to avoid its lie directly under the sterum, to prevent its compression and inadvertent transection during re-sternotomy. (B) Carotid to carotid bypass grafting along with carotid to left subclavian artery bypass. This method of de-branching does not require sternotomy cerebral perfusion, the right radial artery pressure is used as a surrogate for cerebral perfusion pressure. The subclavian artery is not directly cannulated but through an 8 mm Dacron side graft and therefore the right radial artery pressures can be relied upon, unlike direct cannulation, which may hinder flow distally. In case the right common carotid artery is to be used for CPB initiation, the central venous catheter is placed in the left femoral vein, leaving the right groin to the surgeons for femoral artery/vein cannulation. Such a scenario arises in case of massive ascending and arch aneurysm abutting the sternum, where a risk of entering into the aneurysm during sternotomy will be present. The sternotomy is performed after initiation of partial bypass. Pulmonary artery catheter can be inserted as it provides lot of information apart from cardiac output. A transesophageal probe is inserted after tracheal intubation. Careful manipulation of probe is required as the aneurysm may be compressing on the esophagus. The whole of the arch is not visible due to the blind spot as a result of the left bronchus traversing between the esophagus and the arch. Only the distal portion of the arch is visible and therefore the distal anastomosis with the DTA can be evaluated postoperatively. In case of extensive aortic dissection, ascending aorta and arch is repaired and an elephant trunk of length less than 10 cm is left floating in the descending aorta. TEE can be helpful in assessing the flow through the trunk. TEE also provides information regarding biventricular function (systolic and diastolic), regional wall motion abnormality, stroke volume, other valvular function and preload. Temperature measurements are done from two sites, nasopharyngeal and rectal. Since the surgery at our center is performed under mild to low moderate hypothermia (30–32°C), a higher pump flow is kept, and a hematocrit of 30% is the target, to improve oxygen carrying capacity.

Antifibrinolytics are now routinely used in aortic surgery.[35] At present only two antifibrinolytics are being used to prevent excessive postoperative bleeding-tranexamic acid and e-aminocaproic acid. Earlier, aprotinin use was the standard institutional practice, but post Canadian BART (blood conservation using antifibrinolytics in a randomized trial) study in 2007, manufacturer (Bayer Healthcare Pharmaceuticals, Leverkusen, Germany) has withdrawn it from the market, after the study demonstrated increased 30-day morbidity and mortality with its use. In the period post November 2007 when aprotinin was withdrawn, a retrospective study compared aprotinin effect on blood bank resource utilization in patients requiring DHCA between 2006 and 2007 with tranexamic acid. The study concluded that patients treated with tranexamic acid required more clotting factors than aprotinin group and higher incidence of recombinant factor VIIa use.[36] The factor VIIa use is reserved for bleeding not controlled after adequate surgical homeostasis and blood product transfusion. Excessive usage of blood and blood products cause exaggeration of the inflammatory response and therefore should be used with diligence. Rapid transfusion of blood and blood products can cause drift in temperature and chelate calcium, both of which will further impair the coagulation process and cardiac systolic function. Use of blood warmers and Bair hugger will prevent temperature drift.

Post-surgery the first important issue is to assess the cerebral status. Therefore, intraoperatively short acting anesthesia agents are given as infusion along with inhalational agents to avoid awareness. Adequate pain management is also important, as pain may result in systemic hypertension, with the risk of increased bleeding from the suture line. For this purpose dexmeditomidine (central α-2 adrenoceptor agonist) is an ideal agent due to its multifaceted effect.[37,38] Since there is a risk of recurrent laryngeal nerve palsy, post-extubation vocal cord movement should be documented. The left phrenic nerve course is also near the area of surgical dissection and its injury will result in post-operative diaphragmatic palsy, which may cause difficulty in breathing and desaturation due to atelectasis development.

## Anesthesia Management for Hybrid Procedure

The anesthetic management for a hybrid procedure is no less intensive compared to open procedure. As the procedure involves arch vessels, there is always a potential risk of neurological injury, thus rendering neurological monitoring vital. Invasive line placement is also similar. Induced hypotension is required during stent release for proper stent positioning and release. Rapid transfusion system should always be on stand-by, especially in cases of leaking pseudoaneurysm, which has the potential to rupture during stent deployment. TEVAR is less invasive and avoids the need for cardiopulmonary bypass. Morbidity is low and recovery is faster with less need for blood transfusion.

### Strategies to minimize cerebral injury in arch surgery

- Minimize particulate embolization
  - Axillary cannulation
  - Avoid manipulation of diseased vessels
  - Trifurcation graft
  - Aspirate cerebral vessels prior to resuming cerebral perfusion

## Conclusion

Aortic arch surgery is associated with an increased risk of neurological injury either in the form of transient neurological deficit or permanent neurological deficit. These insults are either ischemic or embolic in nature. A careful planning among the team members and use of cerebral monitoring can help in significantly improved outcome.

## REFERENCES

1. Layton KF, Kallmes DF, Cloft HJ, Lindell EP, Cox VS. Bovine aortic arch variant in humans: clarification of a common misnomer. Am J Neuroradiol 2006;27:1541–42.

2. Jakanani GC, Adair W. Frequency of variations in aortic arch anatomy depicted on multidetector CT. Clin Radiol, 2010; 65:481–87.

3. 2014 ESC Guidelines on the diagnosis and treatment of aortic diseases: Document covering acute and chronic aortic diseases of the thoracic and abdominal aorta of the adult. The Task Force for the Diagnosis and Treatment of Aortic Diseases of the European Society of Cardiology (ESC). Eur Heart J 2014;35:2873–2926.

4. Hiratzka LF, Bakris GL, Beckman JA, Bersin RM, et al. 2010 ACCF/AHA/AATS/ACR/ASA/SCA/SCAI/SIR/STS/ SVM guidelines for the diagnosis and management of patients with Thoracic Aortic Disease: a report of the American College of Cardiology Foundation/American Heart Association Task Force on Practice Guidelines, American Association for Thoracic Surgery, American College of Radiology, American Stroke Association, Society of Cardiovascular Anesthesiologists, Society for Cardiovascular Angiography and Interventions Society of Interventional Radiology, Society of Thoracic Surgeons, and Society for Vascular Medicine. Circulation 2010; 121:e266–e369.

5. Brady AR, Thompson SG, Fowkes FG, Greenhalgh RM, Powell JT. Abdominal aortic aneurysm expansion: risk factors and time intervals for surveillance. Circulation 2004; 110:16–21.

6. De Bakey ME, Crawford ES, Cooley DA, et al. Successful resection of fusiform aneurysm of aortic arch with replacement by homograft. Surg Gynecol Obstet 1957; 105:657–64.

7. Griepp RB, Stinson EB, Hollingsworth JF, et al. Prosthetic replacement of the aortic arch. J Thorac Cardiovasc Surg 1975; 70:1051–63.

8. Ueda Y, Miki S, Kusuhara K, et al. Surgical treatment of aneurysm or dissection involving the ascending aorta and aortic arch, utilizing circulatory arrest and retrograde cerebral perfusion. J Cardiovasc Surg (Torino) 1990; 31:553–8.

9. Fox LS, Blackstone EH, Kirklin JW, Bishop SP, Bergdahl LAL, Bradley EL. Relationship of brain blood flow and oxygen consumption to perfusion flow rate during profoundly hypothermic cardiopulmonary bypass. J Thorac Cardiovasc Surg. 1984; 87:658–64.

10. Svensson LG, Crawford ES, Hess KR, et al. Deep hypothermia with circulatory arrest. Determinants of stroke and early mortality in 656 patients. J Thorac Cardiovasc Surg 1993; 106:19–28; discussion 28–31.

11. Michenfelder, JD and Milde, JH. The relationship among canine brain temperature, metabolism, and function during hypothermia. Anesthesiology 1991; 75:130–136.

12. Nemoto EM, Klementavicius R, Melick JA, Yonas H. Norepinephrine activation of basal cerebral metabolic rate for oxygen ($CMRO_2$) during hypothermia in rats. Anesth Analg 1996; 83:1262–7.

13. McCullough JN, Zhang N, Reich DL, et al. Cerebral metabolic suppression during hypothermic circulatory arrest in humans. Ann Thorac Surg 1999; 67:1895–9.

14. Di Eusanio M, Wesselink RM, Morshuis WJ, et al. Deep hypothermic circulatory arrest and antegrade selective cerebral perfusion during ascending aorta-hemiarch replacement: a retrospective comparative study. J Thorac Cardiovasc Surg 2003; 125:849–54.

15. Ginsberg MD, Graham DI, Busto R. Regional glucose utilization and blood flow following graded forebrain ischemia in the rat: Correlation with neuropathology. Ann Neurol 1985; 18:470–81

16. Ye J, Yang L, Del Bigio MR. et al. Neuronal damage after hypothermic circulatory arrest and retrograde perfusion in the pig. Ann Thorac Surg. 1996; 61:1316–22.

17. Griepp RB, Ergin MA, McCullough JN, et al. Use of hypothermic circulatory arrest for cerebral protection during aortic surgery. J Card Surg. 1997; 12:312–21.

18. Mills NL, Oschner JL. Massive air embolism during cardiopulmonary bypass. Causes, prevention and management. J Thorac Cardiovas Surg, 1980; 80:708–17.

19. Coselli JS. Retrograde cerebral perfusion is an effective means of neural support during deep hypothermic circulatory arrest. Ann Thorac Surg, 1997; 64:908–12.

20. Urbanski PP, Lenos A, Blume JC, et al. Does anatomical completeness of the circle of Willis correlate with sufficient cross-perfusion during unilateral cerebral perfusion? Eur J Cardiothorac Surg 2008; 33:402–8.

21. Malvindi PG, Scrascia G, Vitale N. Is unilateral antegrade cerebral perfusion equivalent to bilateral cerebral perfusion for patients undergoing aortic arch surgery? Interact Cardiovasc Thorac Surg 2008; 7:891–7.

22. Hagl C, Ergin MA, Galla JD, et al. Neurologic outcome after ascending aorta-aortic arch operations: effect of brain protection technique in high-risk patients. J Thorac Cardiovasc Surg 2001; 121:1107–21.

23. Griepp RB. Cerebral protection during aortic arch surgery. J Thorac Cardiovasc Surg 2001; 121:425–7.

24. Bakhtiary F, Dogan S, Dzemali O, et al. Mild hypothermia (32°C) and antegrade cerebral perfusion in aortic arch operations. J Thorac Cardiovasc Surg 2006; 132:153–54.

25. Villard J, Froment JC, Milleret R, Dureau G, Amouroux C, Boivin J, et al. Type-I complete acute aortic dissection. Value of arterial perfusion by the axillary artery route (in French). Ann Clir Thorac Cardiovasc 1976; 15:133–5.

26. Sabik JF, Nemeh H, Lyte BW, et al. Cannulation of the axillary artery with a side graft reduces morbidity. Ann Thorac Surg 2004;77:1315–20.

27. Sinclair MC, Singer RL, Manley NJ, Montesano RM. Cannulation of the axillary artery for cardiopulmonary bypass: safeguard and pitfalls. Ann Thorac Surg 2003; 75:931–4.

28. Sabik JF, Lyte BW, Mc Carthy PM, Cosgrove DM. Axillary artery: an alternative site of arterial cannulation for patients with extensive aortic and peripheral vascular disease. J Thoac Cardiovasc Surg, 1995; 109:885–91.

29. First WH, Baldwin JC, Starnes VA, Stinson EB, et al. A reconsideration of cerebral perfusion in aortic arch replacement. Ann Thorac Surg, 1986; 42:273–81.

30. Banbury MK, Cosgrove DM 3rd. Arterial cannulation of the innominate artery. Ann Thorac Surg, 2000; 69:957.

31. Michenfelder JD: Anesthesia and the brain: clinical, functional, metabolic and vascular correlates. New York, Churchill, Livingstone, 1988.

32. Devohurst AT, Moore SJ, Liban JB. Pharmacological agents as cerebral protectants during deep hypothermic circulatory arrest in adult thoracic aortic surgery. Anesthesia, 2002; 57:1016–21.

33. Toner CC, Standford J. general anesthetics as neuroprotective agents In: Bailliere Tidall, editor. Bailliere's clinical Anesthsiology. International practice and research. UK, Saunders, 1996; 10:515–33.

34. Kruger T, Hoffmann I, Blettner M, Borger MA. Intraoperative neuroprotective drugs without beneficial effect? Results of the German Registry for Acue aortic Dissection Type-A (GERAADA). Euro J Cardiothoracic Surg, 2013; 44:939–46.

35. Fergusson DA, Hébert PC, Mazer CD, Fremes S, MacAdams C, Murkin JM, et al. A comparison of aprotinin and lysine analogues in high-risk cardiac surgery. N Engl J Med 2008; 358:2319–31.

36. Sniecinski RM, Chen EP, Makadia SS, Kikura M, Bolliger D, Tanaka KA. Changing from aprotinin to tranexamic acid results in increased use of blood products and recombinant factor VIIa for aortic surgery requiring hypothermic arrest. J Cardiothorac Vasc Anesth 2010; 24:959–63.

37. Bhana N, Goa KL, McClellan KJ. Dexmedetomidine. Drugs 2000, 59:263–68.

38. Barr J, Fraser GL, Puntillo K, Ely EW, Gélinas C, Dasta JF, Davidson JE, Devlin JW, Kress JP, Joffe AM, Coursin DB, Herr DL, Tung A, Robinson BR, Fontaine DK, Ramsay MA, Riker RR, Sessler CN, Pun B, Skrobik Y, Jaeschke R, American College of Critical Care Medicine: Clinical practice guidelines for the management of pain, agitation, and delirium in adult patients in the intensive care unit. Crit Care Med. 2013, 41:263–306.

# CHAPTER 5

# Anesthesia for Descending Thoracic Aorta Repair

Parag Gharde, Shiv Kumar Choudhary

## HISTORY

In the year 1950, the first report of successful replacement of descending thoracic aorta (DTA) came from Swan *et al*.[1] It was a case of coarctation of aorta with 8 cm aneurysm of DTA. The aneurysmal segment was replaced by an arterial homograft. Blalock three months earlier had performed resection of the coarct segment and an end-to-end anastomosis in the same patient. Denton A. Cooley performed the repair of a large pseudoaneurysm of the right subclavian artery by ligating the subclavian artery, proximally and distally.

DeBakey and Cooley[2] were the first to report the use of a graft in a DTA aneurysm via a thoracoabdominal incision. Debakey in 1954 reported the first successful resection of the thoracic aorta aneurysm and its replacement by homograft.[3]

At the time when Swan *et al*[1] first reported replacement of the DTA aneurysm, there was no concept of spinal cord ischemia, paraplegia, abdominal organ ischemia, as these case reports were from CoA related DTA repair, where a rich collateral circulation was already in place and hence the authors did not come across these complications. It was realized later when isolated thoracic aneurysms were repaired.

## PATHOPHYSIOLOGY

The descending thoracic aorta extends from distal to the origin of left subclavian artery up to the diaphragm. Dilatation of any portion of this aortic segment is termed as aneurysm of descending thoracic aorta (Fig. 5.1). When an aorta dilates to a diameter greater than 50% (1.5 times) of normal, irrespective of the segment of aorta (root, ascending, descending, or abdominal aorta), it is

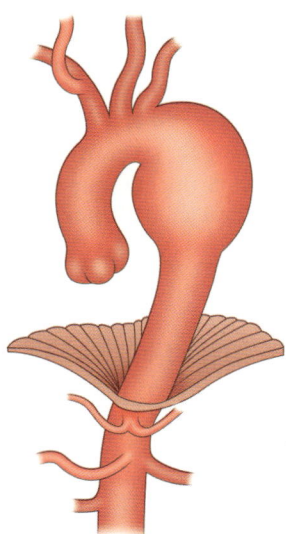

**Fig. 5.1:** Isolated aneurysm of the descending thoracic aorta involving the proximal and part of mid descending thoracic aorta

defined as an aneurysm. Based on the shape of an aneurysm it can be either fusiform or saccular. In a fusiform aneurysm there is a uniform/symmetric dilatation, while a saccular aneurysm appears as a localized out-pouching.[4] An aneurysm can also be classified based on the wall of the aneurysm. A true aneurysm has all the 3 layers—tunica intima, media and adventitia. A pseudoaneurysm on the other hand results from rupture of the aortic wall, which is contained by the surrounding tissue and therefore is a more serious condition. A pseudoaneurysm is always saccular in shape but the reverse is not always true (saccular aneurysms are not always pseudoaneurysms). The weakening in the aortic wall is due to degeneration of the extracellular matrix in the aortic media, consisting of structural protein like collagen and elastin, which results in aneurysm formation and dissection.

TA aneurysm may not always present in isolation and at times have varied extention into the abdominal aorta and the crawford classification helps in grouping such aneurysms appropriately (Fig. 5.2).

Disease of the aorta is an ancient one. The earliest evidence comes from computed tomographic (CT) scans of Egyptian mummies. These scans have revealed that 3500 years ago, atherosclerosis and arterial calcification were relatively common.[5] In the 19th and mid 20th century aortic aneurysm due to syphilis was common in absence of antibiotic therapy. With the discovery of penicillin there was rapid decrease in its incidence, only to be replaced by atherosclerotic aortic disease. Syphilitic aortitis induced dilatation of the aorta has a long latency period from the primary infection to aneurysmal dilatation. Syphilitic aortitis commonly involves the aortic arch, ascending aorta and the descending thoracic aorta, with the sinus of Valsalva often being spared.[6] Vascular involvement in late syphilis is due to lodging of spirochetes in the vasa vasorum, which supplies nutrient to the wall of the aorta during the secondary phase of the disease. The aortic wall weakens over time due to reduced blood supply. This results in the loss of tunica media with subsequent fibrosis and calcification.[7]

Atherosclerosis starts as an intimal lesion called atheroma, which protrudes into the arterial lumen. Abdominal aorta is a more common site for atherosclerosis than thoracic aorta. Atherosclerosis more commonly causes occlusive arterial disease, but aortic aneurysm has also been attributed to it. The reason for this varied presentation has not been fully understood. Aneurysm or the dilatation of aorta occurs due to weakening in the aortic wall structure, mostly in the medial segment of the wall. This is commonly due to medial degeneration, which was earlier termed as cystic medial necrosis. Loss of elastic fibers along with increased deposition of proteoglycans is seen on histological examination of the atherosclerosed aortic segment. Recent evidence suggests that these changes are a form of inflammatory response because of the presence of inflammatory cell infiltration.[8]

Matrix metalloproteinases (MMPs) have been found to be responsible for medial degeneration. MMPs function in the extracellular environment of the cells and degrade both matrix and non-matrix proteins. They play an important role in wound healing, tissue repair and remodeling in response to injury and in progression of diseases such as atheroma, arthritis, cancer and chronic tissue ulcers. Tissue inhibitors of metalloproteinase regulate their activities. Two subsets of MMPs-MMP-2 and MMP-9 have been found in increased levels in the media of thoracic aortic aneurysm. The levels are increased in patients with aneurysm of different etiologies, like-tricuspid, bicuspid and even Marfan's syndrome.[9] In Marfan's and other genetic abnormalities of the connective tissue, there is mutation in fibrillin protein and this defective protein is more susceptible to the proteolytic degeneration. The resulting fragmentation of the aortic

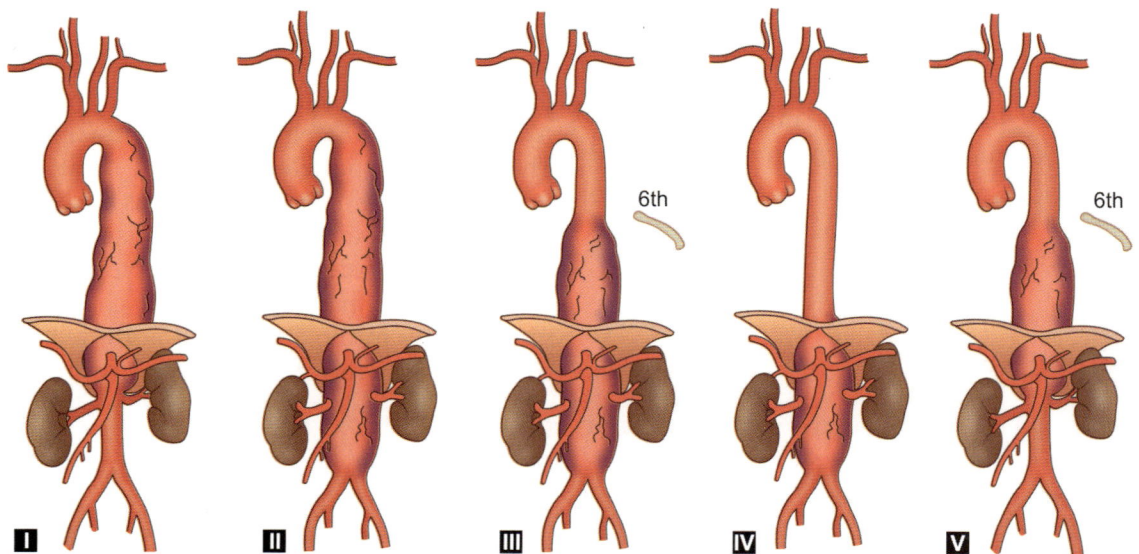

**Fig. 5.2:** Crawford classification of thoracoabdominal aortic aneurysms. The classifical classification was described up to extent IV. The extent V is a later addition to the classification system by safi's group. *Type I*, distal to the left subclavian artery to above the renal arteries. *Type II*, distal to the left subclavian artery to below the renal arteries. *Type III*, from the sixth intercostal space to the renal arteries. *Type IV*, from the 13th intercostal space to the iliac bifurcation (entire abdominal aorta). *Type V*, below the sixth intercostal space to just above the renal arteries

microfibrils and elastic lamellae weakens the aortic wall, making it prone for aneurysmal formation.[10]

## Diagnostic Markers for Acute Aortic Syndrome

With so much of resemblance in the presentation between coronary and aortic syndrome, most of the times a false diagnosis of acute coronary syndrome is reached and treatment is initiated on those lines. Without imaging, it is often difficult to diagnose acute aortic syndrome. Some headway has been made in this direction by means of bioassay. Biomarkers, similar to their diagnostic role in acute coronary syndrome, may help in making an early diagnosis in acute aortic syndrome and proper management strategy can be activated at the earliest. At present there are no reliable circulating biomarkers for thoracic aortic disease and imaging modality is currently the gold standard. But imaging modalities, especially CT angiographyand MRI are not available in all the hospitals, small towns and remote places. An ideal biomarker will be the one that can be performed bedside in a kit form and easily available with good sensitivity and specificity. Making an early diagnosis in both the conditions is the key to survival. Misdiagnosis is common because of common clinical symptoms. There have been instances when acute aortic syndrome patients underwent thrombolytic therapy for being misdiagnosed as an acute coronary event (*Box 5.1*). In up to 40% of cases, the diagnosis of acute aortic syndrome has been missed or overlooked[11], while in others, the diagnosis was made only after postmortem.[12] Among the acute aortic syndrome, it is the type-A aortic dissection, which calls for an early diagnosis and surgery, as it carries nearly 45–50% mortality in the first 48 hours. On the other hand, type-B variant is a less malignant form, mostly treated

| Box 5.1 | Biomarkers for diagnosis of acute aortic syndrome |
|---|---|

- D-dimers
- C-reactive protein (CRP)
- Smooth muscle myosin heavy chain

medically, unless it is complicated by malperfusion syndrome. Some of the biomarkers that are used in clinical practice are mentioned below.

### 1. D-Dimers

In dissection, exposure of the media to blood elements initiates a coagulation cascade and a consumption coagulopathy, depending upon the surface area of tissue exposed. D-dimer is a fibrin degradation product and becomes apparent in circulation following fibrinolysis of thrombus. In acute aortic dissection D-dimer with a cutoff valve of 0.5 µg/ml carries a sensitivity of 100% and a specificity of 68.6%.[13] D-dimer levels will be raised in condition resulting in coagulation, such as, recent trauma or surgery, deep vein thrombosis, pulmonary embolism and disseminated intravascular coagulation. D-dimers help in distinguish between the ACS and AAS but not if the chest pain is due to pulmonary embolism. The other drawback is because of the availability of a variety of assays, which have different cutoff values and sensitivity. D-dimer may give a false negative result in patients with thrombosed false lumen, shorter dissection lengths and younger age groups.

### 2. C-Reactive Protein

The liver in response to inflammatory process produces CRP, an acute phase protein. Schillinger *et al.*[14] have demonstrated CRP as an independent predictor of poor prognosis in patients with AAS, especially when the value of CRP were >6.3 mg/L. Both CRP and white blood cell counts are higher in chest pain patients with dissection versus other diagnosis.

### 3. Smooth Muscle Myosin Heavy Chain

The smooth muscles present in the aortic wall, uterus and intestine have smooth muscle myosin (SMM). Any injury to the smooth muscle cells will result in release of SMM into the circulation. Since aortic dissection involves tearing into the media, which mainly has smooth muscle cells, this will result in release of the SMM. Katoh *et. al*[15] first came up with the finding of rise in the serum SMM heavy chain in patients with aortic dissection. The elevated state was in the first 24 hours. A cutoff level of 2.5 mg/ml has shown to be sensitive. The values are not elevated in the setting of ACS. The unusual finding of Suzuki et al was the higher values of SMM heavy chains in thoracic dissection than in the abdominal dissection. The probable explanation given for this is that the atherosclerotic changes occur more prominently in the abdominal aorta with more of the smooth muscle cells being replaced by fibrotic material.[16]

### Evaluation

Imaging is the basis for diagnosing and following-up of patients with aortic disease.

The consensus is lacking in terms of measuring the aneurysm dimension that is so crucial in decision-making regarding the path to be chosen-whether to undergo an intervention or follow-up. Whether to measure inner edge to inner edge or outer edge to outer edge? Whether to make measurements in systole or diastole?

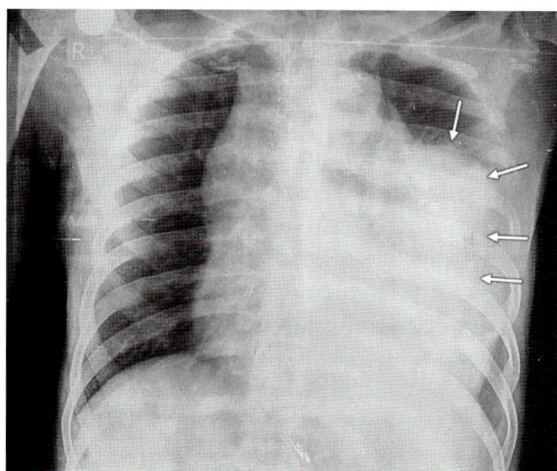

**Fig. 5.3:** Chest-X ray showing enlarged shadow of descending thoracic aortic aneurysm (white arrow heads), along the lateral left heart border. The patient incidentally also has a dilated ascending aorta

| Box 5.2 | Imaging in evaluation of DTA aneurysm |

- Chest X-ray
- Ultrasonography
  - Transthorasic echocardiography
  - Transesophageal echocardiography
- Computed tomography
- Magnetic resonance imaging

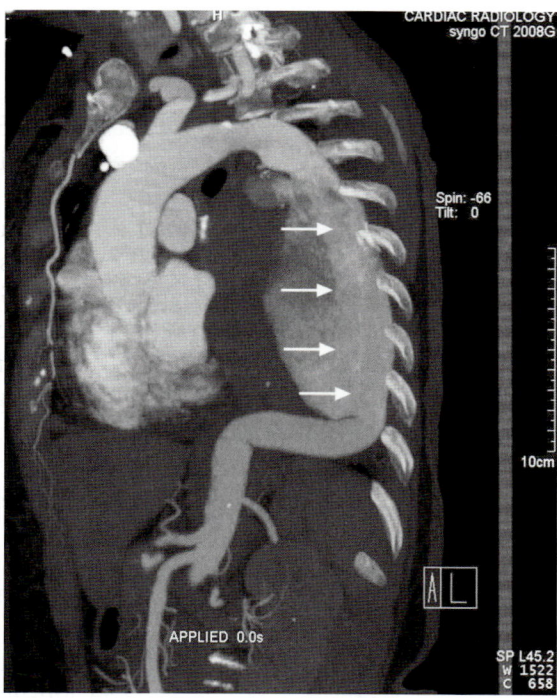

**Fig. 5.4:** Computed tomography angiography of the same patient (chest X-ray) showing a type B dissection with dilated descending thoracic due to enlarging false lumen with smaller true lumen (white arrow heads), starting distal to the left subclavian artery. Note the dilated ascending aorta as well

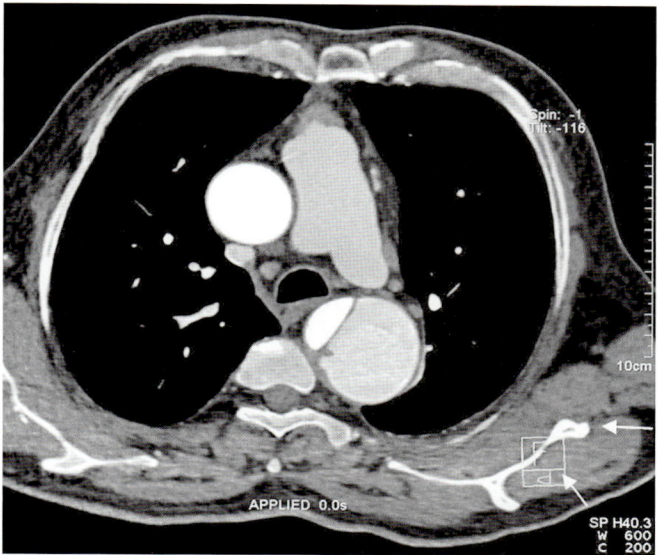

**Fig. 5.5:** The computed tomography angiography shows a type-B aortic dissection in axial cut (white arrow head). The true lumen appears brighter due to presence of more contrast agent compared to the false lumen. There is no dissection in the ascending aorta located next to the main pulmonary artery. The axial cut is taken at the level of pulmonary artery bifurcation and the main stem bronchus is yet to bifurcate

Computed tomography is central to the diagnosis, extension of the disease, risk stratification, management and follow-up (Figs 5.4 and 5.5). The image acquisition should always be gated to electrocardiogram so as to avoid motion artifacts.

## MANAGEMENT

When a patient becomes symptomatic due to aortic aneurysm, an intervention is warranted. Symptoms due to DTA aneurysm are classically of pain related-interscapular pain or chest pain radiating to back. Most often the patients are asymptomatic and the disease is picked on medical examination. As the DTA aneurysm approaches size ≥7 cm there is a rapid increase in the risk of dissection or rupture. This point is referred to as the 'hinge point' (Fig. 5.6). Based on this, the absolute size of >6.5 cm or >6.0 cm in case of connective tissue disorder is an indication for open or endovascular intervention. But the size of the aneurysm needs to be adjusted to body size in case of extremes of body habitus. Two treatment options are available conservative medical management and interventional—endovascular repair and open surgical repair.

### A. Medical Management

Medical management is initiated when the DTA aneurysm size has not reached the trigger point for surgical or closed repair. The aim is to reduce the shear

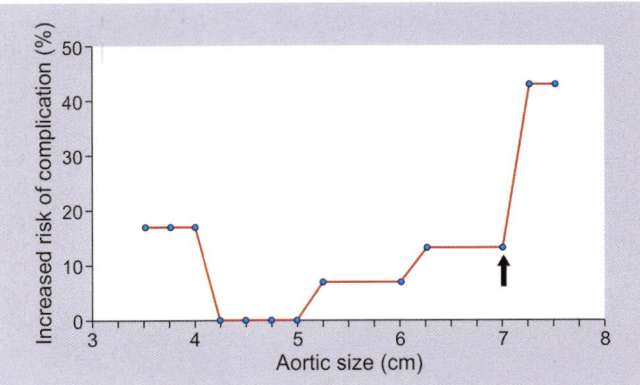

**Fig. 5.6:** The risk of rupture or dissection of descending aortic aneurysm increases proportionally with aortic diameter, with a sudden increase in risk as the aortic diameter reaches 7 cm. This is the 'Hinge point' for the descending thoracic aortic aneurysm, depicted by the bold arrow

stress on the aneurysmal aortic segment by drug therapy to reduce cardiac contractility and systemic hypertension. Aortic disease of other etiologies like connective tissue disorders may not show same efficacy with these medical treatments.

### Risk Modification Strategy and its Perioperative Use

#### 1. Beta-blockers

Patients with thoracic aneurysm are already on beta-blockers and the drug should be continued till the day of surgery. The idea behind this is to decrease the ventricular contractility and control the blood pressure. By doing so, the stress on the dilating aortic segment can be reduced and thus may retard the progression rate of aneurysm expansion. Also since atherosclerosis is the commonest pathology behind aortic aneurysm, these patients may also have underlying coronary artery disease. Beta-blockers may also help the patient on this front by decreasing the myocardial oxygen demand. Whether antihypertensive therapy has any beneficial role in aortic disease apart from atherosclerosis etiology has still not been proven.

The following discussion is for patients who are not on chronic beta-blocker therapy and its perioperative use. Beta-blockers have seen highs and lows in clinical practice as a perioperative drug. Beta-blocker gained attention through small observational studies which showed beneficial effects on major adverse cardiac events in patients undergoing non cardiac surgery.[17] A large multicentric randomized control trial (RCT) by Mangano et al[18] showed encouraging results with atenolol on cardiovascular mortality and morbidity after non-cardiac surgery. This first large randomized trial paved the way for release of guidelines by the American College of Physician in 1997, which advocated the

administration of atenolol to all the patients with or at risk of CAD undergoing non-cardiac surgery. The possible explanation for such a benefit lay in its ability to control the heart rate and contractility, thus decreasing oxygen demand and improving myocardial perfusion by increasing the duration of diastole. In a meta-analysis by Devereaux, et al.[19], questions were raised regarding mortality benefits from perioperative use of β-blocker in non-cardiac surgery. The Pre-operative Ischemic Evaluation (POISE) trial,[20] the largest RCT ever on perioperative use of β-blockers took the sheen out of its regular use in operating room. The trial consisted of 8351 patients with or at risk of CAD, was randomized to placebo or metoprolol succinate extended release 100 mg orally. The therapy was initiated 2–4 hours before surgery and then continued for 30 days. The study showed reduced incidence of perioperative myocardial infarction (MI) but at the same time there were adverse events that increased mortality in the study drug group (3.1% vs 2.3%, p=0.0317). Stroke was also significantly common in the drug group. All this was advocated to the increased incidence of perioperative hypotension. These significant finding dramatically reduced the usage of β-blockers. Though the study was criticized for use of very high dosage of metoprolol and combined with anesthetic agents and perioperative blood loss probably resulted in significantly increased incidence of perioperative hypotension and complications. Then came the Dutch Echocardiographic Cardiac Risk Evaluation Applying Stress Echocardiography (DECREASE-IV) trial,[21] which comprised of 1066 patients with intermittent risk undergoing non-cardiac surgery. These patients were randomised to either bisoprolol, fluvastatin, bisoprolol and fluvastatin combination or a double placebo. The therapy was started 30 days before scheduled surgery. The target heart rate was 50–70 beats per minute. There was no difference in the incidence of stroke between the various groups, but the trial was terminated early due to slow patient recruitment. This trial could have infused life into the practice of perioperative use of β-blockers, but for the reports of scientific misconduct on part of the researchers,[22,23] questions have been raised on the validity of two influential RCT on perioperative β-blocker use.[21,24] This has prompted 2014 ACC/AHA Perioperative Guideline Systematic Review Report,[25] which omitted DECREASE-I and DECREASE-IV trails, but no new RCT trials were included. The report concluded that there is insufficient robust data on efficacy and safety of acute perioperative β-blocker regimens that use agents aside from metoprolol or should initiate treatment 2 to 45 days prior to surgery.

## 2. Nitrates

At present there is no strong evidence available that prophylactic use of intraoperative nitroglycerine has any significant effect on perioperative events of myocardial ischemia, or MI, in high-risk patients undergoing non-cardiac surgery.[26] It is best to continue medications to the patient till the time of surgery. Nitrates may cause some hemodynamic disturbance as it decreases preload through venodilatation. Preoperative fasting and hypotensive effect of anesthetic agents may trigger reflex tachycardia in response to decrease preload. One of the difficult groups to manage is a patient with diabetic mellitus and autonomic nervous system dysfunction. It is a big challenge to attain stable hemodynamics due to unpredictable response to vasodilators or vaso-constrictors, especially in the changing dynamics due to blood loss, aortic cross clamp application and its release. Managing such cases with an invasive arterial pressure monitoring will be of immense help. Invasive monitoring is an integral part of anesthesia management protocol in patients undergoing aortic surgery. A central venous catheter is of utmost importance to deliver vasoactive or vasodilator drugs, because of its early response as compared to peripheral line. Therefore the effect is easier to titrate.

## 3. Statins

Statins (HMG-CoA reductase inhibitors) reduce low-density lipoproteins (LDL) and triglyceride levels, while increasing the high-density lipoproteins. Statins have been shown to be beneficial in patients with hyperlipidemias, history of CAD, coronary calcium score more than 300 Agatston unit, family history of premature acute coronary event (first degree relative—male <65 years, female <55 years). The guidelines[27] grade the therapy intensity based on the degree of LDL-C level lowering required—moderate intensity therapy (lowering LDL-C by 30–50%), or high intensity therapy (lowering LDL-C by >50%) and maximum benefit is seen when the LDL-C levels are <70 mg/dl. Additional benefits of statins have been reported in patients undergoing major vascular surgery apart from its lipid lowering properties.[28] ESC guidelines strongly recommend statins use in vascular surgery patients.[29] There have been reports of significant cardiovascular events when statin therapy was stopped.[27] Hence statins should be continued in patients already taking them and should be restarted as soon as possible post-operatively. A randomized trial is ongoing to evaluate beneficial role of statins in endovascular and open aneurysmal repair. (PROCEDURE study—Prevention of Cholesterol Embolization during Endovascular and Open Aneurysm Repair with Pitavastatin.)[30]

## B. Invasive Intervention Management

### I. Endovascular Repair

With the advent of transcutaneous endovascular aortic replacement (TEVAR), an additional therapeutic choice is available apart from the traditional open surgical repair. In absence of any randomized control trial to guide the choice between open surgery and TEVAR, the selection option is mostly institutional based. TEVAR being expensive and with long-term results lacking, it is mainly reserved for old age patients with severe comorbidities and low life expectancy. In DTA aneurysm due to connective tissue disorder like Marfan disease, surgery is preferred over TEVAR. Evidence is lacking in use of TEVAR in such patients, except in emergency situations to stabilize the condition and then proceed for the definitive open surgical repair.[31] TEVAR can be considered in patients who have DTA aneurysm with maximum diameter ≥5.5 cm (Table 5.1).[32]

Hybrid procedure may be required if the landing zone encroaches upon the supra-aortic vessel takeoff. This may need a branched graft to the innominate and the left common carotid along with a side-to-side graft anastomosis between the left common carotid artery and the left subclavian artery (Fig. 5.8).

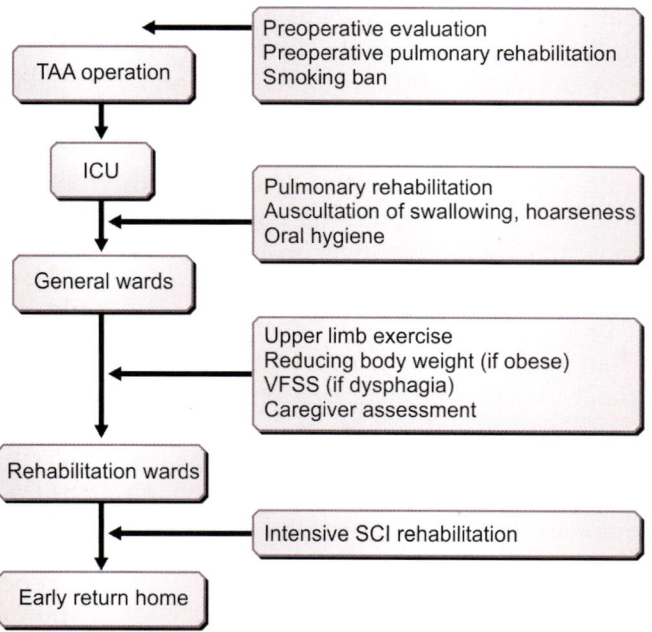

**Fig. 5.7:** The flowchart depicts various measures need to be taken at different levels to ensure a good outcome in a patient of thoraco-abdominal aortic aneurysm

**Table 5.1:** The 2014 European Society of Cardiology (ESC) guidelines on the diagnosis and treatment of aortic diseases recommendation on endovascular thoracic aortic repair

| Recommendations | Class[a] | Level[b] |
|---|---|---|
| It is recommended that the indication for TEVAR or EVAR be decided on an individual basis, according to anatomy, pathology, comorbidity and anticipated durability, of any repair, using a multidisciplinary approach. | I | C |
| A sufficient proximal and distal landing zone of at least 2 cm is recommended for the safe deployment and durable fixation of TEVAR. | I | C |
| In case of aortic aneurysm, it is recommended to select a stent-graft with a diameter exceeding the diameter of the landing zones by at least 10–15% of the reference aorta. | I | C |
| During stent graft placement, invasive blood pressure monitoring and control (either pharmacologically or by rapid pacing) is recommended. | I | C |
| Preventive cerebrospinal fluid (CSF) drainage should be considered in high-risk patients. | IIa | C |

[a]Class of recommendation.
[b]Level of evidence.

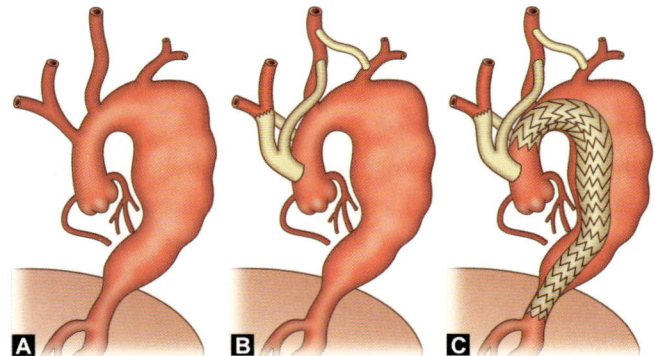

**Figs 5.8A to C:** Endovascular stenting of descending thoracic artery may require revascularization (debranching) of supra-aortic branch vessels if the stent implant is going to cover the origin of arch vessels

## II. Open Surgical Repair

Isolated DTA aneurysm is approached via a left thoracotomy incision between the fourth and seventh intercostal spaces, guided by the location of the aneurysm involvement of the DTA segment. Incision may be extended to paramedian laparotomy if the aneurysm extends into the abdominal aortic segment. The left groin is draped for easy surgical access of the femoral vessels for distal perfusion. With left heart bypass technique the left heart is unloaded from the strain of high proximal clamp just distal to the subclavian artery. Also it provides blood supply distal to the clamp, which reduces the ischemic period of visceral organs and kidney. This strategy provides support to spinal cord perfusion as well. The risk of paraplegia after thoracoabdominal repair ranges between 6 and 8%.[33] The neurological complication incidence were higher with clamp and sew technique. The distal perfusion can be provided by two methods—partial left heart bypass and partial cardiopulmonary bypass. The partial left heart bypass is initiated by using a heparin-coated circuit with the cannula placed either in the left pulmonary vein or the left atrial appendage. A centrifugal pump returns the blood through a cannula either in the abdominal aorta or the left femoral artery. The other approach requires full heparinization with blood drained via a long venous cannula (through femoral vein) into a venous reservoir and returned through a femoral artery cannula.

## ANESTHETIC MANAGEMENT

### A. Preoperative Evaluation

As elaborated in the pathophysiology section of the chapter, atherosclerosis is the commonest cause for aortic disease in the modern era. Atherosclerosis is the disease of the old and thus most patients seeking surgical intervention for their aortic pathology are at increased risk for carrying coronary artery disease and other comorbidities of old age. Like in atherosclerosis of coronary artery, smoking also increases the risk of aortic atherosclerosis. Smoking and old age both also contribute to pulmonary dysfunction. Diabetes and renal dysfunction show increasing presence with age (Fig. 5.7). Hence for a safe conduct of anesthesia and perioperative as well as postoperative period, the patient should be evaluated from all the risk organ perspective, apart from the main pathology, for which the patient requires surgical intervention. Unlike the atherosclerotic aortic disease, the abnormal connective tissue aortic disease patients are younger and hence do not carry the above-mentioned comorbidities.

The atherosclerotic aortic patients are at increased risk of harboring coronary artery disease. Hence, it is of utmost importance that a careful history is taken of patient's physical health status, previous hospital records, and drug history. To decrease perioperative cardiac events, the American Heart Association/American College of Cardiology guidelines on perioperative evaluation for non-cardiac surgery impress upon the following:

a. Exercise capacity.

b. Patient specific clinical variables.

c. Surgery specific risk.

*a. Exercise capacity:* The functional capacity of a patient indirectly reflects on the cardiac status. Physical activity can be expressed in metabolic equivalents (1 MET = 3.5 ml oxygen/kg/min). A patient whose normal daily activity is less than 4 METs, and is unable to perform daily activity because of cardiac restriction, is at increased risk of perioperative event. An important factor that needs to be kept in mind is that the functional restriction may not always reflect upon patient's cardiac status. Restriction in functional activity can also be due to orthopedic cause, residual paralysis post stroke, or pulmonary disease-chronic obstructive pulmonary disease (COPD), interstitial lung disease. If the functional restriction is due to chest pain (angina) then most often it is due to coronary artery disease (CAD). If it is due to cardiac breathlessness then it is probably because of valvular or poor left ventricle (LV) function. Patients with CAD are at increased risk of perioperative myocardial infarction (MI), resulting in acute LV dysfunction and poor outcome. Perioperative MI carries high early mortality ranging from 3.5 to 25%, with higher deaths in patients with marked troponin elevation.[34] There are two distinct mechanisms that can cause perioperative MI. A fixed coronary artery stenosis will cause MI if the supply-demand balance is disrupted. A non-significant plaque may become acutely occlusive if it is unstable. An unstable plaque may rupture, develop fissure and provide an ideal environment for development of acute thrombosis. Coronary angiography may consider these coronary lesions as mild, but this does not guarantee a safe perioperative course. Angiography cannot comment on the stability of the plaque. An intravascular ultrasound may help in differentiating between a stable and an unstable plaque. A vulnerable plaque has a thin fibrous cap, encasing large amount of macrophages and lipids. Rupture of this thin fibrous cap exposes the highly thrombogenic material to the circulation and triggering acute thrombus formation and acute MI[35]. In an angiographic study of patients with perioperative ACS, nearly 50% of the patients had evidence of plaque rupture.[36] As a protocol at the author's center, all patients undergoing aortic CT angiography for pre-surgery aortic workup also have their coronaries evaluated. An ECG gated CT angiography study can give a fair comment on their coronary system. If the calcium score is high, these patients are subjected to coronary angiography.

What If the angiography report suggests of significant CAD? The 2007 ACC/AHA guideline[26] have given Class-I indication to preoperative coronary revascularization with coronary artery bypass graft (CABG) or percutaneous coronary intervention (PCI) in the following, with all carrying level of evidence-A.

1. CABG in patients with stable angina but with significant left main coronary artery stenosis.
2. Coronary revascularization in patients with stable angina but with left main equivalent disease and ejection fraction <50%.
3. Coronary revascularization in patients with stable angina and triple vessel disease. (Survival benefit is greater when LVEF is <50%)
4. Coronary revascularization in patients with high-risk unstable angina or non-ST elevated MI.
5. Coronary revascularization in patients with acute ST elevated MI.

Some of the patients coming for aortic surgery may already have undergone revascularization procedure. Such a case requires detailed information about the type of revascularization procedure performed. The guideline suggests that elective non-cardiac surgery is not recommended within 4 to 6 weeks of bare metal coronary stent implantation or within 12 months of drug eluting stent implantation. As this is the period required for endothelialization of the stent and continuation of antiplatelet therapy. Incomplete endothelialization and discontinuation of antiplatelet therapy in wake of excessive bleeding intraoperatively, along with the hypercoagulable state during surgery further enhances the risk of acute in-stent thrombosis. Elective non-cardiac surgery is not recommended within 4 weeks of coronary revascularization with balloon angioplasty.

The coronary artery revascularization programme trial (CARP)[37] was the first randomized multicentric study to evaluate the role of prophylactic revascularization in patients with significant CAD on coronary angiography, undergoing elective vascular operation. The CARP study selected patients on the basis of coronary angiogram having one or more major coronary arteries with atleast 70% stenosis; suitability for selecting the type of revascularization was based on the angiography. CABG patients underwent vascular surgery 3 month later while the PCI group underwent surgery 2 weeks post PCI. Within 30 days following vascular surgery(abdominal aortic aneurysm or severe symptomatic peripheral vascular disease), mortality was 3.1% in the coronary revascularization group and 3.4% in the non-revascularization group. The PCI performed consisted of bare metal stent and was performed in 59%, while CABG was done in 41% of the cohort. Thus this study showed that revascularization before elective vascular surgery did not alter long-term survival. On further analysis of the results of CARP study, it was revealed that patients with unstable CAD and left main CAD were the ones who benefitted from revascularization. An important limitation in the CARP trial was that most of the patients had single or double vessel disease with normal LV ejection fraction, and thus formed a relatively low risk group, in whom revascularization would not have shown significant benefits. It has been proven beyond doubt that the most severe stenosis are not always responsible for perioperative MI, since the degree of stenosis increases over time, giving enough time for the collaterals to develop. While in milder stenosis, when the vessel is completely occluded, it often results in catastrophe, as collaterals are not developed in them.[38] Preoperative revascularization is not a magic wand or the Holy Grail for perioperative MI prevention. One can reap its benefits only if done in selective patients. Those at significant risk of perioperative MI include, patients with unstable angina, high-risk coronary anatomy and low ejection fraction. This group of patients will show maximum benefit from preoperative revascularization. Also it should be kept in mind that these procedures carry its own risk. The CABG procedure itself carries a mortality risk of 1.4%.

Ageing involves the vasculature, which become less compliant and the patient becomes hypertensive. These patients with aortic disease are already on anti-hypertensive medications to retard the growth of the dilated aortic segment. The anti-hypertensive agents are continued in the perioperative period. Tachycardia and hypertension is due to catecholamine and cortisol release, induced by, pain, surgical trauma, anemia and hyperthermia. This may increase the shear stress on the unstable plaque, which may catapult to acute thrombosis of the coronary artery. Patients are usually on β-blockers and intraoperatively the target heart rate is between 60 and 70 beats per minute. β-blockers should be continued in patients who have been taking them for long time.[26] Acute withdrawal will result in rebound tachycardia and hypertension intraoperatively and initiate ACS. Therefore, AHA/ACC guidelines make it a class-I indication to continue β-blocker therapy in the perioperative period. The POISE trial only studied the acute intraoperative effect of β-blockers. Intraoperatively short acting β-blocker like esmolol (half life-9 minutes) can be started to achieve the target heart rate. Lack of tight heart rate control may be one of the reasons why some of the RCT have failed to show benefit with β-blockers. The evidence is growing with more data suggesting that the best efficacy of β-blocker is seen when the targeted heart rate is less than 65 beats per minute.[39] Caution is warranted with use of β-blockers in patients with LV dysfunction. Vigilance is required

to prevent hypertensive episodes especially during application of aortic cross clamp. In the event of high suspicion of perioperative occurrence of MI, postoperative troponin level measurements will be helpful. In the POISE trial it was the hypotensive episodes, which caused stroke and was the major cause for mortality. The AHA guidelines fail to specify any target systolic blood pressure levels when on β-blocker therapy intraoperatively, while the ESC defines the systolic pressures of more than 100 mmHg as safe level to administer β-blockers. Most of the hypertensive patients are on combination anti-hypertensive regimen. Angiotensin converting enzyme inhibitors (ACEI) or angiotensin receptor blockers (ARB) is commonly used along with β-blockers. ACEI or ARB use have been shown to be associated with increased incidence of intraoperative hypotension[40] and in patients with CAD, this can be detrimental.

*b. Surgery specific risk:* Based on the type of surgery and the 30-day risk of cardiovascular death and MI, it is divided into low risk <1%, intermediate risk 1–5% and high risk >5%.[41] Aortic and major vascular surgery belongs to the high-risk surgery group. Apart from the type of surgery, the type of intervention selected is also important. Endovascular procedures are less invasive compared to the conventional open repairs. Therefore in the presence of severe comorbidities, an endovascular procedure will be an ideal choice.

*c. Patient specific risk*

i. **Pulmonary evaluation:** Patients coming for aortic surgery are often old and suffer from pulmonary disease such as COPD, lung fibrosis and restrictive lung disease. Smokers commonly ail from atherosclerotic disease. An abstinence of at least one month is ideal. These patients need to be carefully evaluated for their pulmonary function and their medication optimized before being taken-up for elective surgery. A preoperative lung function test should be done in all patients, especially those undergoing thoracoabdominal aortic repair surgery, which involves thoracotomy and abdominal incision. A baseline arterial blood gas analysis, if possible, is always encouraged. These patients should pay a visit to the physiotherapist before surgery and learn how to perform incentive spirometry. This helps in the postoperative period, as they are well acquainted with spirometry and know their baseline level and set it as their target. Elective surgery needs to be delayed until pulmonary condition is optimized, as it significantly affects postoperative course. If not, then many remain on the ventilatory support for prolonged period and ultimately succumb to ventilatory-pulmonary complication.

An expanding aortic aneurysm may encroach upon the surrounding structures. The airway-trachea, carina and the left main bronchus share close relation with the aortic arch and the DTA. As these patients undergo CT angiography for the evaluation of the aortic disease, its important for the anesthesiologist to have a look at them for deviation and compression of these structures, both of which have an important bearing on intra-operative as well as postoperative management. Since thoracic aortic disease requires aortic exposure through left thoracotomy, left lung isolation is mandatory. To achieve this a double lumen tube (DLT) placement is needed. Selection between left and right sided DLT greatly depends on how significant is the left bronchus deviation. Left sided DLT is commonly preferred because of the ease of its placement. Chest X-ray or the CT angiography can provide information about pleural effusion and lung collapse. If there is pleural effusion and lung collapse on the right side then its better to drain it and expand the collapsed lung segment before positioning the patient. Otherwise, it becomes difficult to maintain adequate oxygenation and normocapnia with single lung ventilation in right lateral position because of the effusion and mediastinal shift.

Lung isolation is not only for surgeon's comfort. At times the aneurysm is adherent to the lung, and while separating these two, the lung may get injured and in the heparinized environment there may be significant intrapulmonary bleed. In absence of lung isolation the dependent right lung may also get flooded due to gravity drainage.

ii. **Renal function:** A preoperative serum creatinine level >2 mg/dl is identified as a risk factor for postoperative renal dysfunction.[42] Care is needed when these patients undergo CT angiography for aortic evaluation as they are at increased risk of contrast induced nephropathy. Other risk factor is the presence of diabetes mellitus. Adequate hydration and pharmacotherapy can prevent or decrease the severity of contrast induced nephropathy. Beneficial effect of N-acetylcystine has been controversial, and those who have demonstrated good response suggest using higher dosage of N-acetylcystine.[43] Diabetic patients are commonly on oral hypoglycemic agent metformin because of its association with lower cardiovascular morbidity

and mortality, compared to the other oral hypoglycemic agents.[44,45] The major but infrequent complication with metformin is lactic acidosis. Though the drug is not nephrotoxic, its concentration increases in patients with chronic kidney disease and this increases the risk of lactic acidosis. There is also a strong evidence that metformin inhibits the pathway for cardiac ischemic pre-conditioning. Whether this effect holds true for other organs is not known. Delaying elective surgery by more than a week after exposure to radiographic contrast will protect the kidney from double blow-contrast effect and ischemia during application of aortic cross clamp. Avoiding nephrotoxic drugs and dose adjustment of antibiotics according to the renal function will also be helpful. In the perioperative period maintaining high hematocrit and perfusion pressures will reduce intraoperative renal injury. The incidence of renal failure is high in patients undergoing thoraco-abdominal aortic aneurysm (TAAA) repair (22.8%) compared to descending aortic aneurysm (7%), as in TAAA repair the kidney is exposed to periods of ischemia and approximately 30% of them will require dialysis. Pharmacotherapy for renal protection has shown different results, causing confusion as to which agent should be used. Mannitol,[46] low dose continuous furosemide[47] has shown little benefit. Even renal dose dopamine[48–51] (1–3 mg/kg/min) infusion on the pretext of renal protection has been questioned. Also minimizing exposure to blood and blood products will reduce inflammation induced renal injury.[52] Renal perfusion with either cold crystalloid (4°C) or blood will reduce the incidence of renal dysfunction.

## B. Anesthesia Preparation

Pre-anesthetic check-up is the time when the anesthetists gain direct access to the patient. This is an opportunity to build bridges and gain their confidence. Apart from the disease history, enquiring about sleeping habits-like snoring, sleep apnea, position in which the patient sleeps and interest (listening to music, reading, etc.) is also important. All this information goes a long way in making the patient's stay comfortable. An overview of how the things will unfold, from the operating room to the intensive care unit (ICU), will make the patient more comfortable as they will be aware of what to expect next. A video, guiding the patient to the operating room (OR) and the ICU will be highly appreciated by the patient. A good night sleep is of paramount importance and to meet this goal an anxiolytic (alprazolam) or a sedative like diazepam is to be given. Patients are premedicated with intramuscular injection of promethazine (0.5 mg/kg) and morphine (0.1 mg/kg) before being shifted to the OR. The ambient temperature in the OR is kept comfortable. The OR table should have a Bair hugger warming blanket. In case of TAAA repair where a lateral thoracotomy position is required, a beanbag vacuum positioning system is placed on the table. It helps in securing the patient in a desired position. The standard American Society of Anesthesiologist monitoring is applied to the patient, which includes a 5-lead ECG, pulse oximetry and a non-invasive blood pressure. Two large bore intravenous cannula are placed, one under local infiltration, and second inserted after the induction of anesthesia. It is ideal to check pulses in both the arms so as to place an invasive arterial line in the arm with better pulse. As a convention at the author's center, a right radial artery is cannulated, as there is a possibility of the left subclavian artery getting clamped during proximal clamp placement. A right femoral artery should also be cannulated to measure pressure distal to the clamp, leaving the left groin to the surgeon, in case a partial fem-fem CPB is to be initiated. Also monitoring of upper and lower body pressures helps in adjusting the flows during partial CPB. A baseline ABG is taken at room air, which gives an idea of patient's respiratory status, unless the patient is deeply sedated due to premedication. The near infrared spectroscopy sensors (NIRS) are applied over the forehead after proper skin preparation to provide optimal contact and low impedance. The sensors are properly secured to prevent accidental peeling, especially during lateral positioning of the patient. A baseline NIRS values are taken after 5 minutes of applying the sensors with patient breathing on room air, which acts as a reference value to future changes. Anesthesia induction can be achieved in different ways; provided all the roads lead to Rome, i.e. they all achieve the desired set goals. The author prefers an opioid (fentanyl) based anesthesia. Etomidate is reserved for patients with severe LV dysfunction. Tracheal intubation is facilitated by rocuronium. If DLT has to be placed then most often a left sided tube is selected. Once the tube crosses the glottis, fiberoptic bronchoscope (FOB) is introduced through the bronchial end of the tube and advanced into the left bronchus. The DLT is then railroaded over the bronchoscope. The tube position is again checked after positioning the patient in the lateral position (this is the time when tube malposition occur), otherwise repositioning the tube under the drapes is a difficult proposition. One lung ventilation is initiated before left thoracotomy. Post-tracheal intubation, a large nasogastric (NG) tube is inserted, followed by transesophageal echocardiography (TEE) probe. The NG tube helps in gastric decompression; this also helps in gaining good image quality during TEE examination by removing air from the stomach. The NG tube also helps the surgeon to delineate esophagus from the aorta during the dissection period, especially in absence of a TEE probe. TEE is helpful in evaluating the cardiac functional status, the diseased aorta and post repair, the graft status. TEE also helps in proper placement of the long venous cannula through the femoral vein using the midesopahgeal bicaval view for partial CPB. A right internal jugular vein (RIJV) triple lumen catheter and a 8–10 French sheath is introduced into the RIJV. Sheath is life saving when rapid transfusion is required in the wake of torrential bleeding. Usually a cell saver device is always kept active and the processed blood is rapidly transfused by the rapid transfusion system (Belmont-5000). This system also has a heating system that prevents iatrogenic hypothermia during significant volume transfusion. Two temperature probes are used, one is inserted nasopharyngeal and the other is rectal.

## C. Aortic Cross Clamp Associated Physiologic Changes

The hemodynamic effect of aortic clamping depends on the level at which the aorta has been clamped. Supra-celiac clamp placement is associated with maximum hemodynamic perturbation as compared to an infra-celiac aortic clamp. When a supra-celiac clamp is placed there is sudden increase in the LV afterload, resulting in significant proximal hypertension. Though a higher proximal aortic pressure is required to support perfusion distal to the clamp, but at proximal MAP more than 100 mmHg will warrant vasodilatory therapy, as it will also result in increased CSF production and pressure, which will hamper SCPP (Fig. 5.9). Since majority of aortic patients are elderly, very high pressures may increase the risk of intracerebral hemorrhage, and in presence of systemic heparinization the cerebral outcome will be catastrophic. If the pressures distal to the clamp is less than 40 mmHg and the predicted clamp duration is prolonged (more than 20 minutes), as with the complex aortic repair, then a distal perfusion strategy should be instituted before re-applying the clamp (Fig. 5.10). Partial CPB will also prevent upper body hypertension, but close coordination is required between the anesthesiologist and the perfusionist to maintain stable hemodynamics. Since the splanchnic and kidney accounts for 50% of the total cardiac output, a supraceliac clamp will result in collapse of their venous system in absence of any significant arterial flow. This venous collapse shifts blood into the central venous

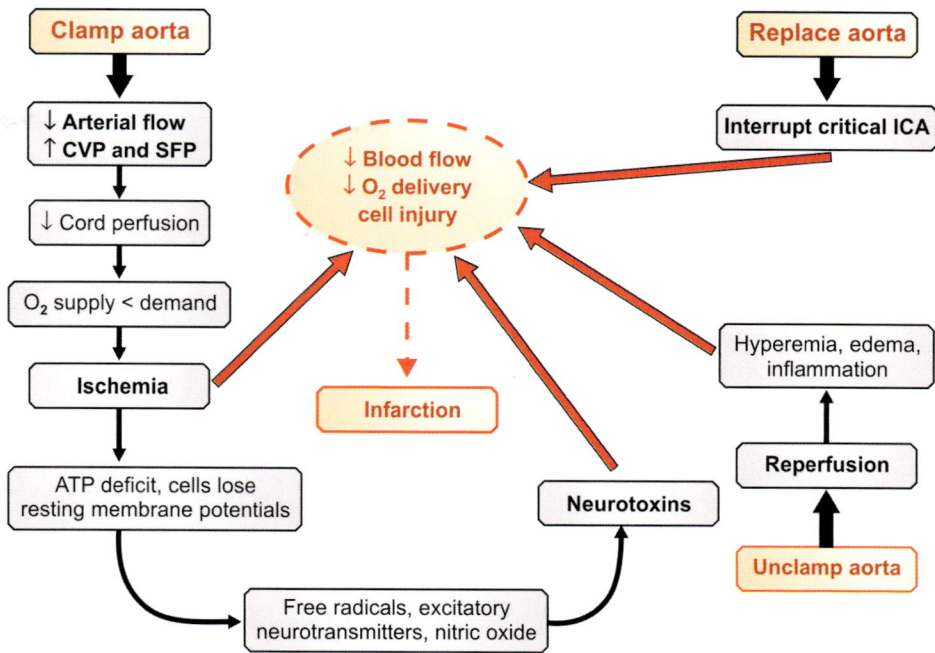

**Fig. 5.9:** The flow diagram depicts the events which results in spinal cord injury starting with application of aortic clamp and replacement of thoracic aorta

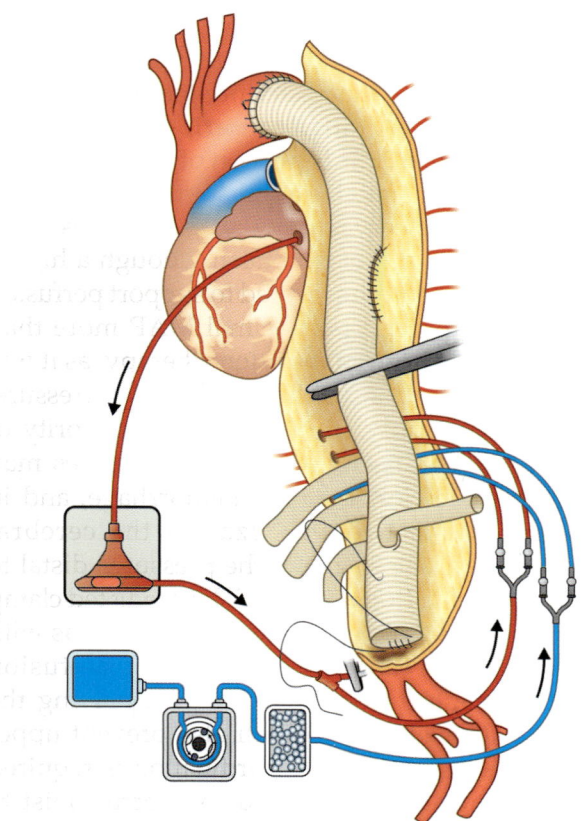

**Fig. 5.10:** Partial left heart bypass. The blood drained from the left lower pulmonary vein and with the help of centrifugal pump, it perfuses the lower body, the major back bleeding intercostals and the visceral arteries. A separate pump tranfuses cord crystalloid solution to the renal arteries for renal protection

circulation, thus increasing cardiac preload, which translates into increased stroke volume and therefore further increase in the proximal pressures. Study by Aadahi et al[53] has shown that during aortic cross clamping the cardiac output increases by 43% from the baseline. The heart rate increases by 38% along with increase in pulmonary capillary wedge pressure (PCWP). The increase in the CO is due to increase in the heart rate or increase in the preload or both.[54] The hemodynamic effect is totally different when aorta is clamped below the celiac artery (for abdominal aortic aneurysm). The splanchnic system has significant capacity to accommodate blood and the shift of blood into the central venous system is not appreciable. Therefore, this results in decrease in preload and the proximal hypertension is relatively less. If with supra-celiac clamping proximal hypertension is not seen then it means that either there is cardiac under-filling or the LV has become dysfunctional due to increased afterload. Such a situation will warrant either inotropic support of institution of partial bypass. Control of proximal hypertension begins with deepening the plane of anesthesia. If this is not sufficient then beta-blocker is added to control reflex tachycardia and increased contractility. Esmolol is a good option because of its short duration of action. Labetalol can also be used for it has both α and β-blockade effects. Vasodilators, especially venodilator like nitroglycerine may prove more beneficial in decreasing the preload by increasing the capacitance of the venous system. Sodium nitroprusside is an attractive choice for hypertension, but is not the first choice, as it causes increase in CSF production, which further decreases SCPP. The vasodilators may worsen the hypoxemia due to one lung ventilation.

## D. Aortic Cross Clamp Release

Acute hemodynamic changes occur due to aortic clamp application, the reverse effect happens when the aortic clamp is released. Sudden clamp release results in significant hypotension, which may warrant reapplication of partial clamp over the aorta. To avoid such a hemodynamic collapse, its best to prepare for the event well before in advance. The preparation involves decreasing the inhalation dial setting, stopping all vasodilatory infusions, increasing the preload and starting a vasoconstrictor. Before the clamp release one should be also ready for the need of rapid transfusion in the event of significant bleeding.

## E. Spinal Cord Protection

Paraplegia is a definite concern whenever long segment of thoracic aorta or thoracoabdominal aorta is to be replaced. For the patient who came walking into the hospital on his own, and post surgery is not be able to walk is both an emotional and physical disaster. Earlier the reported incidence of paraplegia was as high as 40%.[55] With improvement in the surgical approach and our understanding of spinal cord perfusion and collateral network, presently the paraplegia incidence post TAAA repair ranges from 8 to 28%.[56] The wide range of spinal cord injury (SCI) reported reflects upon the differences in surgical practice, the varied extent of aorta replaced, different patient population, etiology, employing different spinal cord protection strategy-intercostal reimplantation, distal perfusion, cerebral spinal fluid (CSF) drainage, epidural cold saline infusion, (Fig. 5.11) and epidural papaverine. The renowned aortic centers follow different philosophies, which also results in almost same outcome, this confuses as to which protocol to adopt. With the advent of endovascular stenting for aortic aneurysms the reported rates for SCI has further been lowered to 3–12%.[57] The expert aortic centers claim SCI incidence in the range of 3 to 6% with open surgical repair. The incidence of SCI has not touched the zero figure even at the best aortic institutes suggests that our understanding of SCI is still not complete. CSF drainage is one of the adjunct methods described to prevent SCI. A systematic review and meta-analysis by Cina' et al[58] support the use of CSF drainage to prevent paraplegia.

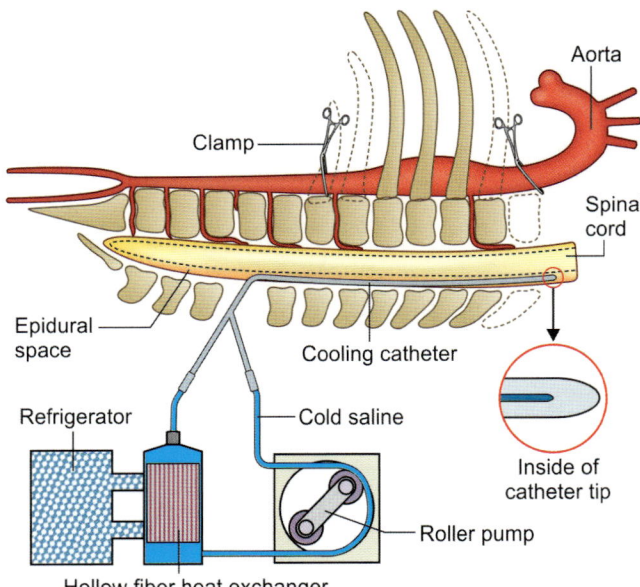

**Fig. 5.11:** Epidural cooling minimizes spinal cord injury by lowering the metabolic requirement during aortic cross clamping period

### 1. Spinal Cord Blood Supply

The reason behind paraplegia incidence during aortic surgery lies in its unique blood supply pattern. The anterior or the ventral portion of the spinal cord carries the motor tract, while the posterior spinal cord carries the sensory tracts. A single anterior spinal artery supplies the anterior 2/3rds portion of the spinal cord, while two posterior spinal arteries supply the posterior portion. It is for this very reason that the anterior spinal cord is at increased risk of ischemia. The anterior spinal artery receives blood supply from collateral system (Fig. 5.12). The thoracic portion of the anterior spinal artery receives blood from the intercostal arteries while the abdominal portion of the anterior spinal artery receives blood supply from the lumbar and pelvic circulation. One of the largest intercostal arteries is the artery of Adamkiewicz or the great radicular artery that usually originates between T8 and L1 vertebral level. Great emphasis has been given to this collateral branch, to the extent that during preoperative imaging workout the origin of this artery is sought for, so that intraoperatively it can be easily located and reimplanted onto the graft. Though it is highly unlikely that a single intercostal will be able to takeover the supply after the other intercostals have been sacrificed. The ischemic time for the spinal cord starts with the application of the aortic clamp, which prevents blood supply from the collateral system, and the anterior spinal cord blood supply solely rests with the anterior spinal artery. Implantation of all the intercostal arteries is an impractical strategy, as it will consume significant

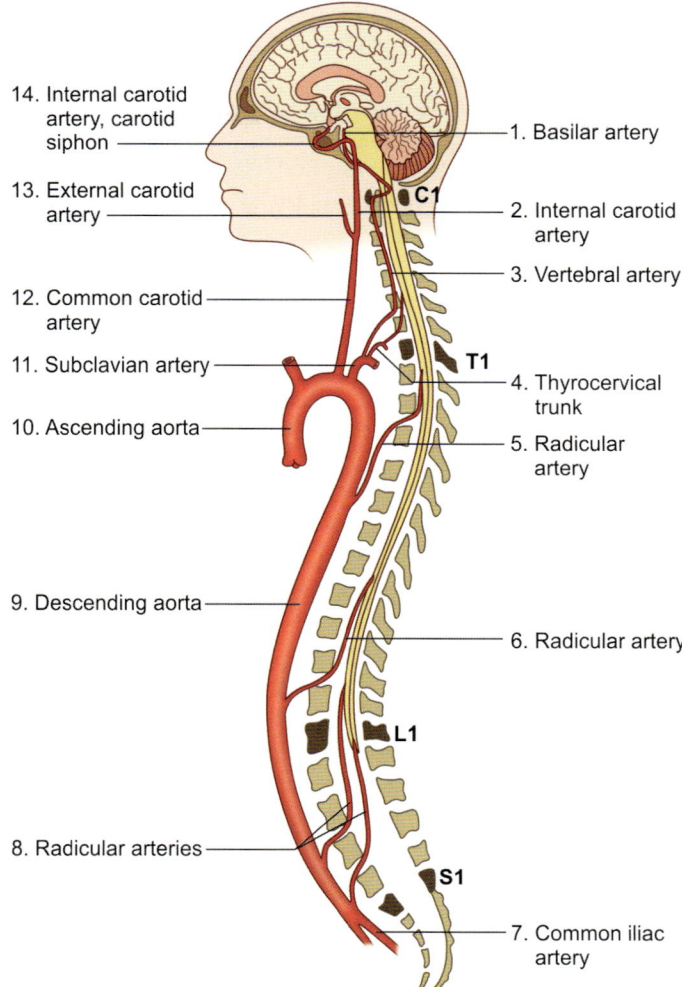

**Fig. 5.12:** Collateral supply from the radicular arteries originating from the descending thoracic aorta and lumbar and sacral collaterals from the abdomen aorta are the key supplemental blood supply to the anterior spinal cord

14. Internal carotid artery, carotid siphon
13. External carotid artery
12. Common carotid artery
11. Subclavian artery
10. Ascending aorta
9. Descending aorta
8. Radicular arteries

1. Basilar artery
2. Internal carotid artery
3. Vertebral artery
4. Thyrocervical trunk
5. Radicular artery
6. Radicular artery
7. Common iliac artery

amount of time on clamp and most of the smaller reimplanted vessels will get thrombosed. Therefore for practical purpose only large back bleeding intercostals are reimplanted which also carries higher degree of patency rates post implantation. The small back bleeding intercostal arteries is ligated, to prevent steal from the anterior spinal cord. During extensive aortic replacement, like type-I and type-II aneurysm repair, distal perfusion will help in preserving spinal cord flow through the collateral network.

## 2. Cerebral Spinal Fluid Drainage

As the aorta is clamped there is significant upper body hypertension. This results in increased CSF production and increased CSF pressure. The spinal cord perfusion pressure (SCPP) is determined by the difference between the mean arterial pressure (MAP) and the CSF pressure.

*SCPP=MAP-CSFP (or CVP, which ever is higher)*

SCPP of more than 40 mmHg is important for spinal cord protection and this will warrant mean distal aortic pressure more than 50–60 mmHg and a central venous pressure less than 10-12 mmHg. Once the aorta is clamped, the fall in distal MAP depends upon the degree of systemic collateral development. Low distal perfusion pressures and no flow from the intercostals, the lumbar collaterals along with increased CSF pressure due to proximal hypertension result into a perfect recipe for paraplegia disaster. The principle behind CSF drainage is that the CSF pressure is reduced which improves SCPP.

CSF drainage is carried out with a 16G Touhy needle inserted into the intrathecal space via L4-5 or L3-4 interspace. An 18G catheter is inserted 4–5 cm into the intrathecal space for CSF drainage (Fig. 5.13). Once clear CSF flow is ascertained, the catheter is fixed to the back and attached to a pressure transducer and a volumetric chamber to measure CSF drainage through a luer lock. The aim is to maintain CSF pressure <10 mmHg. The catheter is usually inserted the day before surgery as the patient will be heparinized during the surgery, and in case of epidural venous plexus injury during needle insertion, it may bleed and form a compressing hematoma causing nerve compression and paraplegia. The catheter is kept for 48–72 hours and then removed in absence of any lower limb motor deficit. If later on the patient complains of loss of lower limb motor power then the catheter is reinserted and CSF is drained. During CSF drainage if the color becomes blood tinged, then the drainage should be stopped, as it may suggest venous bleeding due to excessive CSF drainage. Leaving the catheter for long can increase the incidence of meningitis.

Intraoperative monitoring tools like somatosensory evoked potential and especially motor evoked potential

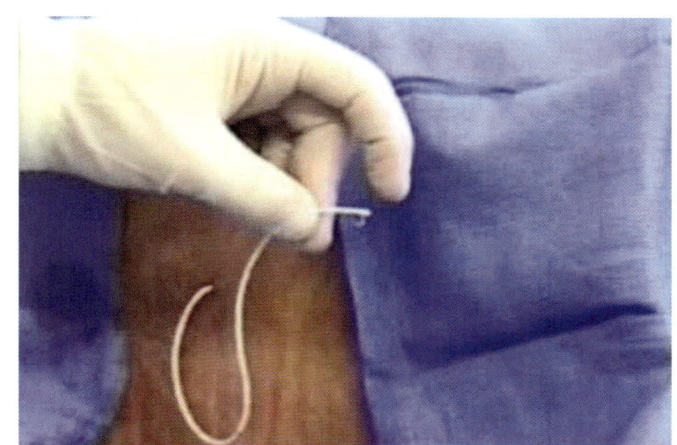

**Fig. 5.13:** Cerebral spinal fluid drainage is used as an adjunct to various ocular methods to decrease spinal cord injury incidence

can help in detection of intraoperative SCI and help in early initiation of interventions to improve spinal cord perfusion. This monitoring tool requires intravenous anaesthetic agents and avoidance of agents which may hamper the interpretation of signals like neuromuscular blocking agents, higher levels of volatile inhalations, nitrous oxide and hypothermia.

## CONCLUSION

Surgical intervention for DTA aneurysm is a challenge for both the surgeon and the anesthesiologist. The challenge is due to the associated comorbidities and the potential risk of postoperative paraplegia. With better understanding of spinal cord perfusion and its collateral blood supply, monitoring, and adjunct therapy, the incidence of paraplegia has been reduced. Endovascular intervention has added a new dimension, but requires long-term follow-up to become an alternative to the conventional open surgical intervention.

A careful planning among the team members and use of cerebral monitoring can help in significantly improved outcome.

## REFERENCES

1. Swan H, Maaske C, Johnson M, Grover R. Arterial homografts. II. Resection of thoracic aortic aneurysm using a stored human arterial transplant. Arch Surg 1950;61:732–7.

2. DeBakey ME, Cooley DA. Successful resection of aneurysm of thoracic aorta and replacement by graft. J Am Med Assoc 1953;152:673–6.

3. Cooley DA, DeBakey ME. Resection of the thoracic aorta with replacement by homograft for aneurysms and constrictive lesions. J Thorac Cardiovasc Surg 1955;29:66–104.

4. Johnston KW, Rutherford RB, Tilson MD, Shah DM, Hollier L, Stanley JC. Suggested standards for reporting on arterial aneurysms. Subcommittee on Reporting Standards for Arterial Aneurysms, Ad Hoc Committee on Reporting Standards, Society for Vascular Surgery and North American Chapter, International Society for Cardiovascular Surgery. J Vasc Surg 1991;13:452–8.

5. Slaney G. A history of aneurysm surgery. In: Greenhagl RM, Mannick JA, Powell JT (Eds). The cause and management of aneurysms. London: WB Saunders, 1990;1–18.

6. Roberts WC, Ko JM, Vowels TJ. Natural History of Syphilitic Aortitis. Am J Cardiol 2009;104(11):1578–87.

7. He R, Guo DC, Estrera AL, Safi HJ, Huynh TT, Yin Z, et al. Characterization of the inflammatory and apoptotic cells in the aortas of patients with ascending thoracic aortic aneurysms and dissections. J ThoracCardiovasc Surg 2006;131:671–8.

8. Segura AM, Luna RE, Horiba K, et al. Immunohistochemistry of matrix metalloproteinases and their inhibitors in thoracic aortic aneurysms and aorticvalves of patients with Marfan's syndrome. Circulation 1998;98(Suppl II):II-331–II-337.

9. LeMaire SA, Wang X, Wilks JA, et al. Matrix metalloproteinases in ascending aortic aneurysms: Bicuspid versus trileaflet aortic valves. J Surg Res 2005;123:40–48.

10. Dietz HC, Cutting GR, Pyeritz RE, et al. Marfan syndrome caused by a recurrent de novo missense mutation in the fibrillin gene. Nature 1991;352:337–9.

11. Olin JW, Fuster V. Acute aortic dissection: The need for rapid, accurate, and readily available diagnostic strategies. Arterio-scler Thromb Vasc Biol 2003;23:1721–3.

12. Van Arsdell GS, David TE, Butan J. Autopsies in acute type A aortic dissection (surgical implications). Circulation 1998; 98:299–302.

13. Weber T, Högler S, Auer J, et al. Ddimer in acute aortic dissection. Chest 2003;123:1375–8.

14. Schillinger M, Domanovits H, Bayegan K, et al. Creactive protein and mortality in patients with acute aortic disease. Intensive Care Med 2002;28:740–745.

15. Katoh H, Suzuki T, Hiroi Y, Ohtaki E, Suzuki S, Yazaki Y, Nagai R. Diagnosis of aortic dissection by immunoassay for circulating smooth muscle myosin. Lancet 1995;345:191–2.

16. Suzuki T, Katoh H, Tsuchio Y, Hasegawa A, Kurabayashi M, Ohira A, Hiramori K, Sakomura Y, Kasanuki H, Hori S, Aikawa N, Abe S, Tei C, Nakagawa Y, Nobuyoshi M, Misu T, Sumiyoshi T, Nagai R. Diagnostic implications of elevated levels of smooth-muscle myosin heavy-chain protein in acute aortic dissection. Ann Intern Med 2000;133: 537–41.

17. Smulyan H, Weinberg SE, Howanitz PJ. Continuous propranolol infusion following abdominal surgery. J Am Med Assoc 1982;247:2539–42.

18. Mangano DT, Layug EL, Wallace A, Tateo I. Effect of atenolol on mortality and cardiovascular morbidity after noncardiac surgery. Multicenter Study of Perioperative Ischemia Research Group [see comments] [published erratum appears in N Engl J Med 1997 Apr 3;336(14):1039]. N Engl J Med 1996;335:1713–20.

19. Devereaux PJ, Beattie WS, Choi PT, et al. How strong is the evidence for the use of perioperative beta blockers in noncardiac surgery? Systematic review and meta-analysis of randomised controlled trials. Br Med J 2005;331:313–21.

20. Devereaux PJ, Yang H, Yusuf S, et al. POISE Study Group. Effects of extended-release metoprolol succinate in patients undergoing non-cardiac surgery (POISE trial): A randomised controlled trial. Lancet 2008;371:1839–47.

21. Dunkelgrun M, Boersma E, Schouten O, et al. Bisoprolol and fluvastatin for the reduction of perioperative cardiac mortality and myocardial infarction in intermediate-risk patients undergoing noncardiovascular surgery: A randomized controlled trial (DECREASE-IV). Ann Surg 2009;249:921–6.

22. Erasmus Medical Centre. Follow-up Investigation Committee: Investigation into possible violation of scientific integrity. Report Summary. November 16, 2011.

23. Erasmus Medical Centre. Report on the 2012 follow-up investigation of possible breaches of academic integrity. September 30, 2012.

24. Poldermans D, Boersma E, Bax JJ, et al. The effect of bisoprolol on perioperative mortality and myocardial infarction in high-risk patients undergoing vascular surgery. Dutch Echocardiographic Cardiac Risk Evaluation Applying Stress Echocardiography Study Group. N Engl J Med 1999; 341:1789–94.

25. Wijeysundera DN, Duncan D, Nkonde-Price C, et al. Perioperative Beta Blockade in Noncardiac Surgery: A Systematic Review for the 2014 ACC/AHA Guideline on Perioperative Cardiovascular Evaluation and Management of Patients Undergoing Noncardiac Surgery: A Report of the American College of Cardiology/American Heart Association Task Force on Practice Guidelines. J Am Coll Cardiol 2014 online.

26. Fleisher LA, Beckman JA, Brown KA. ACC/AHA 2007 guidelines on perioperative cardiovascular evaluation and care for noncardiac surgery: Executive summary: A report of the American College of Cardiology/American Heart Association Task Force on Practice Guidelines (Writing Committee to Revise the 2002 Guidelines on Perioperative Cardiovascular Evaluation for Noncardiac Surgery). J Am Coll Cardiol 2007;50:1707–32.

27. Stone NJ, Robinson J, Lichtenstein AH, et al. 2013 ACC/AHA guideline on the treatment of blood cholesterol to reduce atherosclerotic cardiovascular risk in adults: a report of the American College of Cardiology/American Heart Association Task Force on Practice Guidelines. Circulation. 2014;129:S1–S45.

28. Schouten O, Boersma E, Hoeks SE, Benner R, van Urk H, van Sambeek MR, et al. Fluvastatin and perioperative events in patients undergoing vascular surgery. N Engl J Med 2009; 36:980–9.

29. Poldermans D, Bax JJ, Boersma E, et al. Guidelines for pre-operative cardiac risk assessment and perioperative cardiac management in non-cardiac surgery. Eur Heart J 2009;30: 2769–812.

30. Hoshina K, Nemoto M, Hashimoto T, Miura S, Urabe G, Nakazawa T, Hosaka A, Kato M, Ohkubo N, Miyairi T, Okamoto H, Shigematsu K, Miyata T. Study Design of PROCEDURE Study. A Randomized Comparison of the Dose-Dependent Effects of Pitavastatin in Patients with Abdominal Aortic Aneurysm with Massive Aortic Atheroma: Prevention of Cholesterol Embolization during Endovascular and Open Aneurysm Repair with Pitavastatin (PROCEDURE) Study. Ann Vasc Dis 2013;6:62–66.

31. Waterman AL, Feezor RJ, Lee WA, Hess PJ, Beaver TM, Martin TD, Huber TS, Beck AW. Endovascular treatment of acute and chronic aortic pathology in patients with Marfan syndrome. J Vasc Surg 2012;55:1234–40; discussion 1240–41.

32. Erbel R, Aboyans V, Boileau C, Bossone E, Di Bartolomeo R, Eggebrecht H, et al. 2014 ESC Guidelines on the diagnosis and treatment of aortic diseases: Document covering acute and chronic aortic diseases of the thoracic and abdominal aorta of the adultThe Task Force for the Diagnosis and Treatment of Aortic Diseases of the European Society of Cardiology (ESC). Eur Heart J 2014;35:2873–2926.

33. Lemaire SA, Jones MM, Conklin LD, Carter SA, Criddell MD, Wang XL, Raskin SA, Coselli JS. Randomized comparison of cold blood and cold crystalloid renal perfusion for renal protection during thoracoabdominal aortic aneurysm repair. J Vasc Surg 2009;49:11–19; discussion 19.

34. Le Manach Y, Perel A, Coriat P, Godet G, Bertrand M, Riou B. Early and delayed myocardial infarction after abdominal aortic surgery. Anesthesiology 2005;102:885–91.

35. Priebe HJ. Perioperative myocardial infarction-aetiology and prevention. Br J Anaesth 2005;95:3–19.

36. Gualandro DM, Campos CA, Calderaro D, et al. Coronary plaque rupture in patients with myocardial infarction after noncardiac surgery: Frequent anddangerous. Atherosclerosis 2012;222:191–5.

37. McFalls E, Ward H, Moritz T, Goldman S, Krupski W, Littooy F, Pierpont G, Santilli S, Rapp J, Hattler B, Shunk K, Jaenicke C, Thottapurathu L, Ellis N, Reda D, Henderson W, Coronary-Artery Revascularization before Elective Major Vascular Surgery, N Engl J Med 2004;30,351(27):2795–804.

38. Landesberg G. The pathophysiology of perioperative myocardial infarction: facts and perspectives. J Cardiothorac Vasc Anesth 2003;17:90–100.

39. Raby KE, Brull SJ, Timimi F, et al. The effect of heart rate control on myocardial ischemia among high-risk patients after vascular surgery. Anesth Analg 1999;88:477–82.

40. Bertrand M, Godet G, Meersschaert K, Brun L, Salcedo E, Coriat P. Should the angiotensin II antagonists be discontinued before surgery? Anesth Analg 2001;92:26–30.

41. Glance LG, Lustik SJ, Hannan EL, et al. The Surgical Mortality Probability Model: derivation and validation of a simple risk prediction rule for noncardiac surgery. Ann Surg 2012;255:696–702.

42. Brosius FC III, Hostetter TH, Kelepouris E, et al. Detection of chronic kidney disease in patients with or at increased risk of cardiovascular disease: A science advisory from the American Heart Association Kidney and Cardiovascular Disease Council; the Councils on High Blood Pressure Research, Cardiovascular Disease in the Young, and Epidemiology and Prevention; and the Quality of Care and Outcomes Research Interdisciplinary Working Group: developed in collaboration with the National Kidney Foundation. Circulation 2006;114:1083–7.

43. Thiele H, Hildebrand L, Schirdewahn C, et al. Impact of High-Dose N-Acetylcysteine Versus Placebo on Contrast-Induced Nephropathy and Myocardial Reperfusion Injury in Unselected Patients With ST-Segment Elevation Myocardial Infarction Undergoing Primary Percutaneous Coronary Intervention: The LIPSIA-N-ACC (Prospective, Single-Blind, Placebo-Controlled, Randomized Leipzig Immediate Percutaneous Coronary Intervention Acute Myocardial Infarction N-ACC) Trial. J Am CollCardiol 2010;55(20):2201–9.

44. Inzucchi SE, Bergenstal RM, Buse JB, Diamant M, Ferrannini E, Nauck Metal. Management of hyperglycaemia in type 2 diabetes: A patient centered approach. Position statement of the American Diabetes Association (ADA) and the European Association for the Study of Diabetes (EASD). Diabetologia 2012;55:1577–96.

45. Holman RR, Paul SK, Bethel MA, Matthews DR, Neil HAW. 10-year follow-up of intensive glucose control in type 2 diabetes. N Engl J Med 2008;359:1577–89.

46. Nicholson ML, Baker DM, Hopkinson BR, et al. Randomized controlled trial of the effect of mannitol on renal reperfusion injury during aortic aneurysm surgery. Br J Surg 1996;83: 1230–3.

47. Hager B, Betschart M, Krapf R. Effect of postoperative intravenous loop diuretic on renal function after major surgery. Schweiz Med Wochenschr 1996;126:666–73.

48. Baldwin L, Henderson A, Hickman P. Effect of postoperative low-dose dopamine on renal function after elective major vascular surgery. Ann Intern Med 1994;120:744–7.

49. Marik PE. Low-Dose dopamine: A systematic review. Intensive Care Med 2002;28:877–83.

50. Kellum JA, Decker JM. Use of dopamine in acute renal failure: a meta-analysis. Crit Care Med 2001;29:1526–31.

51. Lassnigg A, Donner E, Grubhofer G, Presterl E, Druml W, Hiesmayr M. Lack of renoprotective effects of dopamine and furosemide during cardiac surgery. J Am SocNephrol. 2000;11:97–104.

52. Godet G, Fleron M-H, Vicaut E, et al. Risk factors for acute postoperative renal failure in thoracic or thoracoabdominal aortic surgery (a prospective study). Anesth Analg. 1997;85: 1227–32.

53. Aadahl P, Saether OD, Aakhus S, Strømholm T, Myhre HO. The importance of echocardiography in thoracic aortic surgery. Eur J Vasc Endovasc Surg 1996;12:401–6.

54. Gelman S, Khazaeli MB, Orr R, Henderson T. Blood volume redistribution during cross-clamping of the descending aorta. Anesth Analg 1994;78:219–24.

55. McGarvey ML, Cheung AT, Szeto W, Messe SR. Management of neurologic complications of thoracic aortic surgery. J Clin Neurophysiol 2007;24:336–43.

56. Greenberg R, Resch T, Nyman U, Lindh M, Brunkwall J, Brunkwall P, Malina M, Koul B, Lindblad B, Ivancev K. Endovascular repair of descending thoracic aortic aneurysms: An early experience with intermediate-term follow-up. J Vasc Surg 2000;31:147.

57. Feezor RJ, Martin TD, Hess PJ Jr, et al. Extent of aortic coverage and incidence of spinal cord ischemia after thoracic endovascular aneurysm repair. Ann Thorac Surg 2008;86: 1809–14.

58. Cina CS, Abouzahr L, Arena GO, et al. Cerebrospinal Fluid Drainage to Prevent Paraplegia During Thoracic and Thoraco abdominal Aortic AneurysmS urgery: A Systematic Review and Meta-Analysis. Journal of Vascular Surgery 2004:40:36–44.

# CHAPTER 6

# Anesthesia for Abdominal Aorta Disease

Sambhunath Das

## INTRODUCTION

Abdominal aortic aneurysms (AAA) are a substantial burden on health care system. It occurs mostly among men older than 65 years of age. Presently patients are presenting with AAA even at the age less than 45 year. In 1990, the global age-specific prevalence rate per 100,000 ranged from 8.43 in the 40 to 44 years age group to 2,422.53 in the 75 to 79 years age group; the corresponding range in 2010 was 7.88 to 2,274.82.[1] Prevalence was higher in developed versus developing nations, and the rates within each development stratum decreased between 1990 and 2010. Globally, the age-specific annual incidence rate per 100,000 in 1990 ranged from 0.89 in 40 to 44 years age group to 176.08 in the 75 to 79 years age group. In 2010, this range was 0.83 to 164.57.[1] The disorder is the thirteenth leading cause of death in the USA.[2] Although some patients have vague symptoms, such as back pain or abdominal pain, most abdominal aneurysms are asymptomatic until rupture. The rupture of AAA leads to death in 65% of patients.[3]

## DEFINITION

An aneurysm occurring in any portion of the infra-diaphragmatic aorta could be termed as an abdominal aortic aneurysm. Common practice restricts this definition to an aneurysm of the infrarenal aorta. Aneurysms involving the renal ostia (*intrarenal, suprarenal aorta*) are also included under this term. In adult, the infrarenal abdominal aortic diameter is between 15 mm and 24 mm.[4] McGregor and colleagues[4] proposed the definition of an abdominal aortic aneurysm as an aorta with an infrarenal diameter greater than 30 mm. In 1991, the society for vascular surgery and the international society for cardiovascular surgery adhoc committee on standards in reporting proposed as a criterion that the infrarenal diameter should be 1.5 times the expected normal diameter.[5] There is no definite consensus on the definition of abdominal aortic aneurysm; however, the disorder is conventionally diagnosed if the aortic diameter is 30 mm or more. Aneurysms affect three layers of the vascular tunic; otherwise, the dilatation is called a *pseudo-aneurysm.* Most aneurysms are fusiform since the whole circumference of the artery is affected, whereas an aneurysm that includes only a part of the circumference is termed *saccular.* An inflammatory aneurysm is characterized by extensive perianeurysmal and retro-peritoneal fibrosis and dense adhesions to adjacent abdominal organs.

**Classification of AAA** (according to site) (Fig. 6.1):

I. Infrarenal
II. Juxtarenal
III. Intrarenal or pararenal
IV. Suprarenal

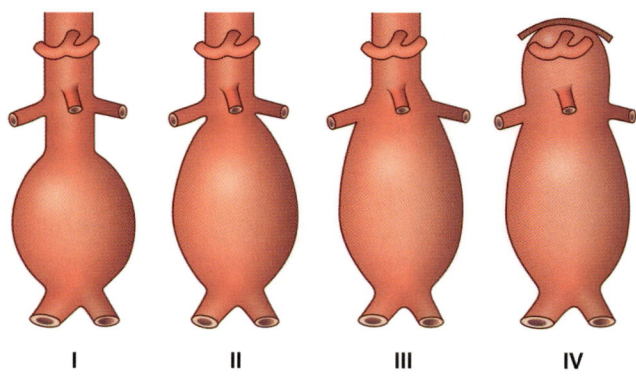

Fig. 6.1: Different types of abdominal aneurysm

## ETIOLOGY AND RISK FACTORS

There are many causes of aneurysmal dilatation, but few abdominal aortic aneurysms are the direct consequence of specific causes such as trauma, acute infection (brucellosis, salmonellosis), chronic infection (tuberculosis), inflammatory diseases (Behçet and Takayasu disease)[6,7] and connective tissue disorders (Marfan syndrome, Ehlers-Danlos type IV).[8] Thus, most abdominal aortic aneurysms are called non-specific. Moreover, because this disorder is invariably associated with severe atherosclerotic damage of the aortic wall, it has been traditionally regarded as a consequence of atherosclerosis.[9] This conventional view has been increasingly challenged in recent years.

### Etiology for abdominal AA

1. Trauma
2. Acute infection (brucellosis, salmonellosis)
3. Chronic infection (tuberculosis)
4. Inflammatory diseases (Behçet and Takayasu disease)
5. Atherosclerotic damage of the aortic wall
6. Non-specific causes

## RISK STRATIFICATION

Tables 6.1 and 6.2 shows the method of stratifying perioperative risk for AAA surgery.

| Table 6.1: Glasgow aneurysm score-points | |
|---|---|
| Age | (points = no. of yrs) |
| Shock | 17 points |
| MI | 7 points |
| CVA | 10 points |
| Renal disease | 14 points |

\# score >84 => 65% mortality

| Table 6.2: Hardman index-points | |
|---|---|
| Age >76 years | 1 |
| Creatinine >1.9 mmol/L | 1 |
| Hb < 9 gm% | 1 |
| MI on ECG | 1 |
| H/O loss of consciousness | 1 |

\# score ≥ 2 => 80% mortality

### Pathophysiology

- Alteration in aortic wall connective tissue—elastin and collagen
- Degradation of elastin appears to be an early feature of aneurysm
- Collagen disruption is the ultimate cause of rupture
- Collagen/elastin (C/E) ratio equilibrium is maintained by *matrix metalloproteinase* (MMP) and tissue inhibitors
- Imbalance of C/E ratio → proteolysis → aneurysm formation

## METHODS OF DIAGNOSIS PROCEDURE

The examination for a pulsatile mass should be done by bimanual palpation of the supraumbilical area. Sensitivity of abdominal palpation for detection of abdominal aortic aneurysms increases with the diameter of the lesion: 61% for aneurysms 3.0–3.9 cm, 69% for those 4.0–4.9 cm, and 82% for those 5.0 cm and larger. The palpation sensitivity also depends inversely on the size of the abdominal waist line.[10] Abdominal standard radiography can incidentally be diagnostic, mainly in the transverse view, if calcifications are present in the aortic wall, which allows visualization of dilatation. However, standard radiography is not the method of choice for the diagnosis of abdominal aortic aneurysms. Ultrasonography is the simplest and cheapest diagnostic procedure and can accurately measure the size of the aorta in longitudinal as well as in anteroposterior and transverse directions with an accuracy of 3 mm.[11] Ultrasonography is largely used not only for the initial assessment and the follow-up surveillance, but also for population screening. If the diameter of the aneurysm is such that surgical procedureis contemplated, CT is the next step to help determine which treatment should be used (endovascular or open surgery). Serial CT scans can be used to visualize the proximal neck (the transition between the normal and aneurysmal aorta), the extension to the iliac arteries, and the patency of the visceral arteries (Figs 6.2A and B). They can also measure the thickness of the mural thrombus. Venous anomalies that can be hazardous during the access to the neck are also clearly indicated (left venacava, posterior left renal vein). CT can also display the presence of blood within the thrombus (crescent sign), which has been regarded by some groups as a predictive marker of imminent rupture.[12,13] In case of inflammatory aneurysm, CT allows estimation of the thickness of the aortic wall outside of the calcified deposits and visualisation of the presence of para-aortic fibrosis potentially associated with uretero-hydronephrosis. Extravasation of contrast material is diagnostic of aneurysm rupture. With three-dimensional imaging, helical CT and CT angiography can provide additional anatomical details, especially useful if endovascular procedure is considered (Fig. 6.3).[14] MRI, combined with magnetic resonance angiography (MRA), is of little harm since non-nephrotoxic contrast material (e.g. gadolinium) is used, whereas conventional arteriography uses nephrotoxic contrast material, which can lead to renal failure and distal embolization. Because of the steady development of MRA and CT angiographies, there will be hardly any place left for conventional aortography during preoperative assessment of

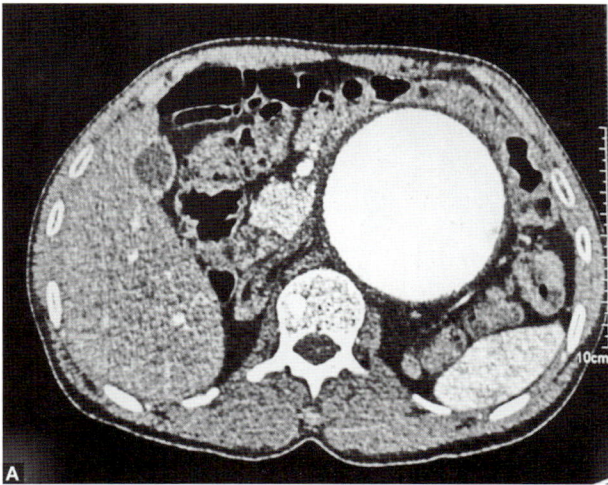

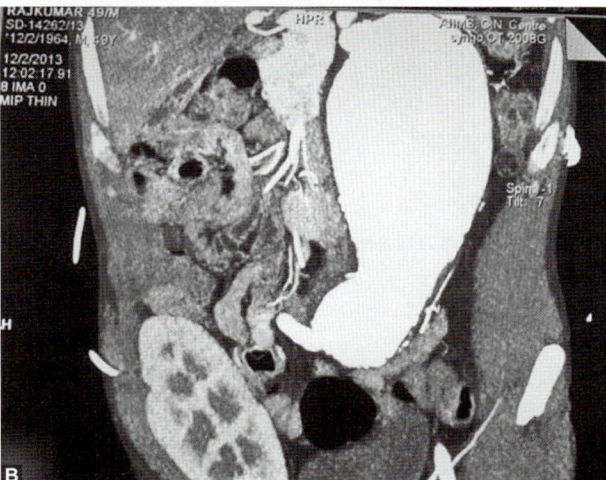

**Figs 6.2A and B:** (A) Cross-section axial, (B) Sagittal

**Fig. 6.3:** CT angio 3D construction

the disorder. The use of conventional aortography is mainly restricted to the placement of endovascular devices or when a horse-shoe kidney is diagnosed.

## Clinical Presentation

### Unruptured Abdominal Aortic Aneurysms

Non-ruptured aneurysms are generally asymptomatic in most patients. They are essentially diagnosed incidentally during extensive clinical examination, especially in patients who complain of coronary, peripheral, or cerebrovascular diseases, or during population screening. Fleming and co-workers[15] reported that population screening in men aged 65–74 years significantly reduces mortality related to the disorder. Non-ruptured aneurysms might exceptionally be diagnosed after complications, such as distal embolization and, even more rarely, acute thrombosis. Minor and less specific symptoms include chronic vague abdominal and back pain, which can result from direct pressure or distension of adjacent structures. Recent onset of severe lumbar pain has been deemed to indicate impending rupture. Ureteric hydronephrosis might also take place, especially if the aneurysm is inflammatory or involves the iliac bifurcation.

### Ruptured Abdominal Aortic Aneurysms

Rupture of abdominal aortic aneurysms is heralded by the triad of sudden-onset pain in the mid-abdomen or flank (that may radiate into the scrotum), shock, and the presence of a pulsatile abdominal mass. However, the degree of shock varies according to the location and size of the rupture and the delay before the patient is examined. Rupture from the anterolateral wall into the peritoneal cavity is usually dramatic and most often associated with death at the scene. Most patients with a rupture who reach the clinic alive have a rupture of the posterolateral wall into the retroperitoneal space; a small tear can temporarily seal the rupture and the initial blood loss might be small. This initial event is systematically followed within hours by a larger rupture. This biphasic evolution emphasizes the importance of the intermediate period after the initial event, which should be used for medical transfer and emergency repair.

Anecdotally, the first episode of rupture could be definitely contained and become a chronic pulsatile extra-aortic hematoma. Very rarely, the aneurysm might spontaneously rupture into the duodenum); an incidence rate at necropsy of 0.04 to 0.07% has been reported.[16–18] More often, aorto-duodenal fistula can occur after previous repair, with an incidence rate of 0.5 to 2.3%.[19] Rupture into the vena cava can also take place with an apparent pattern of lower extremity edema erroneously attributed to cavoiliac thrombophlebitis.

However, the development of high output congestive heart failure and the perception of continuous abdominal noise is pathognomonic. The overall prevalence of aortocaval fistula is 3 to 6% of all ruptured aortic aneurysms.[20,21]

## Management

**The management of AAA can be divided into 4 categories:**

1. Medical management to control hypertension, cardiac dysfunction and stabilization of renal and other concommitted diseases.
2. Endovascular graft placement across the AAA segment. It avoids the complications related to open surgical techniques.
3. Open surgical treatment
4. Hybrid procedure, i.e. combined endovascular graft and surgery

During open surgical treatment, the abdomen is entered either through a long midline or a wide transverse incision. A retroperitoneal approach has been recommended in patients with chronic obstructive pulmonary disease. Disadvantages of this approach include: first that the intraperitoneal content cannot be inspected; and second, access to the right iliac artery can frequently be difficult, especially if there is a large right iliac aneurysm. Once the abdominal cavity is opened, the neck of the aneurysm needs to be identified to control it. In the cases of a suprarenal or intrarenal neck, a clamp above the renal arteries might be needed briefly. The iliac arteries are controlled in much the same way. The inferior mesenteric artery is tied close to the aortic wall to keep it collateral to the superior mesenteric artery; in some instances, encircling the inferior mesenteric artery with a rubber to re-implant it on the aortic prosthesis via a Carrell patch could be wise to maintain direct flow for sigmoid and rectum. The vascular graft is a knitted synthetic textile sealed with collagen or albumin. The upper anastomosis is of the end-to-end type and the distal anastomosis is located on the aortic bifurcation, the iliac bifurcations, or the common femoral arteries depending on the extent of aneurysmal transformation and the patency of the external iliac arteries (Fig. 6.4). Care is taken to preserve at least one internal iliac artery and to detect perioperatively a potential left colonic-ischemia. In sexually active male patients, the recommendation is not to dissect the lateral left aortic wall and the common left

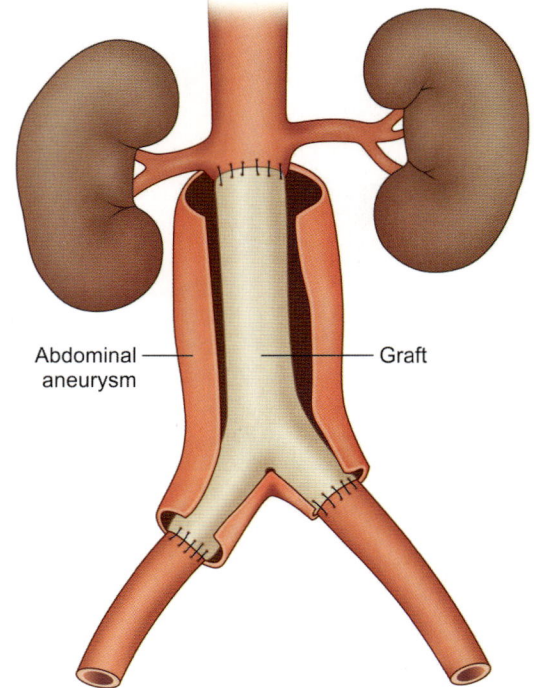

**Fig. 6.4:** Aorto-bifemoral graft at aneurysmal segment

iliac artery. Whenever possible, iliac anastomosis should be the preferred choice instead of common femoral anastomosis because anastomosis in the groin is more prone to infection. Specific morbidities linked to surgery are left colon ischemia and renal failure (eventually due to thromboembolic events in renal arteries). Postoperative paraplegia, a huge concern with thoracoabdominal surgery, is infrequent with abdominal aortic aneurysm surgery. The incidence of paraplegia after endovascular repair or open surgery has been reported to be 0.21% and 0.25–0.9%, respectively. Since the very beginning of surgery for abdominal aortic aneurysms, survival after successful elective aneurysm repair has been reported to be less than the survival of the matched population for age and sex; 5-year survival after abdominal aortic aneurysm repair was about 70%, whereas the expected survival of a matched population was close to 80%. *Coggia and co-workers* showed, in a preliminary study, the feasibility of repair by total laparoscopic surgery.[23] Even if this technique is minimally invasive and reduces surgical trauma, more experience and further assessment are needed to ensure that the real benefit of this technique is realized compared with open repair.

## ANESTHESIA CONSIDERATIONS

Anesthesia techniques AAA surgical repair may be 3 types. It may be general aaesthesia, regional anesthesia with epidural or spinal and combination of GA and RA. The anesthetic concerns are:

· Long duration anesthesia
· Comorbidities like diabetes, hypertension, tuberculosis, COPD, CAD, etc.
· Geriatric age group
· Aspiration pneumonitis in emergency surgery
· Electrolyte management
· Acid base management

The special considerations of AAA surgery depend on the site of the aneurysm. The extra care must be emphasized on:
1. Ischemia or aortic cross clamp related problems like renal injury and postoperative renal failure, paraplegia, gut ischemia, hepatic injury and *reperfusion injury*.
2. Intravascular fluid shift
3. Hypothermia
4. Hemodynamic fluctuations
5. Bleeding and coagulopathy
6. Postoperative pain

## 1. Ischemia or Aortic Cross Clamp Related Problems

The application of aortic cross clamp (ACC) deprives the blood flow to the abdominal viscera, spinal cord and lower limb. The longer period of ACC produces more ischemia. The level or site of ACC also determines ischemia burden. Infrarenal ACC produces minimum ischemic injuries.

*Prevention of renal injury*: Stabilization of hemodynamics, adequate preload, maintenance of afterload and cardiac output throughout the AAA surgery is prime importance. The ACC time is to be kept as minimum as possible. Selective perfusion of renal, arteries during the period of ischemia is very useful. The use of diuretics and mannitol are controversial but occasionally effective to correct renal blood flow and urine output.

*Prevention of paraplegia*: Paraplegia or paraparesis can be prevented by minimizing cross clamp time, stable perfusion pressure, selective perfusion of artery of Adamcrutz and spinal arteries, CSF drainage and spinal cord cooling.

## 2. Intravascular Fluid Shift

Blood loss is to be replaced with homologous and autologous blood. The fluid shift at reperfusion after release of cross clamp do necessitate large amount of fluid and blood infusion. The use of rapid infusion system is useful in moments of massive blood loss.

## 3. Hypothermia

The open aneurysm surgery exposes the body cavity to the atmosphere for long duration. The massive blood transfusion and fluid infusion also produce hypothermia. The use of warming blanket and fluid warmer is helpful to maintain normothermia (Figs 6.5 and 6.6).

## 4. Hemodynamic Fluctuation

Optimum intravascular volume, vasopressors and vasodilators are useful to treat this problem.

## 5. Bleeding and Coagulopathy

Multiple anastomosis through the high pressure aorta and its branches make prone for bleeding. The unanticipated opening of the vessels ruptured of aneurysm and adhesions also contribute to blood loss

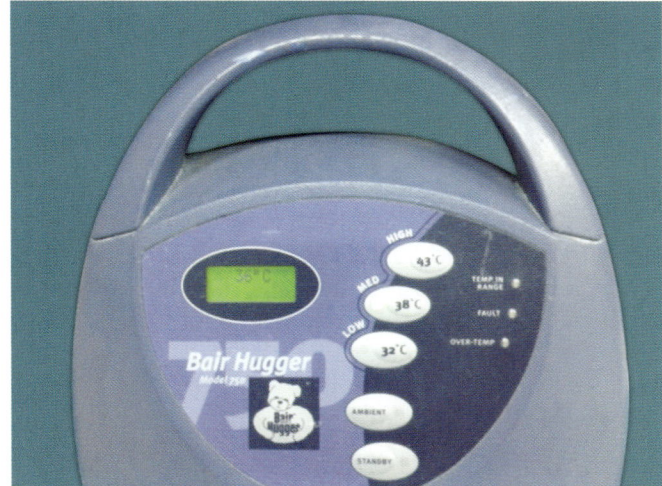

**Fig. 6.5:** Warming blanket device to maintain the temperature from hypothermia

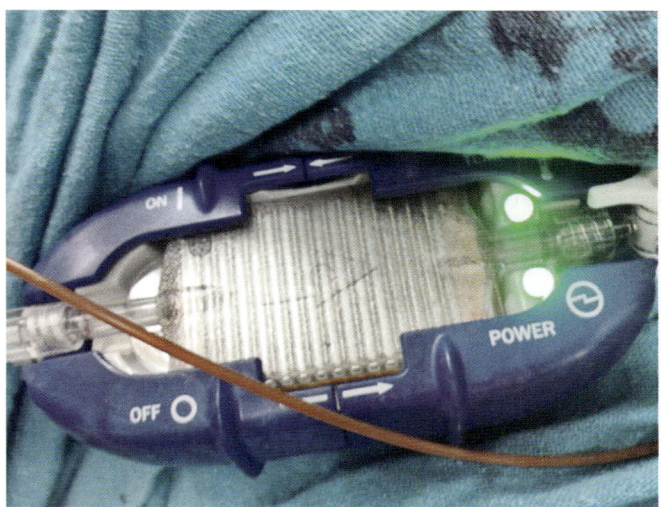

**Fig. 6.6:** Blood warming device

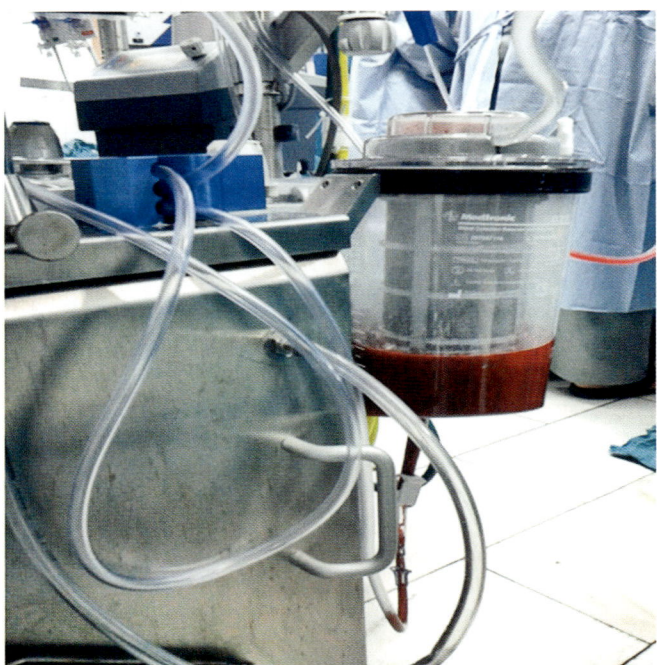

**Fig. 6.7:** Cell saver use for blood conservation during aneurysm surgery

and activation of coagulation system. Blood, crystalloid, colloid, platelet concentrations, fresh frozen plasma, antifibrinolytics and factor VII are useful to correct the haemoglobin and coagulation factors. Blood conservation by cell saver and autologous blood donation are also useful methods (Fig. 6.7).

## 6. Postoperative Pain Management

The extensive surgery requires satisfactory analgesia with single or combined analgesics like narcotics, NSAID, local infiltration, nerve block and epidural analgesia.

## Anesthesia for Ruptured AAA

### Preoperative Management

Ruptured AAA is a surgical emergency and a rapid preoperative evaluation is required. There are certain situations where surgery may be in appropriate, e.g. those who have already suffered a cardiac arrest or patients with terminal illnesses. In the past, patients with severe cardiorespiratory disease may have been refused elective surgery but with the increasing availability of endovascular techniques many of these patients are now receiving surgery.

Successful anesthetic management often requires two experienced anesthetists. A brief and targeted preoperative assessment should be made. Most patients will have extensive atherosclerotic and smoking related diseases. Many patients have significant coronary artery disease which is not always obvious from history and examination. Diabetes, hypertension and renal impairment are also common. Blood pressure should be checked non-invasively in both arms as there may be brachiocephalic and subclavian artery stenosis. If there is a difference in readings, the higher reading should be used. While this is occurring, the second anesthetist must over see the preparation of drugs, equipment and theatre ensuring an adequate supply of blood and coagulation products. We would recommend at least 10 units of red blood cells as well as platelets, fresh frozen plasma, and cryoprecipitate. Hospitals should have a system for issuing these blood products without delay (e.g. without waiting for laboratory coagulation results); near-patient testing may also have a role. The first response of many anesthetists confronted with a patient with a ruptured AAA is to administer intravenous fluids rapidly to restore blood pressure to near normal levels. However, excessive administration of fluids prior to clamping of the aorta will increase bleeding through thrombus dislodgement and dilution of clotting factors. It is reasonable to avoid any form of blood transfusion preoperatively unless the patient is unconscious or displays signs of myocardial ischemia. If pain is severe, small increments of intravenous morphine may be administered whilst arrangements for surgery are being made. It is worth considering siting an epidural catheter preoperatively in patients with a contained leak provided that coagulation results are satisfactory and the patient is hemodynamically stable. The advantage of this is that epidural analgesia may facilitate weaning. The presence of postoperative coagulopathy may contraindicate epidural insertion for 48–72 h.

### Anesthetic Induction

Induction of anesthesia in patients with a ruptured AAA may be associated with cardiovascular collapse because of:

  i. The cardiodepressant effects of intravenous and inhalational agents;
 ii. Relaxation of the abdominal muscles reducing the tamponed effect;
iii. Intermittent positive pressure ventilation reducing venous return; and
 iv. A reduction in sympathetic tone.

Therefore, induction of anesthesia should be performed with the patient on the operating table, fully prepared for surgery and with blood for transfusion present in theatre. In the absence of cross-matched blood, group specific or group O blood should be used. Large volumes of intravenous fluids may be required rapidly; therefore, warmed circuits should be primed with fluids and/or cross-matched blood, preferably using a rapid infusion device. Direct arterial pressure monitoring is preferably instituted before induction of anaesthesia but central venous access can be deferred at this stage unless no other venous access has been secured. No specific anesthetic agent or technique has been shown to significantly improve outcome; the main objectives are to maintain anesthesia with cardiovascular stability and normothermia. Modified rapid sequence induction using a carefully titrated dose of induction agent followed by succinylcholine is appropriate. In an effort to reduce the required dose of induction agent, opioids (e.g. fentanyl, alfentanil) may be administered.

## Maintenance

Anaesthesia is usually maintained with a balanced technique using volatile agents/opioids and neuromuscular blockade. Nitrous oxide will reduce arterial pressure in patients who have reduced myocardial contractility or increased levels of sympathoadrenal activity, both of which are frequently present in patients with a ruptured AAA. For these reasons, some anesthetists avoid its use. High dose opioids (e.g. fentanyl 5–20 mg kg) are often used.[22]

## Aortic Cross-clamping

The physiological response to aortic cross-clamping depends on a number of variables, including preoperative left ventricular function, collateral circulation and the level of the cross-clamp. Once the aorta is cross-clamped, increased after load may cause hypertension proximal to the clamp. This may be attenuated by increasing the depth of anesthesia, or the administration of vasodilators (e.g. NTG). This also allows intravascular fluid loading in preparation for clamp release. Restoration of the circulation at cross-clamp release is accompanied by a sudden decrease in after load and severe ischemia-reperfusion injury. This can cause profound hypotension, lactic acidemia, myocardial ischemia, and cardiovascular collapse. These may be attenuated by maintaining mean arterial pressure and expanding the circulating volume, facilitated by administration of vasodilators during cross-clamp application. Even so, hypotension normally occurs and vasoconstrictors and/or inotropic drugs are usually required.

## Monitoring, Blood Transfusion, and Thermoregulation

Minimum standards of monitoring recommended for ruptured AAA repair include ECG (CM 5 configuration), CVP, arterial line, body temperature and urine output. Pulmonary artery flotation catheters are rarely used. Every hospital should have a protocol for the administration of blood products in these cases because it is not practical to wait for the results of coagulation tests before requesting them. Because of the limitations of standard coagulation tests, many centers are assessing the role of thromboelastography (TEG) in emergency vascular surgery. TEG reliably demonstrates both hypercoagulability and fibrinolysis, both of which are frequently under estimated with conventional coagulation tests; it is potentially useful in any situation where there is a rapidly changing hemostatic profile and is widely used to determine transfusion practice for liver and cardiac surgery. In the UK, 55% of hospitals are now using red cell salvage techniques for elective aortic surgery. In emergency cases cell salvage technique may be lower because of practical difficulties in the emergency situation. Perioperative hypothermia occurs frequently because of the open abdomen, patient exposure, blood loss, and the large volumes of fluids transfused. All attempts should be made to maintain patient temperature intraoperatively by the use of warming blankets and warmed fluids.

## Maintenance of Renal Function

Patients are at risk of developing renal impairment because of preoperative hypotension and hypovolemia; aortic clamping causing direct renal ischemia; a large embolic load; and postoperative blood loss. To avoid postoperative renal impairment, every effort should be made to maintain adequate perfusion pressure and limit the duration of supra-renal clamping. Many anesthetists administer drugs such as mannitol, furosemide or dopamine to prevent renal failure but there is no convincing evidence that they improve outcome. The main priority is to maintain an adequate extracellular fluid volume intra- and postoperatively.

## Postoperative Care

All patients should be transferred to ICU postoperatively where supportive care includes optimization and maintenance of circulating volume. Re-warming will continue until normal body temperature is achieved and respiratory support is usually required for up to at least 24 h and frequently several days. Renal function, coagulation, hemoglobin, and acid–base balance are monitored closely. Renal replacement therapy is required in a significant proportion of patients and those with a coagulopathy may require continuing blood product transfusion. Other important issues include an anticipated prolonged ileus and analgesia. Patients are particularly prone to developing intra-abdominal hypertension (intra-abdominal pressure IAP > 12 mmHg) and abdominal compartment syndrome (ACS) defined as IAP > 20 mmHg. Factors which contribute to the development of ACS include anemia, prolonged hypotension, cardiopulmonary resuscitation, hypothermia, severe acidosis (base deficit >14 mEq) and aggressive fluid resuscitation. These patients may benefit from laparotomy or mesh closure of the abdominal wall with delayed secondary surgical closure after 2–3 days. Performing a mesh closure initially in these patients reduces the incidence of multi-organ failure when compared with patients who require a second operation for ACS in the postoperative period. Monitoring of IAP should be considered in all patients and consideration given to parenteral nutrition if ileus is prolonged.

## Summary

The abdominal aorta aneurysm surgery involves multiple challenges in the perioperative period. The special consideration for ischemic and reperfusion injury to different organs at aortic cross clamp, bleeding at surgery or rupture, hemodynamic alterations, hypothermia and postoperative analgesia are mandatory for successful anesthetic management. The different techniques of renal and spinal cord protection are to be learnt and adopted as per necessity to prevent postoperative morbidity. Blood conservation strategies during AAA surgery are helpful to reduce transfusion related injury.

### Key Notes

- Abdominal aortic aneurysm is the aneurysm of aorta occurring in any portion of the infra-diaphragmatic aorta starting from the exit point at diaphragm to the division into iliac arteries.
- *Types*: Broadly AAA is classified into 4 types with relation to renal artery like suprarenal, juxtarenal, pararenal and infrarenal. According to shape AAA can be classified to fusiform and sacular.
- *Problems*: Unruptured AAA presents with pain and gradually increases in size to have compressive signs. The larger aneurysms are vulnerable to rupture and if not managed promptly, patient may lead to death.
- *Management options*: Small size AAA (<4 cm diameter) is managed medically and examined every 6 monthly. Aneurysm >4 to 6 cm diameter is treated with open surgery or endo-vascular graft.

- *Precautions and anesthesia management*: The operation room or radiological suit must be equipped with blood, emergency drugs, rapid transfusion system, warming blankets and cell saver. Anesthesia may be regional like continuous epidural or spinal and general anesthesia with endotracheal intubation. Anesthesia goal is to maintain stable blood pressure and cardiac output. The consideration for renal, spinal cord and gastrointestinal protection is essential.
- *Monitoring*: Apart from routine hemodynamic monitors, the use of sensory and motor evoke potential, cerebrospinal fluid pressure monitoring, transesophageal echocardiography, temperature, bispectral index and thromboelastography are helpful for better perioperative outcome in the management of AAA patients

## REFERENCES

1. Sampson UK1, Norman PE2, Fowkes FG, et al. Estimation of global and regional incidence and prevalence of abdominal aortic aneurysms 1990 to 2010. Glob Heart 2014; 9(1):159–70.

2. Gillum RF. Epidemiology of aortic aneurysm in the United States. J ClinEpidemiol 1995; 48:1289–98.

3. Kniemeyer HW, Kessler T, Reber PU, Ris HB, HakkiH, Widmer MK. Treatment of ruptured abdominal aortic aneurysm, a permanent challenge or a waste of resources? Prediction of outcome using a multi-organ-dysfunction score. Eur J VascEndovascSurg 2000; 19:190–96.

4. Liddington MI, Heather BP. The relationship between aortic diameter and body habitus. Eur J VascSurg 1992; 6:89–92.

5. 4 McGregor JC, Pollock JG, Anton HC. The value of ultrasonography in the diagnosis of abdominal aortic aneurysm. Scott Med J 1975; 20:133–37.

6. Johnston KW, Rutherford RB, Tilson MD, Shah DM, Hollier L, Stanley JC. Suggested standards for reporting on arterial aneurysms. Subcommittee on Reporting Standards for Arterial Aneurysms, Ad Hoc Committee on Reporting Standards, Society forVascular Surgery and North American Chapter, International Society for Cardiovascular Surgery. J Vasc Surg 1991; 3:452–58.

7. Erentug V, Bozbuga N, Omeroglu SN, et al. Rupture of abdominal aortic aneurysms in Behçet's disease. Ann Vasc Surg 2003;17:682–85.

8. Matsumura K, Hirano T, Takeda K, et al. Incidence of aneurysms in Takayasu's arteritis. Angiology 1991;42:308–15.

9. Towbin JA, Casey B, Belmont J. The molecular basis of vascular disorders. Am J Hum Genet 1999;64:678–84.

10. Reed D, Reed C, Stemmermann G, Hayashi T. Are aortic aneurysms caused by atherosclerosis? Circulation 1992; 85:205–11.

11. Fink HA, Lederle FA, Roth CS, Bowles CA, Nelson DB, Haas MA. The accuracy of physical examination to detect abdominal aortic aneurysm. Arch Intern Med 2000;160:833–36.

12. Quill DS, Colgan MP, Sumner DS. Ultrasonic screening for the detection of abdominal aortic aneurysms. Surg Clin North Am 1989;69:713–20.

13. Mehard WB, Heiken JP, Sicard GA. High-attenuating crescent in abdominal aortic aneurysm wall at CT: a sign of acute or impending rupture. Radiology 1994;192:359–62.

14. Siegel CL, Cohan RH, Korobkin M, Alpern MB, Courneya DL, Leder RA. Abdominal aortic aneurysm morphology: CT features in patients with ruptured and nonruptured aneurysms. AJR Am J Roentgenol 1994;163:1123–29.

15. Arita T, Matsunaga N, Takano K, et al. Abdominal aortic aneurysm: rupture associated with the high-attenuating crescent sign. Radiology 1997;204:765–68.

16. Sprouse LR, Meier GH, Parent FN, et al. Is three-dimensional computed tomography reconstruction justified before endovascular aortic aneurysm repair? J Vasc Surg 2004; 40:443–47.

17. Fleming C, Whitlock EP, Beil TL, Lederle FA. Screening for abdominal aortic aneurysm: A best-evidence systematic review for the US Preventive Services Task Force. Ann Intern Med 2005;142:203–11.

18. Parry DJ, Waterworth A, Kessel D, Robertson I, Berridge DC, Scott DJ. Endovascular repair of an inflammatory abdominal aortic aneurysm complicated by aorto duodenal fistulation with an unusual presentation. J Vasc Surg 2001; 33:874–79.

19. Kane JM, Meyer KA, Kozoll DD. An anatomical approach to the problem of massive gastrointestinal hemorrhage. AMA Arch Surg 1955;70:570–82.

20. Hirst AE Jr, Affeldt J. Abdominal aortic aneurysm with rupture into the duodenum; a report of eight cases. Gastroenterol 1951;17:504–14.

21. Lemos DW, Raffetto JD, Moore TC, Menzoian JO. Primary aortoduodenal fistula: a case report and review of the literature. J Vasc Surg 2003;37:686–89.

22. Davis PM, Gloviczki P, Cherry KJ Jr, et al. Aorto-caval and ilio-iliac arteriovenous fistulae. Am J Surg 1998;176:115–18.

23. Coggia M, Dicenta I, Javerliat I, Colacchio G, Goeau-Brissonniere O. Total laproscopic aortic surgery: transperitoneal left retrorenal approach. Eur J Vasc Endovasc surg. 2004; 28:619–22.

# CHAPTER 7

# Anesthesia for Aortic Dissection

Poonam Malhotra Kapoor

## INTRODUCTION

Aortic dissection, particularly ascending aortic dissection is the most fatal catastrophe of the aorta. Aortic dissection is an event which results from separation of the layers of the tunica media by entrance of blood, producing a false lumen with variable proximal and distal extension (Fig. 7.1). The vessel lumen is not dilated and often is compressed by the advancing hematoma. In contrast, an aortic aneurysm involves dilation of all three layers of the vessel wall and has a highly different pathophysiology and implications for management.

As the layers of the wall of the aorta separate or are torn, blood flows between the layers causing wider separation of the two walls. This is the phase when aortic dissection occurs, which prevents blood from flowing and the aortic wall thus bursts (Fig. 7.2).

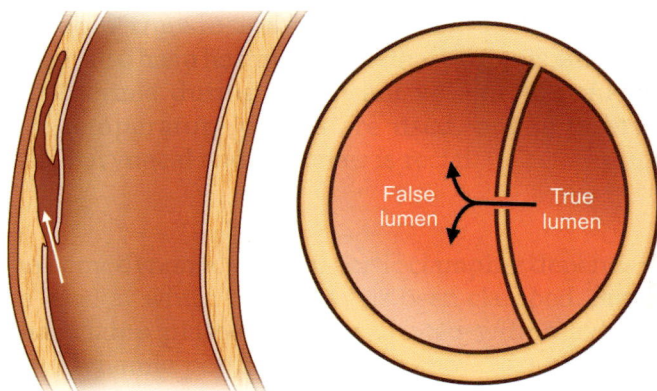

Fig. 7.2: The false and true lumen in acute aortic dissections

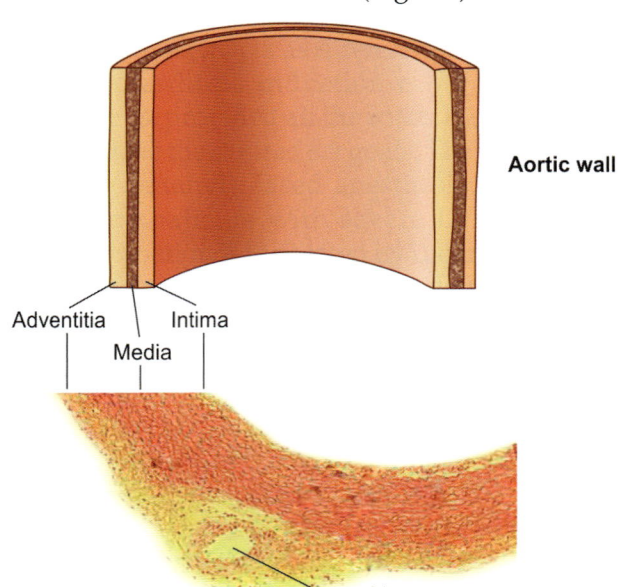

**Aortic wall**

Fig. 7.1: The anatomy of aorta

| Definitions of aorta |
|---|
| **Aortic aneurysm (or true aneurysm)** |
| Focal permanent aortic dilation with a diameter greater than 50% the normal diameter for that aortic segment. Although a true aneurysm has all three aortic wall layers, the intima and media may be so attenuated in giant aneurysms that they are undetectable |
| **Aortic pseudoaneurysm (or false aneurysm)** |
| Results from aortic rupture, and its wall consists of periarterial connective tissue rather than all the aortic wall layers. *Aortic ectasia*: Defined as aortic dilation less than 150% of the expected diameter for that aortic segment. *Aortomegaly*: Defined as aneurysmal involvement of two or more aortic segments. |
| **Acute aortic dissection** |
| Primary tear in the aortic intima, with blood from the aortic lumen penetrating into the diseased media leading to dissection and creating a true and false lumen. Rupture of the vasa vasorum leads to hemorrhage in the aortic wall with subsequent intimal disruption, creating the intimal tear. |

| Anatomy of aorta | |
|---|---|
| Aortic wall | Outer adventitia<br>Middle media<br>Inner intima |
| Aortic dissection | It results from internal tear that exposes media to pulsatile blood |
| Aortic atherosclerosis | Injures the intima to cause thickening, calcification, and ulceration |

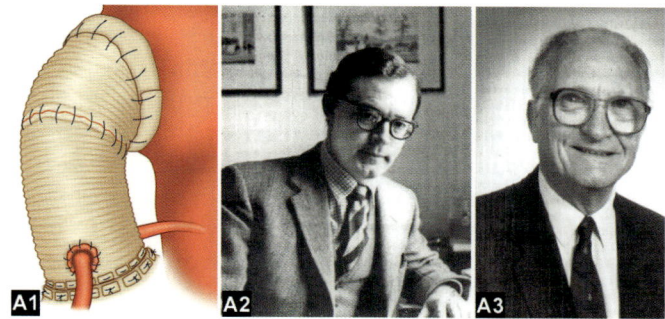

**Fig. 7.4A:** Shorter cross clamp, the standard technique by Dr Hugh Bentall

## HISTORICAL NOTE

King George 2 of Great Britain died (October 25, 1760) while straining on the commode and was the first well documented case of an aortic dissection, but a number of other well-known figures have been diagnosed as well, including Lucille Ball, John Ritter, Prince Diana and Dr. Michael DeBakey. Lannaec (French physician) introduced the term Dissection aneurysm in 1819. First successful outcome of modern treatment of aortic dissection was attributed to Dr. DeBakey in his report, in the first year 1955 and later he devised a classification that is widely used today as DeBakey (Fig. 7.3) classification.

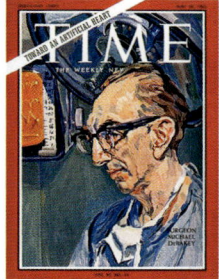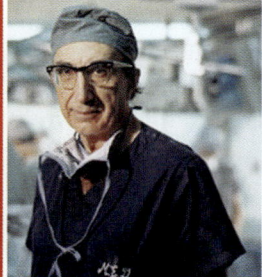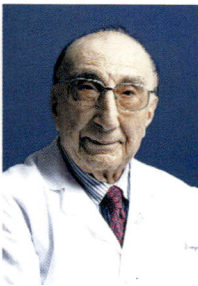

**Fig. 7.3:** Different faces of Dr DeBakey—the man who classified aortic dissections

*Technological and surgical technical improvement followed in the form of:*

- Cardiopulmonary bypass circuit
- Synthetic placements
- Hypothermic circulatory arrest in 1960s to 1975 (Barnard, Schrire, Borst and Griepp with colleaques)
- Open distal anastomosis technique by Livesay in 1982.
- Bioglue has been approved by US FDA to strengthen the disrupted layer
- **Bentall aortic valve surgery**

The standard technique done is straight forward. It has the advantage of a shorter cross-clamp and bypass time compared to valve sparing operations (Fig. 7.4A).

## ETIOLOGY AND PATHOGENESIS

Aortic dissections have varied etiology.[1] Hypertension is present in more than 75% of individuals with aortic

dissection. It is often associated with Marfan syndrome, Loeys-Dietz aneurysm syndrome, Ehlers-Danlos syndrome, bicuspid aortic valve, Turner syndrome and familial thoracic aortic aneurysm/dissection syndrome. Patients at risk are those with previous cardiac surgery especially those on the aorta or the aortic valve, the thoracic aortic aneurysm are most at risk for developing an aortic dissection.

| Acute aortic syndrome |
|---|
| Describes a collection of life-threatening acute injuries to aorta |

| Types |
|---|
| - Aortic dissection (AD)<br>- Intramural hematoma (IMH)<br>- Penetrating atherosclerotic ulcer (PAU)<br>- Traumatic transaction |

| Consequences |
|---|
| - Death caused by Aortic rupture or associated complications<br>- Type A – mortality – 1–2%/hr for first 48 hrs after presentation |

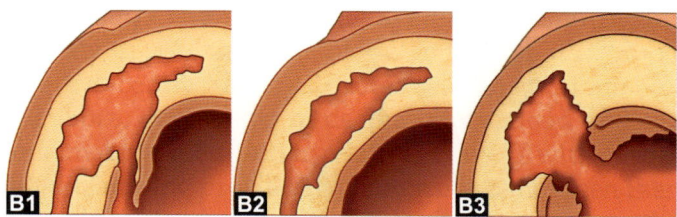

**Fig. 7.4B:** The acute aortic syndrome

| Acute aortic dissection |
|---|
| - Acute aortic dissection is the most common aortic catastrophe<br>- Incidence—5 to 30 per 1 million people per year<br>- Nearly 10,000 cases per year in the USA<br>- May mimic other more common conditions like coronary ischemia, pleurisy, heart failure, stroke and acute abdominal illness<br>- Rapidly fatal<br>- Diagnosis—TEE, CT or MRI |

## CLINICAL FEATURES

A high index of suspicion must be maintained, especially when risk factors for dissection are present and also clinical signs and symptoms suggest this possibility. Severe chest pain or pain radiating to back/abdomen is characteristic of aortic dissection pain. In some instances, the pain resolves and symptoms may be due to other complications such as heart failure from acute aortic regurgitations, shortness of breath, neurological deficits, syncope, or vascular insufficiency.

**Type B patients** are always hypertensive, whereas **Type A patients** do not have hypertension generally.[2] Hypotension complicating acute aortic dissection is usually related to cardiac tamponade, aortic rupture, or heart failure associated with severe aortic regurgitation. Many a times, acute aortic dissection may present with malperfusion syndromes related to malperfusion of gut and lower extremity. The symptoms of acute aortic dissection may be highly variable.

Stastical data show that the mortality rate reaches 50–68% during the first 48 hours after an acute event, with a mean mortality of up to 1% per hour.[3] Nearly 75% of the patients die of aortic rupture of complications related to aortic dissection in the first month of life. After a month, the aortic dissection is termed as chronic aortic dissection. These patients require careful surveillance, optimal medical therapy, and timely intervention.

## CLASSIFICATION OF AORTIC DISSECTION

*Aortic dissection is of two types*—acute or chronic depending on time of presentation as shown in Table 7.1.

**Table 7.1:** Types of aortic dissection

| Pathology | Time of presence |
| --- | --- |
| Acute aortic dissection | Less than two weeks |
| Chronic aortic dissection | Greater than two weeks |

Several different classifications have been used to describe aortic dissections, acute or chronic are based on time frame, and the others are based on anatomical sites.

DeBakey, Stanford and Crawford are the most commonly used classification. The Stanford classification is based on the ascending aortic involvement (Fig. 7.5). Description of the two is given below.

### DeBakey Classification

*Type I* involves ascending aorta, aortic arch, and descending aorta.

*Type II* is confined to ascending aorta only.

*Type III* is confined to descending aorta distal to the left subclavian artery only; IIIa extends up to diaphragm, IIIb extends beyond the diaphragm (Figs 7.5A and B).

### Stanford Classification

The Stanford classification is based on the involvement of the ascending aorta. Type A dissections involve the ascending aorta. Dissections that involve the ascending aorta are much more often lethal than those limited to the distal aorta and call for a different therapeutic approach (Fig. 7.6).

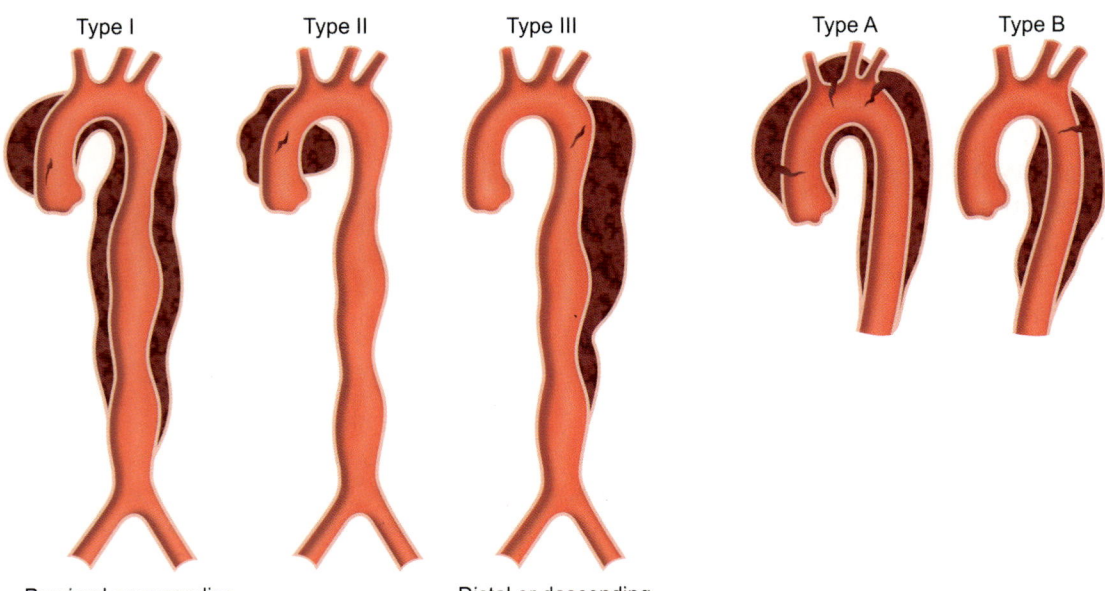

| Type I | Type II | Type III | | Type A | Type B |

Proximal or ascending          Distal or descending

**Fig. 7.5A:** The DeBakey and Stanford classification of aortic aneurysms, type A involves the ascending aorta but may extend into the arch and descending aorta (DeBakey types I and II)

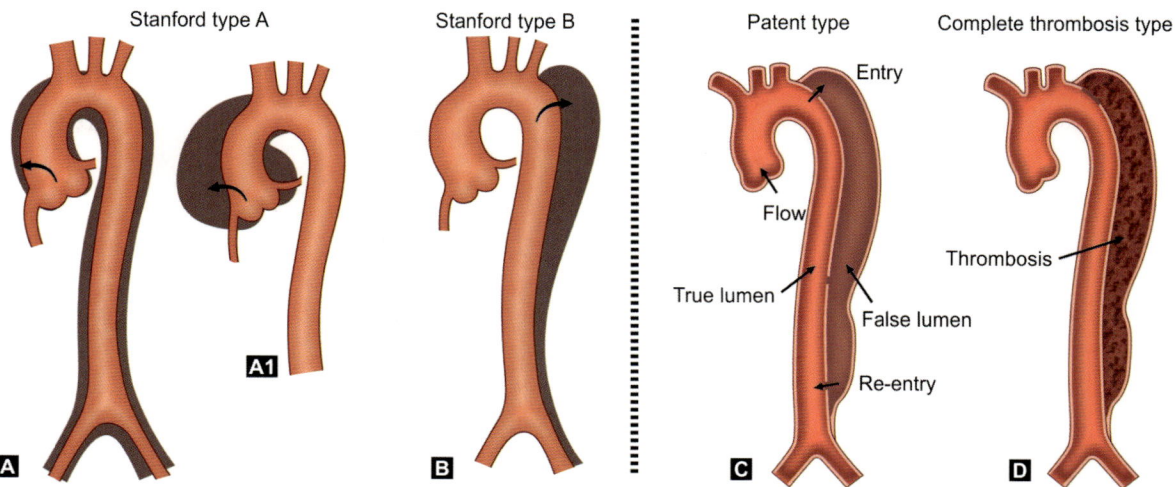

**Fig. 7.5B:** The DeBakey and Stanford classification of aortic aneurysms. Type B involves the descending aorta only (DeBakey type III)

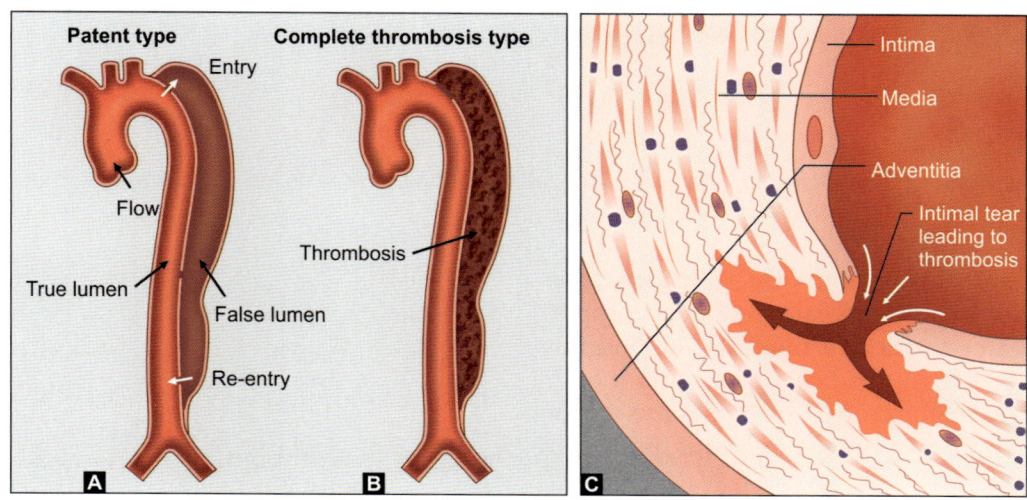

**Figs 7.6 A to C:** Patent and complete thrombosis type

In Stanford type B, the dissection is distal to the origin of the left subclavian artery (Figs 7.5B and Fig. 7.6). The Stanford system also helps to delineate two distinct risk groups for management. Usually, type A dissections require surgery, while type B dissections are best managed conservatively with medical treatment under most conditions (Fig. 7.7).

## Crawford Classification

This classification is also as famous as Stanford and DeBakey. The Crawford classification defines aneurysms as types I, II, III, and IV according to their anatomic location (Fig. 7.8). Type I includes aneurysms involving most of the descending thoracic and the upper abdominal aorta. Type II includes aneurysms involving most of the descending thoracic and most of the abdominal aorta. Type III involves the lower portion of the thoracic aorta and most of the abdominal aorta, and type IV includes most or the entire abdominal aorta.

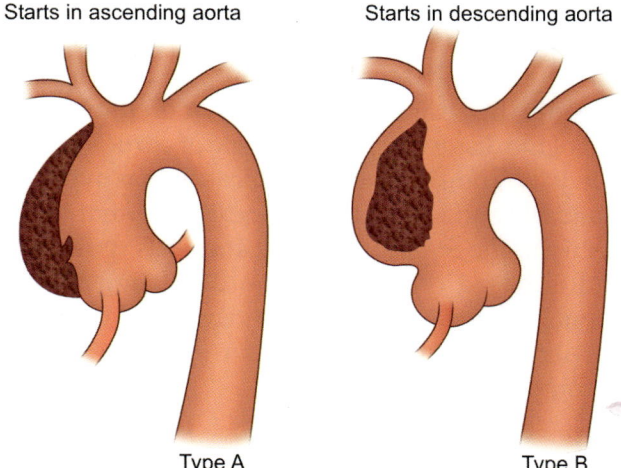

**Figs 7.7A and B:** Types A and B of aortic dissection

Types II and III are most difficult to repair because they involve both the thoracic and the abdominal segments of the aorta. Patients with Crawford type II aneurysms are at greatest risk for paraplegia and renal failure from

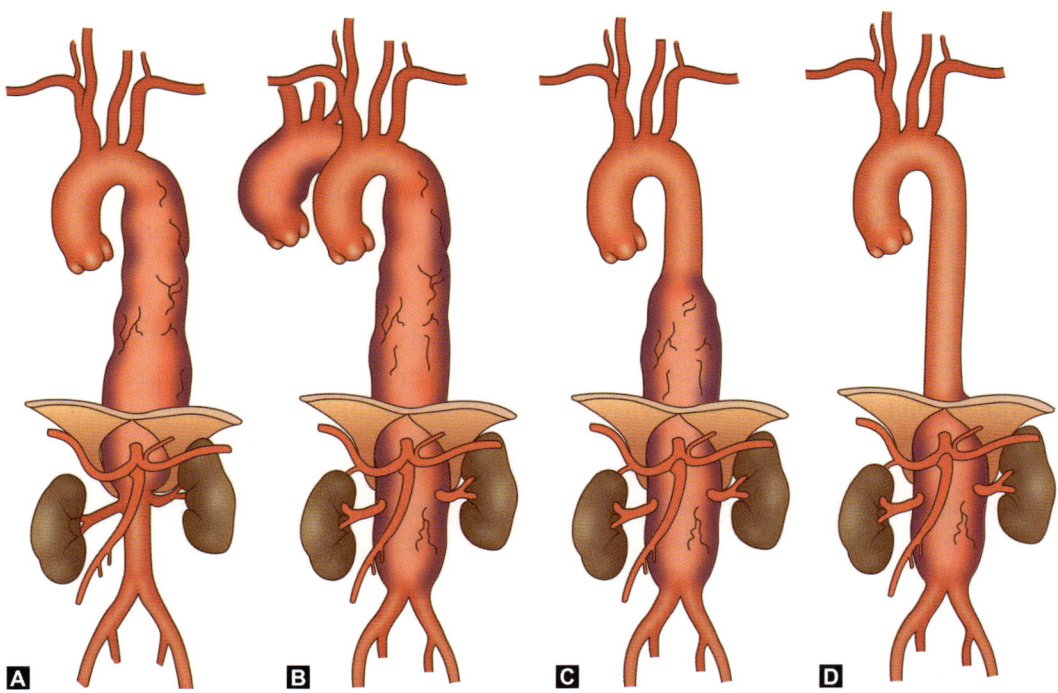

**Figs 7.8A to D:** The Crawford classification of thoracoabdominal aortic aneurysms is defined by anatomic location and the extent of involvement

ischemia to the spinal cord and kidneys during cross-clamp. Even with extracorporeal circulatory support, there is an obligatory period of time when blood flow to these organs is interrupted because the origin of the blood flow is between the cross-clamps. For this reason, protective measures to prevent ischemic injury are important in reducing morbidity.

## SUMMARY OF AORTIC DISSECTION CLASSIFICATION

Several classification systems have been developed to describe aortic dissections. There are three systems commonly in use and are based either on the location/extent of the dissection or on the type of aortic syndrome (Table 7.2). The DeBakey classification has types I, II, IIIa, and IIIb and is based on the location/extent of aortic dissection. The Stanford classification has types A and B and is based on whether the dissection is in the proximal or distal aorta. The Svensson classification has classes 1–5 and is based on the type of aortic syndrome.

## ASCENDING AORTIC ANEURYSMS

Localized dilatation of the aorta 50% over the normal diameter includes all three layers of the vessel (intima, media, and adventitia). Ascending aortic aneurysms arise anywhere from the aortic valve to the innominate artery (Fig. 7.9A and B).

**Table 7.2:** Classification systems for acute aortic dissection/syndromes

| DeBakey classification | Region of aorta involved |
| --- | --- |
| **Type I** | Ascending, arch, descending |
| **Type II** | Ascending only |
| **Type IIIa** | Descending (above diaphragm) |
| **Type IIIb** | Descending (below diaphragm) |
| *Stanford classification* | *Region of aorta Involved* |
| **Type A** | Ascending (proximal to left subclavian artery) |
| **Type B** | Descending (distal to left subclavian artery) |
| *Svensson classification* | *Type of aortic syndrome* |
| **Class 1** | Classic intimal flap (2 lumens) |
| **Class 2** | Intramural hematoma (no intimal flap) |
| **Class 3** | Localized intimal flap |
| **Class 4** | Penetrating aortic ulcer |
| **Class 5** | Iatrogenic/post-traumatic |

## DESCENDING AORTIC DISSECTION

A thoracic aortic aneurysm can be a very serious health risk depending on its size and location within the thoracic aorta. In general, an aneurysm is of greatest concern when it is 5 cm or larger in diameter or if it increases in size more than 0.5 cm every 6 months. A thoracic aortic aneurysm has the potential to either

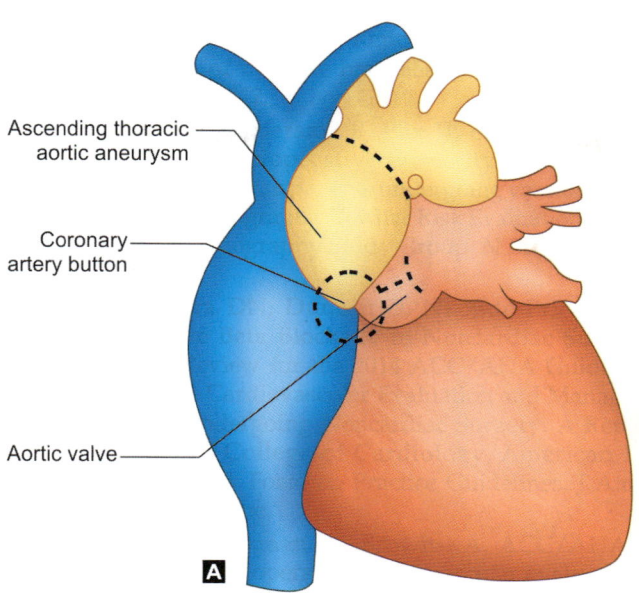

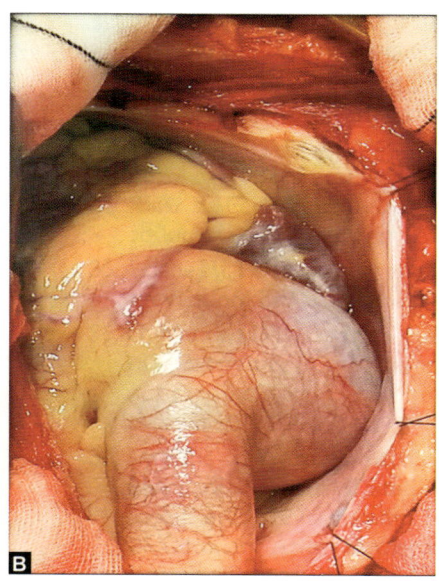

**Figs 7.9A and B:** (A) Ascending aortic aneurysm before surgery. It is closely related to the coronary artery as shown in the dotted lines. (B) Gross picture of ascending aortic aneurysm

rupture (burst) or dissect (layers of the thoracic aortic wall separate) which can cause life-threatening, uncontrolled internal bleeding (Figs 10A and B).

Thoracic aortic aneurysms detected in a timely manner can be treated with either medical management (monitoring of the aneurysm's development and control of risk factors) or surgery.

## ABDOMINAL AORTIC ANEURYSM

An abdominal aortic aneurysm affects the aorta in the abdomen. Symptoms include pain in the lower back,

abdominal swelling, nausea, vomiting, rapid heart rate (tachycardia), sweating and the sensation of a pulse in the abdomen. The types of abdominal aortic aneurysms are shown in Fig. 7.11. An abdominal aortic dissection should be differentiated from an intramural hematoma and a penetrating ulcer as shown in Fig. 7.12.

## NATURAL HISTORY OF AORTIC DISSECTION

a. *Untreated mortality:* Mortality of ascending aortic aneurysms is very high, if left untreated, with two month mortality as high as up to 50% and a 3-month

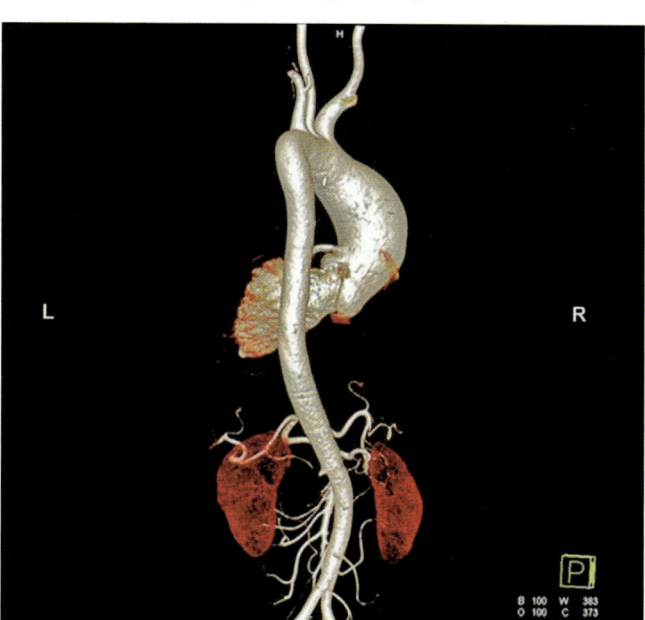

**Figs 7.10A and B:** (A) Descending aortic aneurysms, (B) Aortic aneurysm TEE vs CT scan underestimates aortic diameter by several millimeters as compared to CT

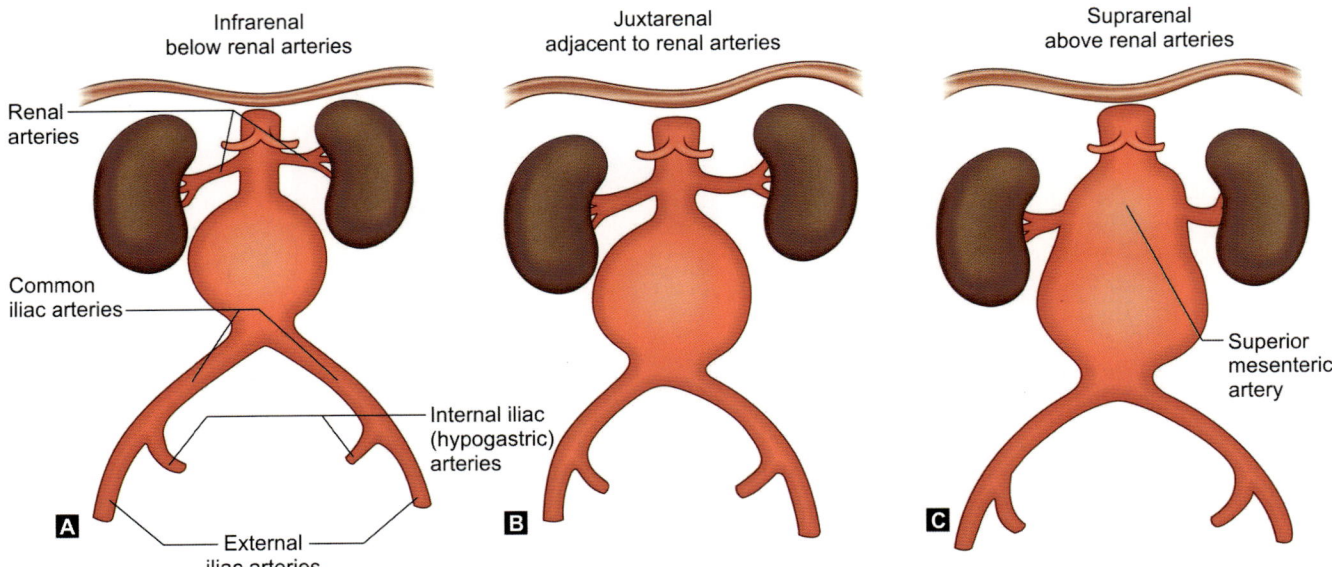

**Figs 7.11A to C:** Types of abdominal aortic aneurysms

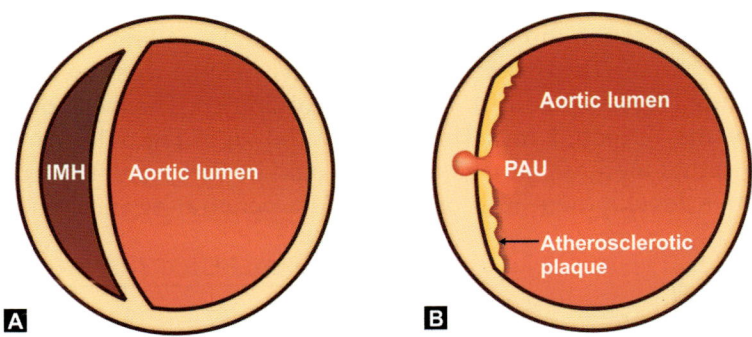

**Figs 7.12A and B:** (A) Aortic dissection intramural hematoma, (B) Aortic dissection penetrating ulcer

mortality reach 90%. The DeBakey type III and Stanford type B have a better prognosis. Rupture of the false lumen into the pleural space or pericardium, progressive heart failure, myocardial infarction, stroke and bowel gangrene are some of the important causes of death in these patients, i.e. aortic valve coronary arteries cerebral or mesenteric vessels involvement primarily.

b. *Surgical mortality:* Overall mortality ranges from 3% to 24% and varies with the section of aorta that is affected. Dissections involving the aortic arch carry the highest mortality, while those confined to the descending thoracic aorta carry the lowest.[4]

## DIAGNOSIS OF AORTIC DISSECTION

Aortic dissections usually present with a dramatic onset and a fulminant course. Aneurysms of the ascending arch, or descending thoracic aorta are often asymptomatic until late in their course. In many circumstances,

the presence of an aneurysm is not diagnosed until medical evaluation is conducted for an unrelated problem or for a problem related to a complication of the aneurysm. Rupture most commonly occur just distal to the left subclavian artery. If the patient survives the initial trauma, signs and symptoms are similar to those seen with aneurysms of the descending thoracic aorta. Diagnosis is best done by the following tests, but the definitive diagnosis is reached on TEE, CT or MRI.

## DIAGNOSTIC TESTS

*Electrocardiogram:* A normal ECG is present in one-third of patients with coronary involvement and most of these patients have non-specific ST–T segment changes.[5] About 20% of patients with type A dissection have ECG evidence of acute ischemia or acute myocardial infarction (Fig. 7.13). These patients with suspected aortic disease and ECG evidence of ischemia

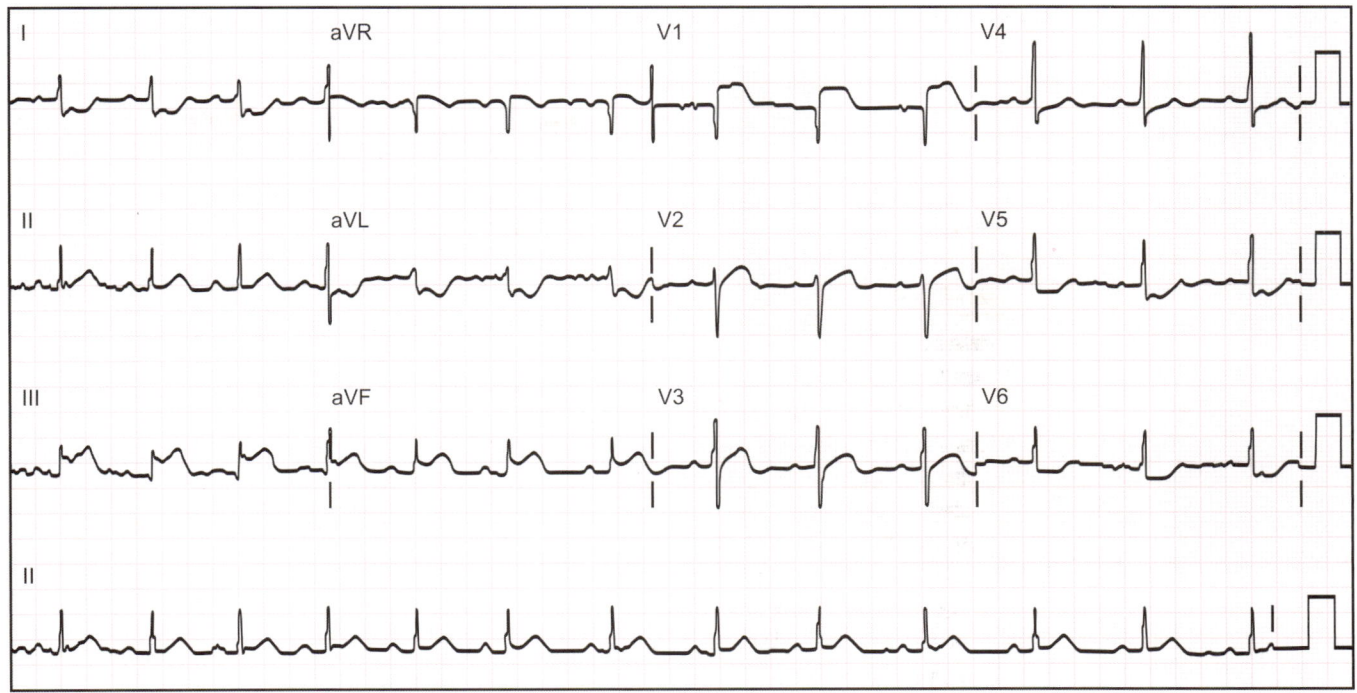

**Fig. 7.13:** ECG of a patient with aortic dissection showing signs of ischemia

must undergo diagnostic imaging before thrombolytic therapy is administered. An ECG helps distinguish acute myocardial infarction, for which thrombolytic therapy may be life saving, from aortic dissection, in which thrombolytic therapy may be detrimental.[5]

*X-ray:* The aortic knuckle changes are seen alongwith intimal calcification more than 6 mm from the end. A widened mediastinum, cardiomegaly (pericardial effusion), and loss of costo-phrenic angle secondary to the presence of a hemothorax may also be noted. A widened mediastinum is a classic X-ray finding with thoracic aortic pathology (Fig. 7.14). Widening of the aortic knob is often seen once the false lumen begins to form.

*CT scan:* A CT Scan should not be done if the patient is unstable. It is relatively rapid and non-invasive and with contrast image enhancement the extent of the dissection along with the true and false lumens can be identified. MRI takes a longer time and with a contrast it can give very high resolution images. An MRI too, is not advocated in hemodynamically unstable patients (Fig. 7.15).

CT is also useful for following the progression of aortic disease. Digital images can be manipulated into a three-dimensional form, which may make it easier to

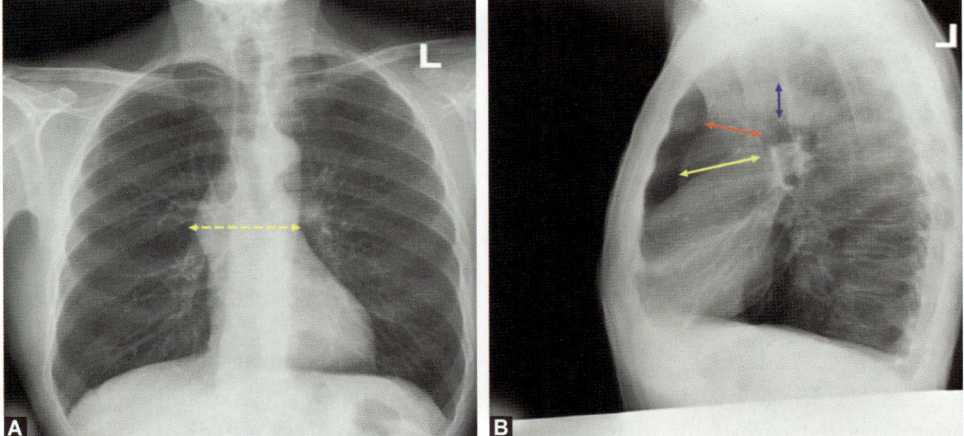

**Figs 7.14A and B:** (A) The CXR of ascending aortic aneurysms in figure showing widening of the mediastinum as a result of the prominence of the ascending aorta. Mass effect can be an indicator of ascending aortic aneurysms. (B) Dilated proximal ascending aorta

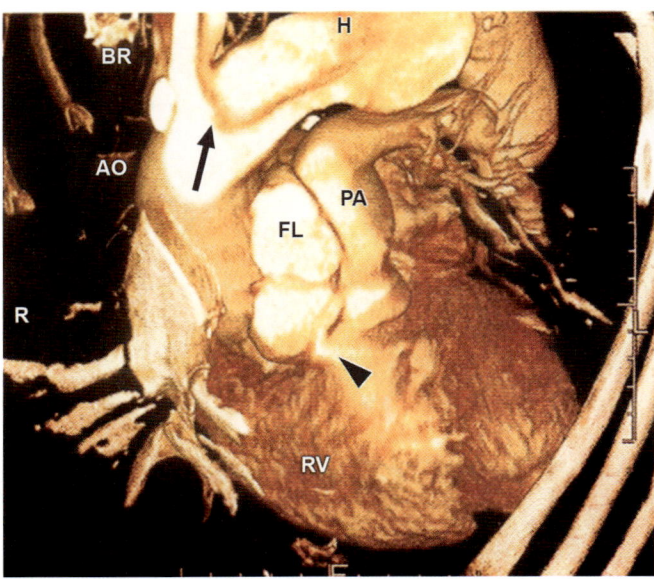

**Fig. 7.15:** Computed tomography angiogram assessment of aortic dissection rupture into the right ventricular outflow tract. Left anterior oblique (LAO) view demonstrating the communication (arrowhead) between the false lumen (FL) and right ventricular outflow tract (RVOT)

assess the lesion and plan repair. Magnetic resonance imaging is extremely sensitive and specific in identifying the entry tear location, presence of false lumen, aortic regurgitation, and pericardial effusion accompanying aortic dissection.[6]

*Magnetic resonance imaging (MRI):* MRI is an appealing option in the detection of low-grade aortic dissection in stable patients in whom the diagnosis is uncertain. MRI shows the site of intimal tear, type and extent of dissection, presence of aortic insufficiency, and differential flow velocities in the true and false channels and in the aortic side branches. It requires no contrast material or ionizing radiation and is noninvasive.[7]

TEE is highly effective in the diagnosis of aortic dissection of the proximal ascending aorta and descending thoracic segment, with reported sensitivity and specificity close to 100%. However, visualization of the aortic arch, distal thoracic aorta, and abdominal segment can be variable with TEE. CT, angiography, MRI, and TEE can all provide the diagnosis, and the modality of choice at your institution will depend on factors such as hemodynamic status and availability of various modalities.

## MEDICAL MANAGEMENT OF AORTIC DISSECTIONS

Immediate management of aortic dissection includes stabilizing the patient with prompt attention to BP reduction. Beta-blockers are the first drugs of choice because of their mechanism of lowering the rate of rise

of ventricular force (dP/dt) and stress on the aorta. The systolic BP should be lowered to about 100 mmHg. In many instances, multiple BP agents are required. In patients in whom refractory hypertension exists, renovascular hypertension related to the dissection flap must be considered. Emergency surgery is recommended for acute Type A dissection; initial medical management is recommended for uncomplicated acute Type B dissection. Surgery or endovascular treatment is recommended for complicated acute Type B dissection or malperfusion syndrome.

The first attempts to treat this condition surgically involved wrapping of the dissected aorta to prevent rupture[8] or treatment of the complications of dissection without definitive repair. This usually resulted in a catastrophic outcome and death. Debakey and colleagues pioneered the surgical treatment of aortic disease, including dissection, and first reported graft replacement of dissected aorta as definitive treatment.[9] Surgical management of Type A dissection is based on a principle of sealing the entry point of the tear and diverting the flow into the true lumen (elephant trunk operation) with the aim to expand the true lumen and to aid thrombosis/obliteration of false lumen. Dissections of ascending aorta, which involve the aortic valve, may require a vasculature or coronaries is managed by bypass grafting.

Most cardiothoracic surgeons prefer to do surgery for Stanford Type A dissections and endovascular treatment for Type B dissection because of significantly lower morbidity and mortality in endovascular treatment. The endograft, once in place, seals the internal tear (entry point) and acts as an artificial lumen for the blood to flow into the true lumen, and not into the surrounding aneurysm sac or false lumen. This reduces the pressure in the aneurysm and false lumen, which eventually shrinks in size over time.

Recent innovations and stent design to tackle endoleak have come in the form of Nellix sac sealing devices, which aim at filling the aneurismal sac with a sealing so that there is no space for an endoleak or stent migration. This device is currently undergoing FDA-investigational device exeption (IDE) trial (Fig. 7.16).

Stent graft placement aims at remodeling of the thoracic descending aorta, typically in Stanford Type B dissection, by sealing one (or multiple) proximal entry tears with a Dacron or PTFE-covered stent, thus initiating thrombosis of the false lumen.[10–13] In addition, reconstruction of a collapsed true lumen might result in re-establishment of side branch flow. If the malperfusion still persists, the true lumen can be expanded with a large, non-covered self expanding

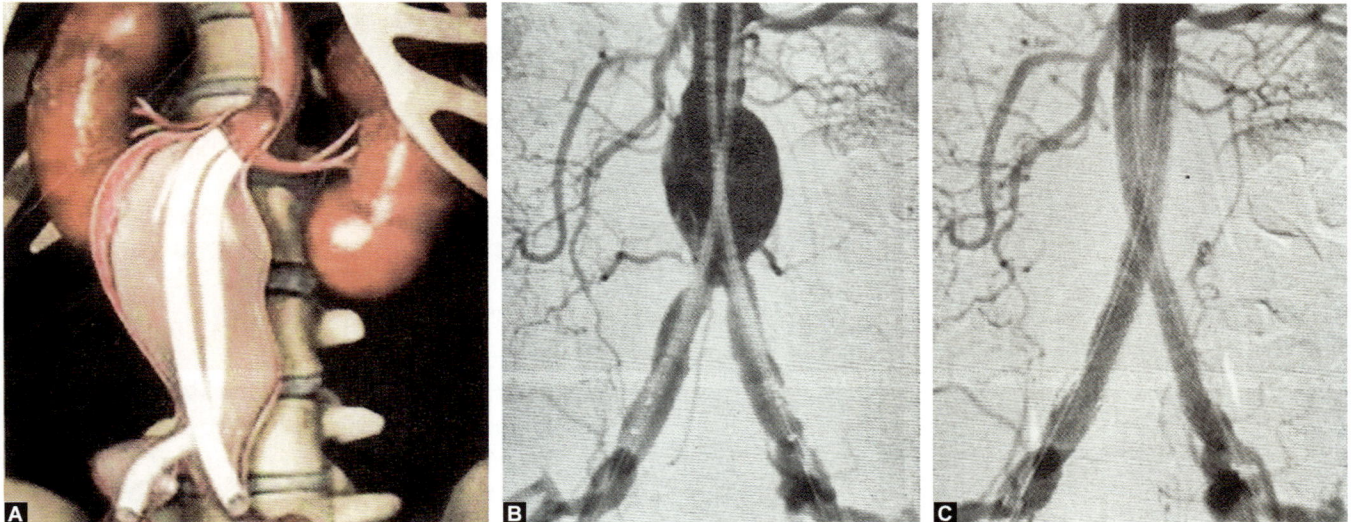

**Figs 7.16A to C:** (A) Principle of Nellix sac sealing device; (B) Abdominal aortic aneurysm–endovascular aortic repair (EVAR) using Nellix devicve; (C) Post EVAR using Nellix device

nitinol stent which is now available (Cook Medical). This aids in rapid expansion of true lumen, faster obliteration and thrombosis of false lumen and ability to access/stent the visceral vessels or do fenestrations. Various scenarios of malperfusion syndrome are amenable to endovascular management (Fig. 7.17).

## PREOPERATIVE MONITORING IN AORTIC DISSECTION SURGERY

Aside from providing vital information with regard to haemodynamic status and conduct of the operation, one of the primary reasons for continuous and detailed

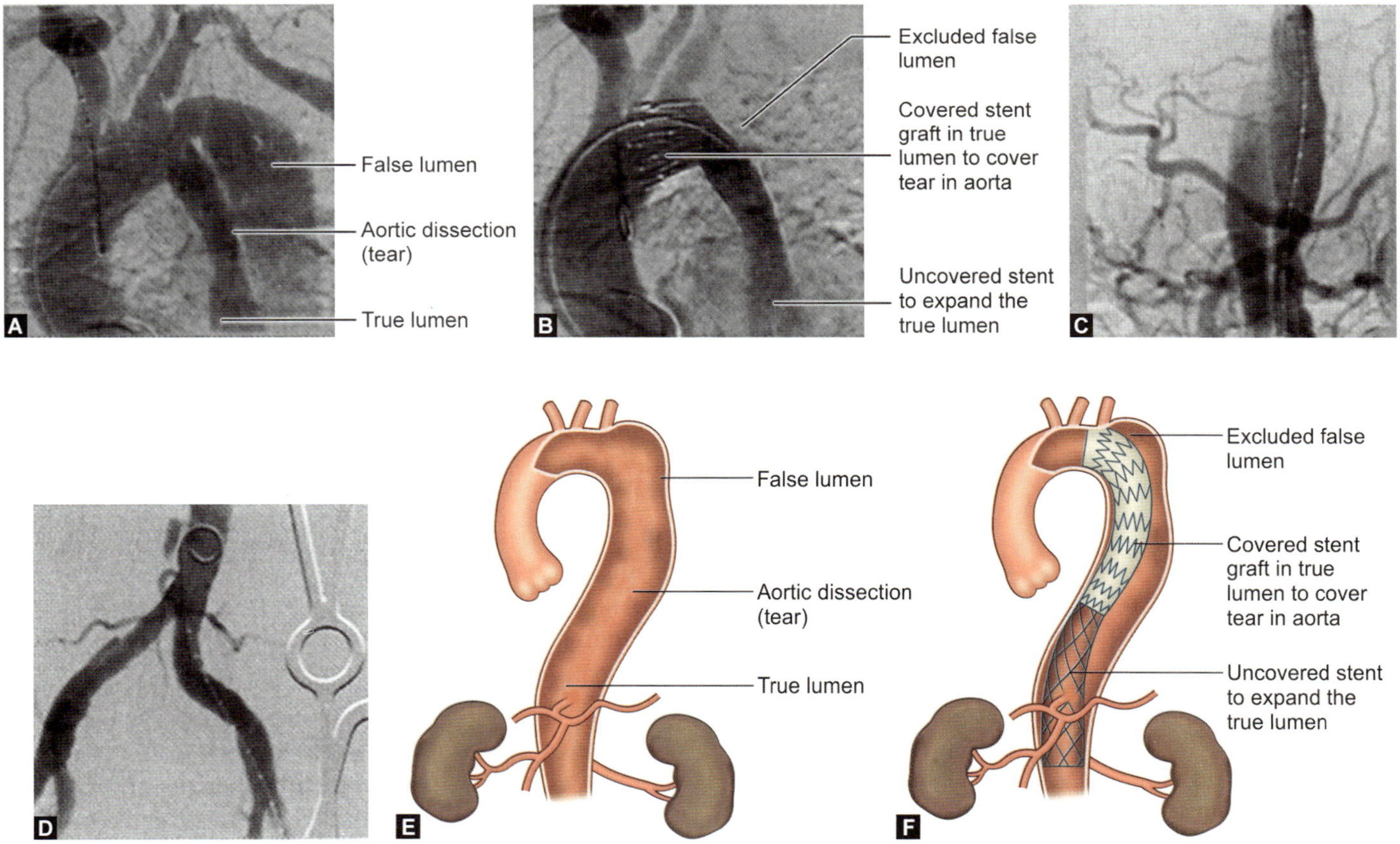

A — False lumen
— Aortic dissection (tear)
— True lumen

B — Excluded false lumen
— Covered stent graft in true lumen to cover tear in aorta
— Uncovered stent to expand the true lumen

C

D

E — False lumen
— Aortic dissection (tear)
— True lumen

F — Excluded false lumen
— Covered stent graft in true lumen to cover tear in aorta
— Uncovered stent to expand the true lumen

**Figs 7.17A to F:** Interventional management of acute aortic dissection monitoring in patients undergoing surgery for acute type A aortic dissection (ATAAD) is to alert anesthetic, surgical, and perfusion staff to ongoing events and potential catastrophes that may occur during surgery. This enables the teams involved to be aware of potential complications, formulate plans for their management, and be alerted once the patient leaves the operating theatre to problems that may be encountered in the intensive care unit.

## Renal Check-up before Aortic Dissection Surgery

Abnormal preoperative renal function has been clearly defined as a risk factor postoperative renal dysfunction. This association is consistent across many studies.[14] Comparatively little is known about the kinetics of renal decline and recovery in the acute postoperative period. Most would suggest transient warm renal ischemia in the setting of normal preoperative function is well tolerated, and recovers in hours. In support of this notion, any renal dysfunction after AAA repair was predicted by renal ischemia times >23 minutes.[14] When warm renal ischemia time exceeds 30 minutes, recovery of function may take 3 to 9 days.[15]

There are a number of monitoring techniques employed during the operative management showing in Table 7.3.

## MONITORING IN MANAGEMENT OF SURGICAL CORRECTION OF AORTIC DISSECTIONS

### Echocardiography

*Transthoracic echocardiography:* Transthoracic echocardiography (TTE) is easily available and the ascending aorta and aortic arch can be visualized well. In obese or chest trauma patients, image quality may be inadequate due to poor echo windows. Transesophageal echocardiography (TEE) has become more popular as experience and availability increase. It is useful perioperatively in the hemodynamically unstable patient. TEE images the entire thoracic aorta except for the most distal ascending aorta and a part of the arch obscured by the trachea or right main bronchus. Echocardiography can be used with high accuracy for decision-making in acute dissection. Echo and acoustic artifacts can be misleading and should be differentiated from the intimal flap by examining the pathology in several image planes.[16] Intravascular ultrasound is a catheter-based imaging study which provides dynamic imaging of the aortic wall and intimal flap.

**Table 7.3:** Essential and desirable monitoring techniques for use in repair of Aortic dissections surgical repair

*Essential monitoring*

- Electrocardiogram
- Pulmonary artery flotation catheter
- Arterial oxygen saturations
- Jugular venous oxygen saturations
- Peripheral and core temperatures
- Transcranial Doppler
- Central venous pressure
- Electroencephalography
- Continuous intra-arterial blood gas monitor
- Transoesophageal echocardiogram
- Near infrared spectroscopy (cerebral and peripheral)

**Aorta imaging TEE: Key Points**

- Proximity of the oesophagus and the thoracic aorta permits high resolution images.
- Emergency evaluation of clinically unstable patients with acute aortic syndromes.
- Detect complications of aortic dissection such as pericardial tamponade, aortic regurgitation, and myocardial ischemia.
- Guide surgical decision making before and after aortic intervention.

**Table 7.4:** The monitoring strategies and their uses

| *Haemodynamic monitoring* | *Neurophysiologic monitoring* (To monitor for intraop spinal ischemia) |
|---|---|
| - ECG | - SSEP |
| - IBP: Proximal aortic pressure | - MEP |
| - Right radial- Innominate A, BP: Repair of arch/prox | - EEG |
| - Left radial A: ACP | - Jugular venous oxygen saturation |
| - Femoral: Distal aortic pressure, avoided in PVD | - Lumbar CSF pressure |
| - CVP: RAP, vasoactive drugs | - Body temperature |
| - PAC: PAP, CO, mixed Svo2 (CPB, DHCA, partial LSHB, aortic-cross clamping) | |
| - TEE for ventricular function and detection of MI with renal wall abnormalities | |

## TRANSESOPHAGEAL ECHOCARDIOGRAPHY

TEE is highly sensitive in the diagnosis of aortic dissection.[17] The proximity of the esophagus to the aorta and the ability to use higher transducer frequencies help to visualize the entire aorta and to detect pericardial effusion and aortic regurgitation.[18] TEE can be quickly performed at the patient's bedside with sedation or light anesthesia and requires no radiation or contrast agent injection. Visualization of the distal ascending aorta and proximal arch used to be difficult because of the interposition of the air-filled trachea and left mainstem bronchus, but evaluation of this "blind spot" has been aided by biplane and multiplane probes (Fig. 7.18).

### Role of TEE in Aneurysms of Sinus of Valsalva (SOV)

A dissection in the sinus of valsalva near the aortic valve, at the beginning of aorta is uncommon.[19] John Thurnam first described sinus of Valsalva aneurysm (SVA) in 1840. Hope further described it in 1939. Aneurysms of left aortic sinus of Valsalva rupturing into left ventricle are relatively rare. In a series of 49 cases reported by Sawyers et al.[20] 34 arose from the right coronary sinus, 13 from the posterior (non-coronary) sinus and only 2 from the left. SVA is caused by dilation, usually of a

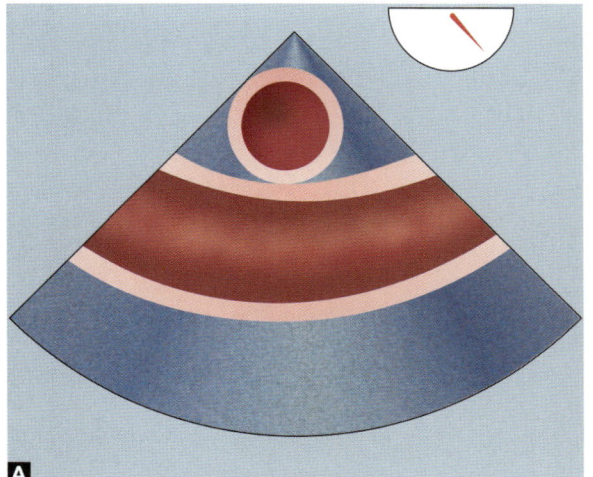
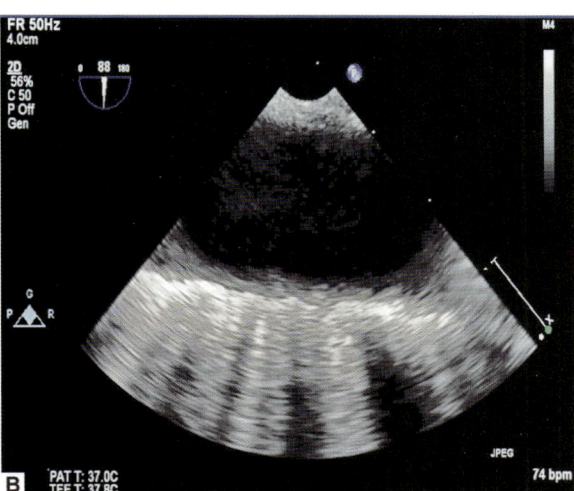

**Video 7.1:** TEE imaging—standard views ME ascending aortic long-axis view

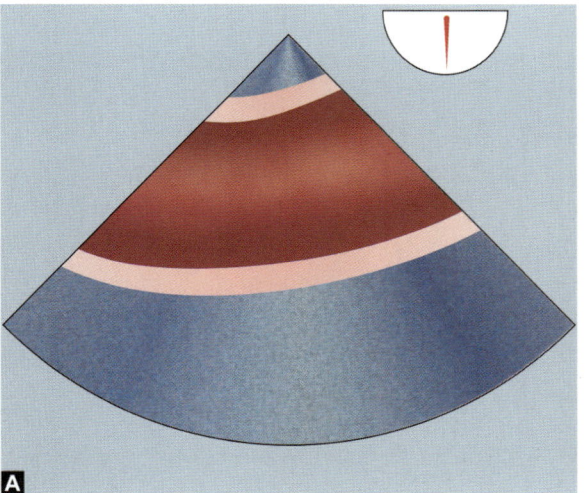
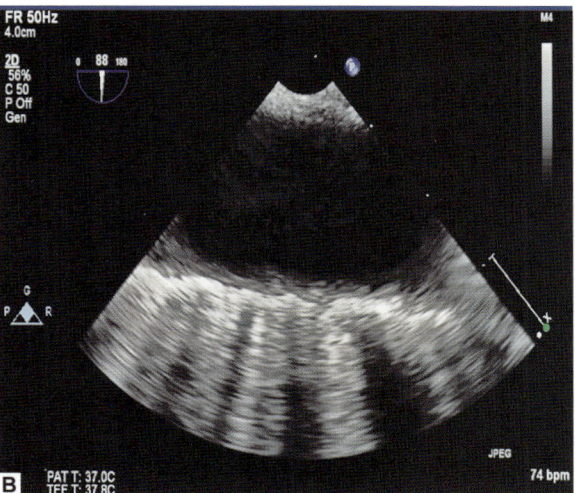

**Video 7.2:** TEE imaging—standard views descending thoracic aorta long-axis view

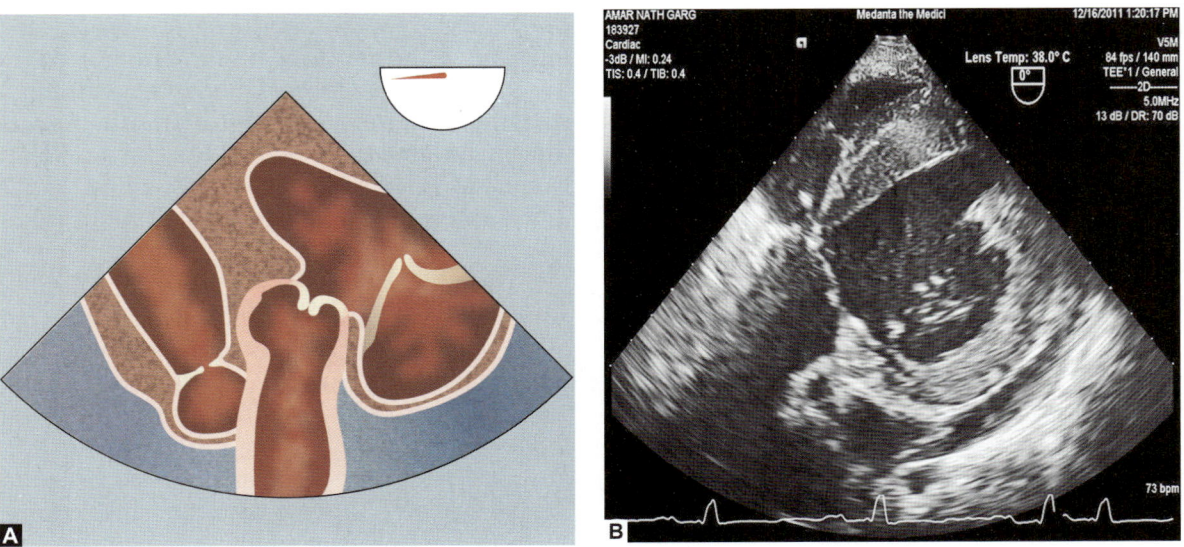

**Video 7.3:** TEE imaging—standard views deep TG 5 chamber view

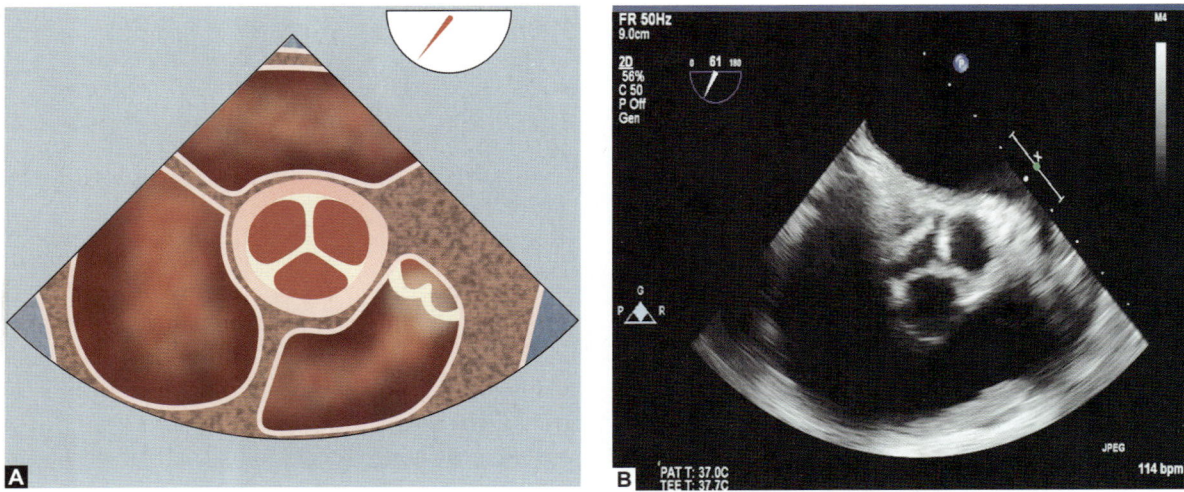

**Video 7.4:** TEE imaging—standard views ME short-axis aortic valve view

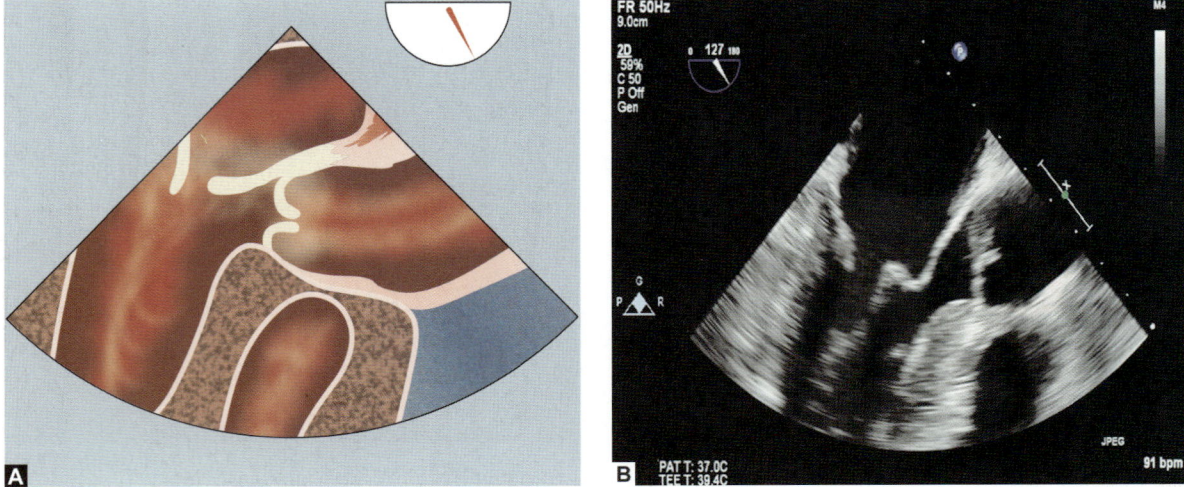

**Video 7.5:** TEE imaging—standard views ME long-axis aortic valve view

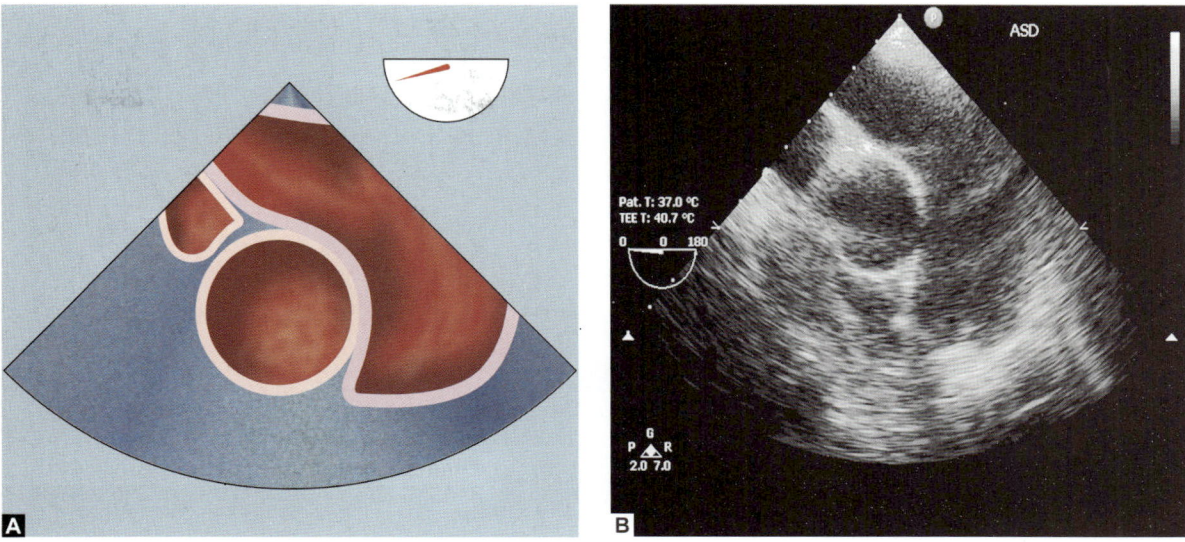

**Video 7.6:** TEE imaging—standard views ME ascending aortic short-axis view

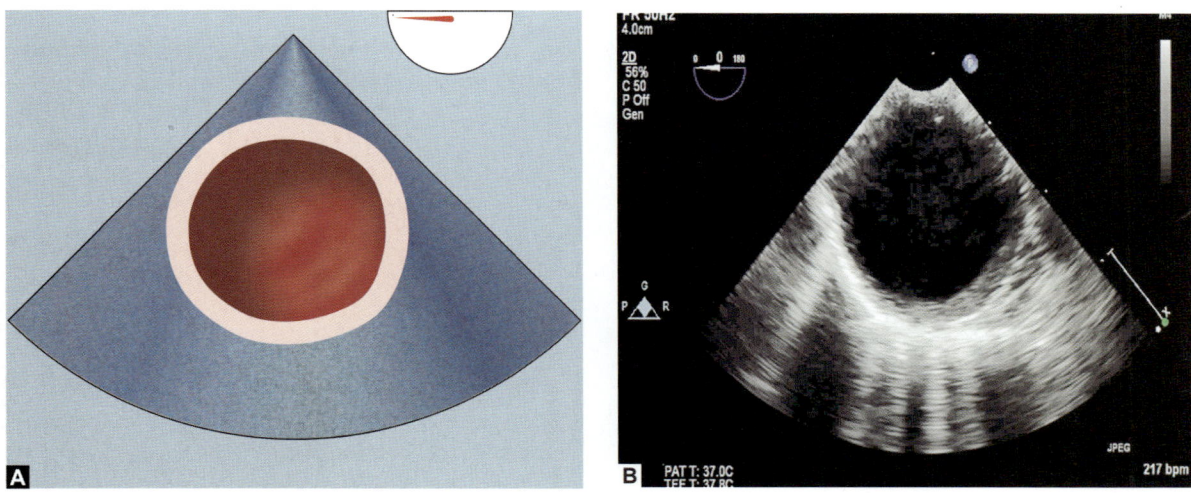

**Video 7.7:** TEE imaging—standard views descending thoracic aorta short-axis view

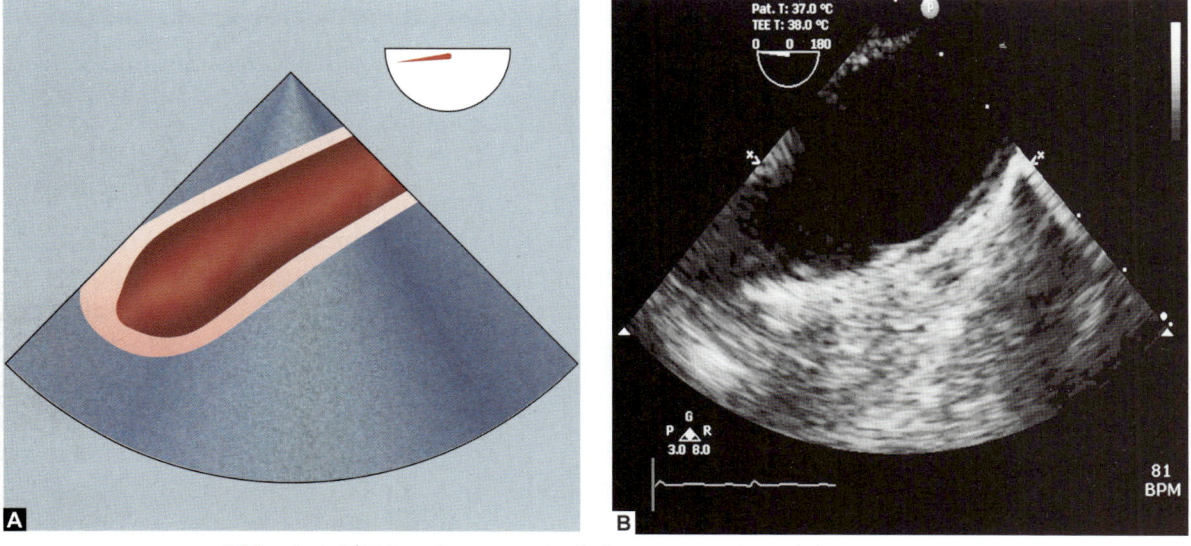

**Video 7.8:** TEE imaging—standard views UE aortic arch long-axis view

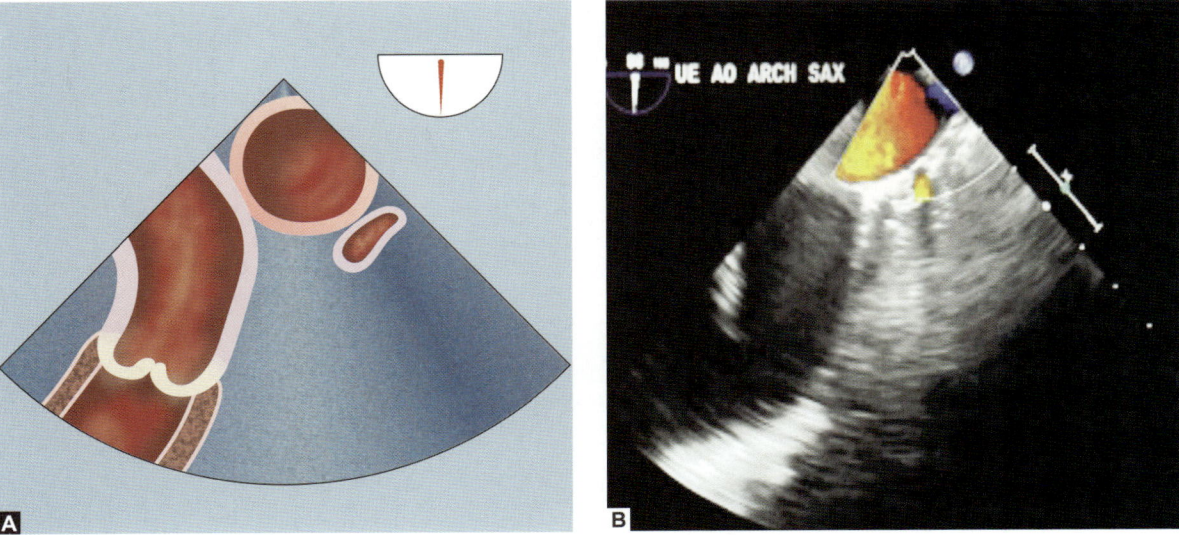

Video 7.9: TEE imaging—standard views UE aortic arch short-axis view

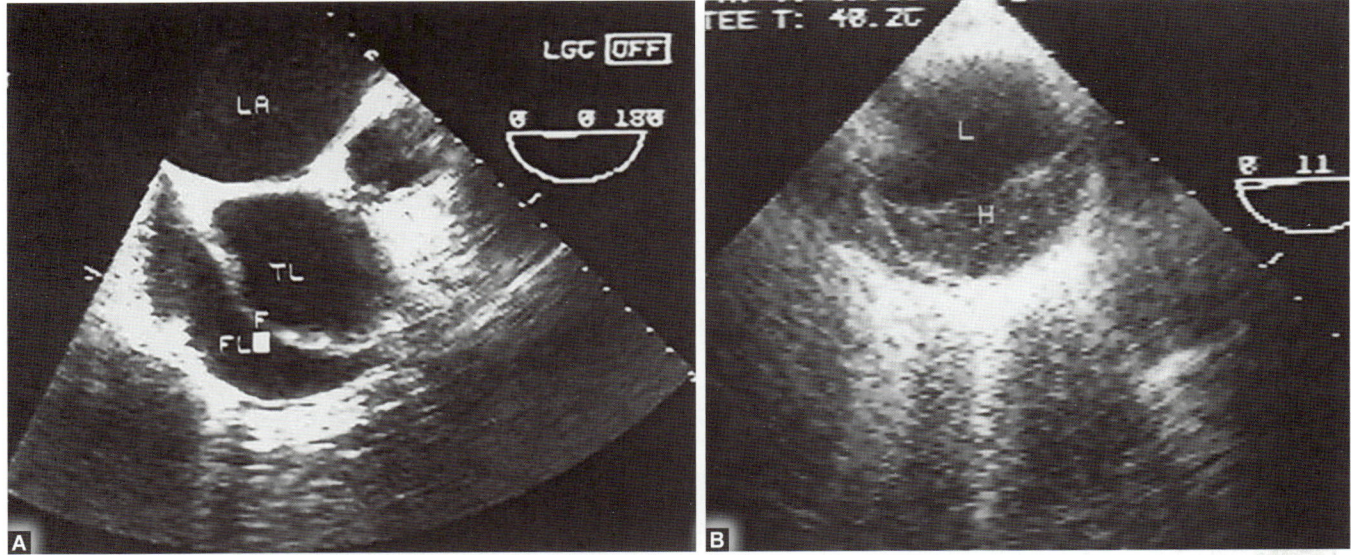

**Figs 7.18A and B:** (A) TEE imaging views of the descending thoracic aorta in the horizontal plane. An aortic dissection is manifested by the presence of a true lumen. (B) TEE view of the descending thoracic aorta in the horizontal plane. An aortic intramural hematoma is manifested by the presence of a hematoma (H) in the aortic wall without an intimal flap

single sinus of Valsalva, from a separation between the aortic media and the annulus fibrosus. A deficiency of normal elastic tissue and abnormal development of the bulbus cordis have been associated with the development of SVA due to the high pressure at the root of the aorta (Figs 7.19 to 7.22).

## Transthoracic Echocardiography for Aortic Dissection

Transthoracic echocardiography (TTE) is an insensitive tool for detecting aortic dissection because it does not visualize the aortic arch or much of the descending aorta,

and imaging quality may not be optimal because of the patient's body habitus (Fig. 7.23). While more sensitive imaging tests are being scheduled, however, TTE can provide valuable information about pericardial effusion or aortic regurgitation[21] and can help determine whether cardiac tamponade is the cause of hypotension in a patient with aortic dissection.

Transesophageal echocardiographic examination in addition to transthoracic echocardiography provides more powerful information about SVAs and coexistent cardiac malformations. This may be additional value for

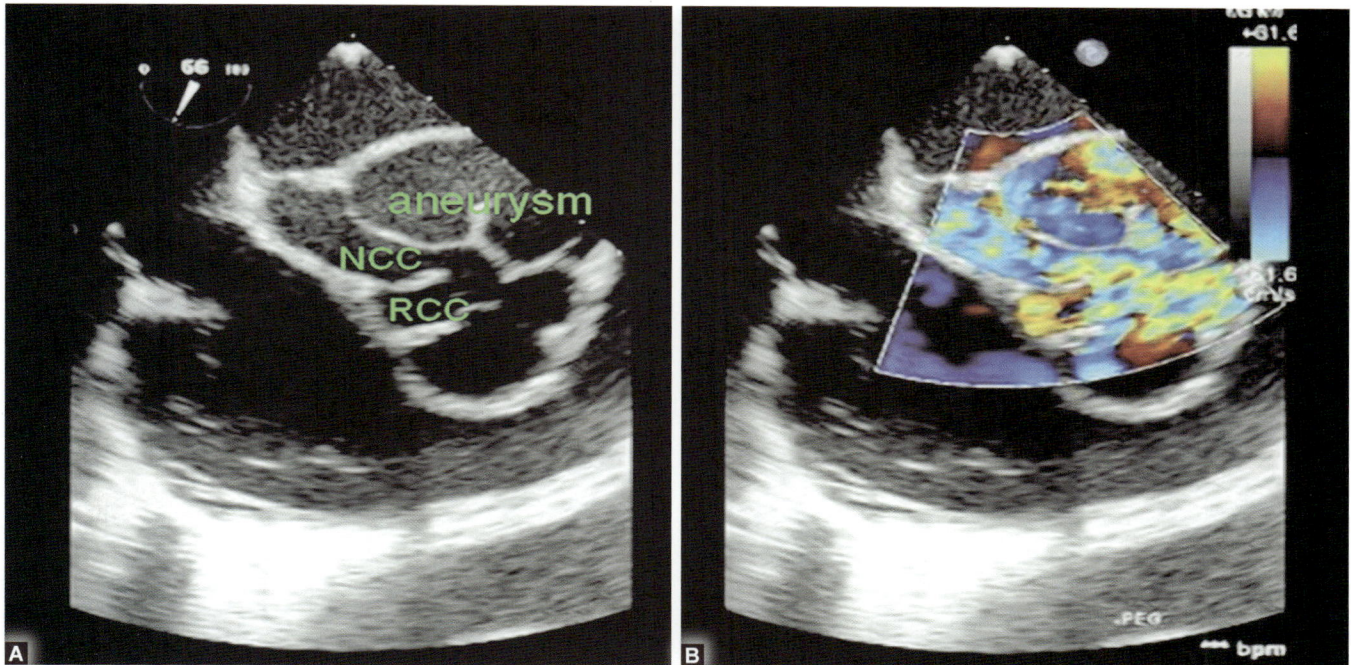

**Figs 7.19A and B:** Mid-esophageal aortic short-axis view showing aneurysm arising from left coronary sinus, normal noncoronary sinus and dilated right coronary sinus[19]

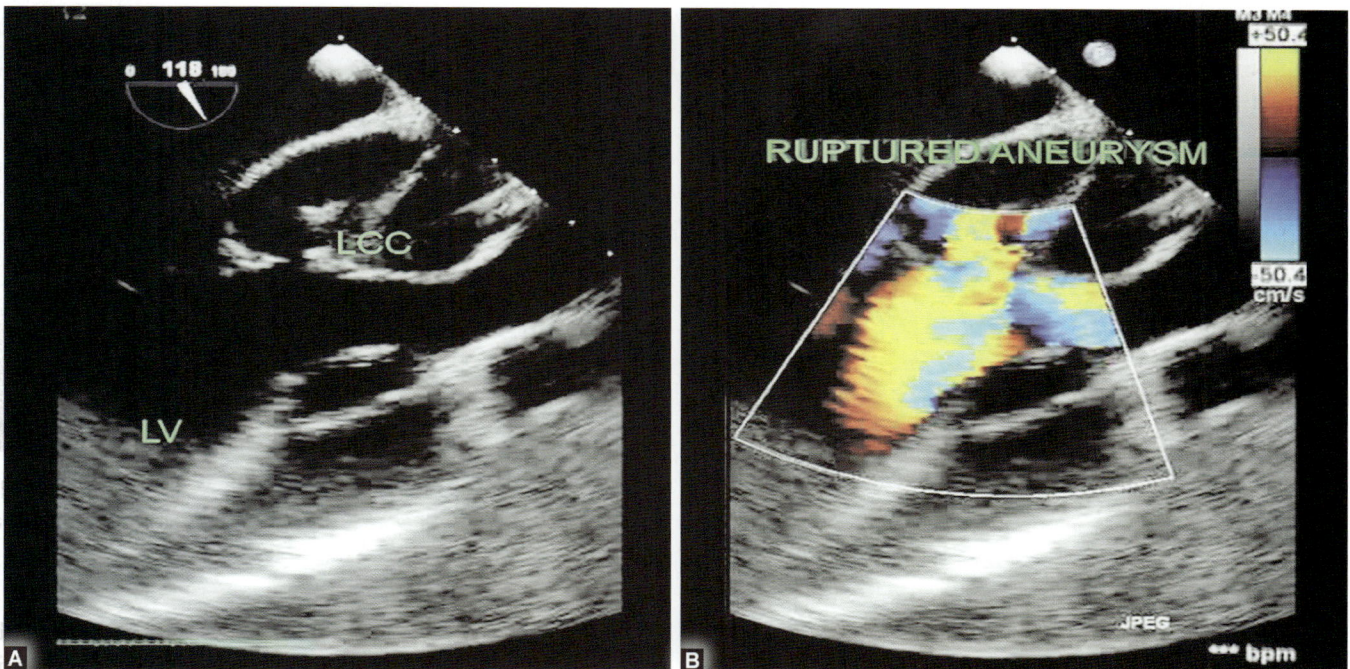

**Figs 7.20A and B:** Mid-esophageal aortic long-axis color Doppler view showing ruptured aneurysm from left coronary sinus into left ventricular cavity

the cardiac surgeon planning resection of the lesion. Multiplane TEE provides conclusive information regarding the origin and size of the aneurysm and presence of thrombotic material and allows precise identification of structural anomalies and shunt locations for perioperative assessment.[23,24] Prognosis is poor with progressive aneurysmal dilatation or rupture unless early surgery is done.

## Pulmonary Artery Catheter (PAC) vs TEE: Imaging of Aortic Dissections

A PAC provides pulmonary artery occlusion pressures (PAOPs) to assess left sided filling, continuous pulmonary arterial pressures and mixed venous oxygen saturations. Continuous or intermittent cardiac output measurement and derived values for systemic and

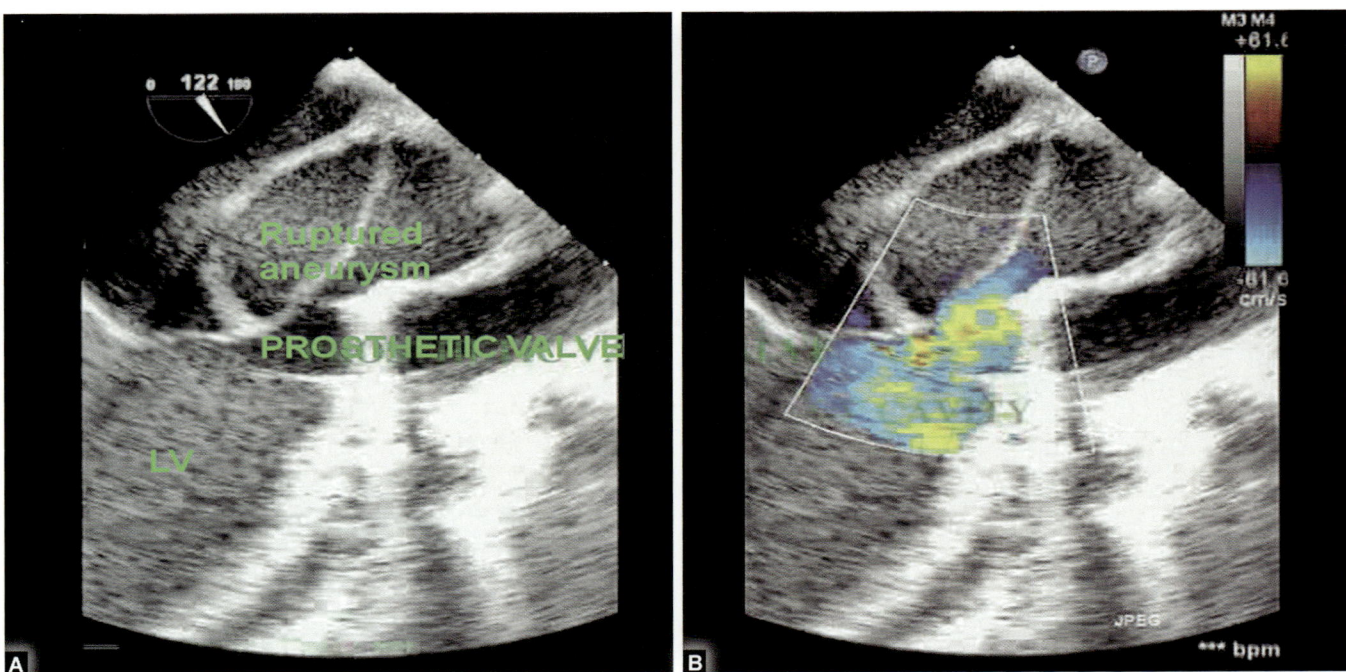

**Figs 7.21A and B:** Post-aortic valve replacement mid-esophageal aortic short-axis view showing prosthetic valve with residual aneurysm[17]

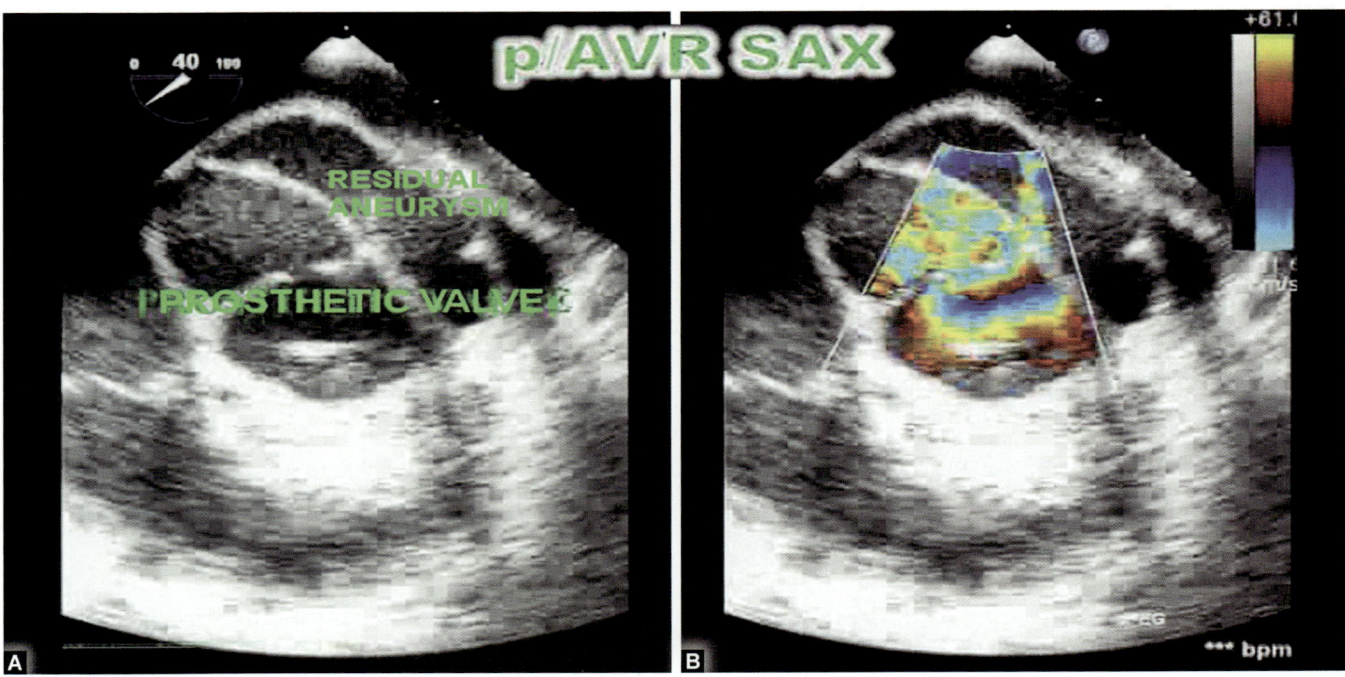

**Figs 7.22A and B:** Post-aortic valve replacement mid-esophageal aortic long axis color Doppler view showing prosthetic valve with residual ruptured aneurysm into left ventricular cavity[19]

pulmonary vascular resistances can also be calculated. Acute myocardial ischemia detection is reflected in PAC data by the acute appearance of C waves, an unexplained increase in PAOP, or a decreased cardiac output. All of these may precede ST and T wave changes on the ECG.

TEE provides an index of preload via the left ventricular end-diastolic area. This may be a more accurate index than the PAOP. The TEE also provides continuous left and right ventricular functional assessment, in addition to myocardial ischemia detection, as reflected by regional wall motion abnormalities. This information can provide invaluable data, particularly during phases of significant hemodynamic strain, e.g. aortic cross-clamping and release. Its limitations include the need

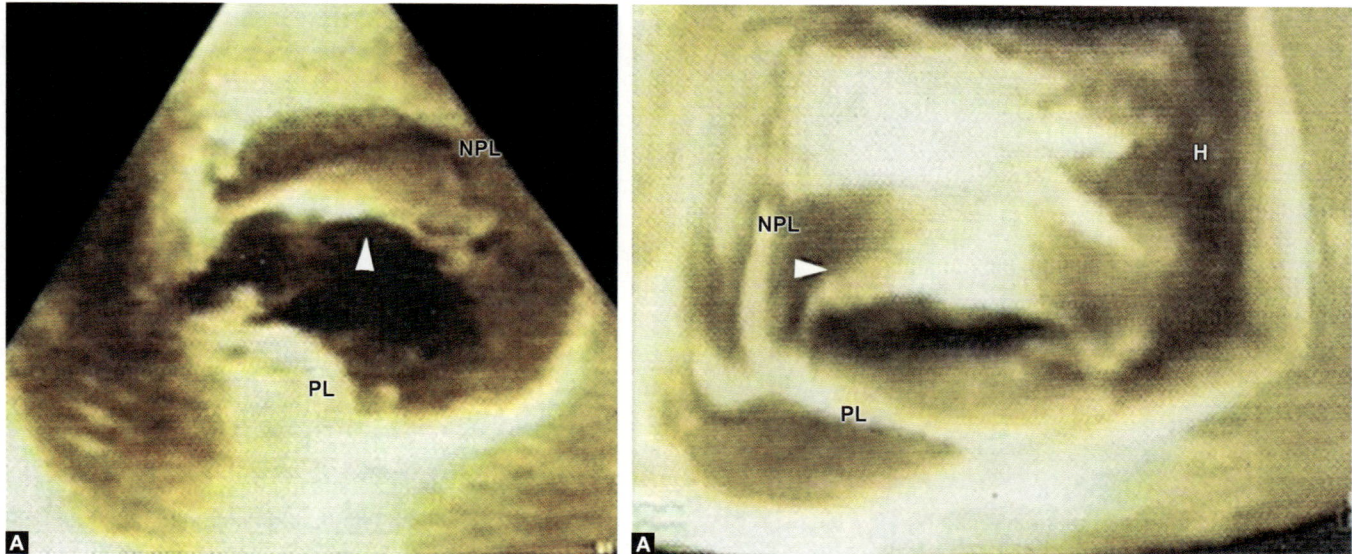

**Figs 7.23A and B:** The live real time 3D transthoracic echocardiography in a patient with aortic valve prosthesis and dissection. Aorta is dissected shortly following by aortic valve replacement with St. Jude prosthesis[22]

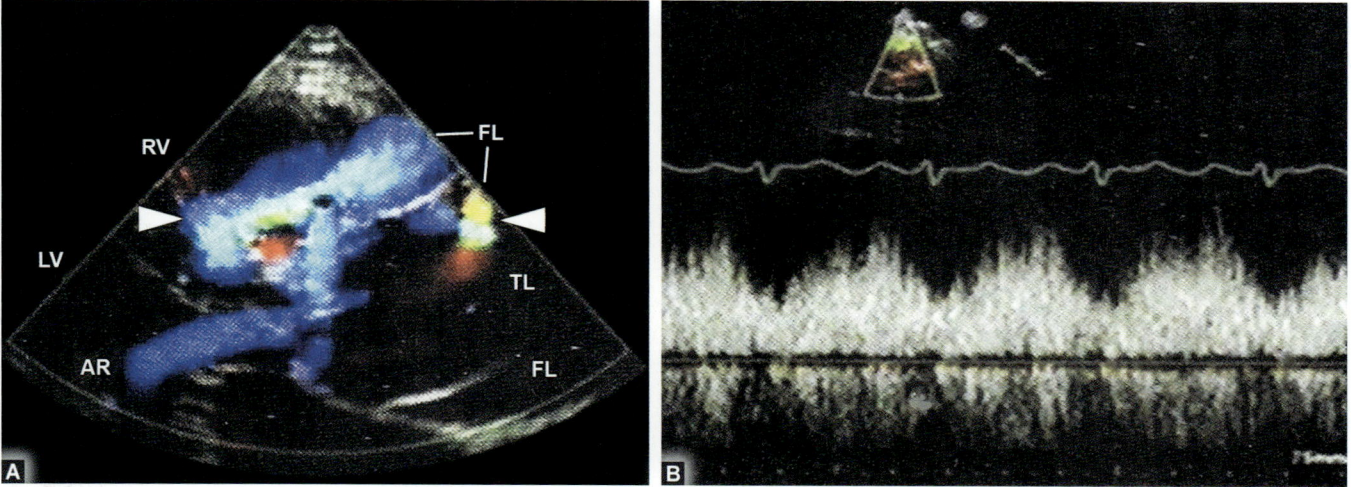

**Figs 7.24A and B:** (A) The parasternal long-axis view. The arrowhead points to the site of rupture of the false lumen (FL) into the right ventricular outflow tract (RVOT). (B) Shows the color Doppler examination. The arrowhead on the rights points to a communication between the true lumen (TL) and FL. The arrowhead on the left shows flow signals moving from the FL to the RVOT. Moderate aortic regurgitation is also displayed. Also shows the continuous wave spectral Doppler interrogation of the rupture site showing continuous flow throughout the cardiac cycle[22]

for expert interpretation and continuous observation and the possibility of probe interference in the surgical field, as well as high purchase and maintenance costs.

Double-lumen endobronchial tubes are recommended not only to improve surgical exposure but also to provide an element of patient safety. By collapsing the left lung, trauma to that lung is decreased. If manipulation during surgery causes hemorrhage into the airway, the contralateral (right) lung is protected from blood spillage. A left-sided tube is technically easier to place and is used often, but it may be impossible to insert in some patients because of aneurysmal distortion of the trachea or left main stem bronchus. Patients with aortic rupture may have a distorted left main stem bronchus. Right-sided tubes may be used, but proper alignment with the right upper lobe bronchus should be checked with a fiberoptic bronchoscope. Alternatively, tubes with an endobronchial blocker should be considered in cases where adequate placement of a double-lumen tube cannot be achieved.

## USE OF TEE TO DETECT AORTIC ARTIFACTS

Aortic dissection, a surgical emergency of the aorta, is caused by a single or multiple tears in the intimal wall.

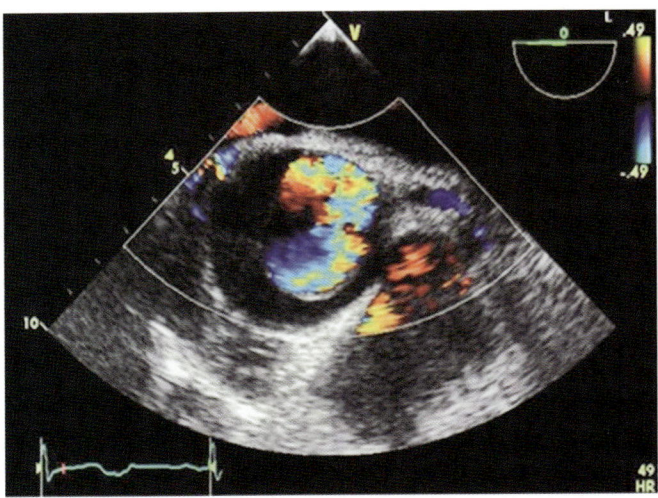

**Fig. 7.25:** The modified mid-esophageal aortic valve long-axis view, color Doppler

Blood under pressure can then dissect the layers from the media to produce a false lumen and an intimal flap. An example of such a flap is shown in Fig. 7.25 and Videos 7.1 to 7.9. Grade 5 atheromas are defined as protruding plaques >5 mm with mobile components. They are seen extending into the aorta from the vessel wall and would not have a linear aspect. One must be vigilant when making the diagnosis of aortic dissection as reverberations and side-lobe artifacts can mimic its appearance. Aortic aneurysm is defined as an abnormal dilation of the aortic diameter, which is not the case here.

## USE OF TEE TO DIFFERENTIATE THE FALSE AND TRUE LUMEN

In Fig. 7.26, the true lumen is identified as number 1 and the false lumen as number 2. Typically, in the ME LAX, the intimal flap will move such that it expands in systole. Furthermore, flow velocity will be higher in the true lumen and colour Doppler interrogation will show

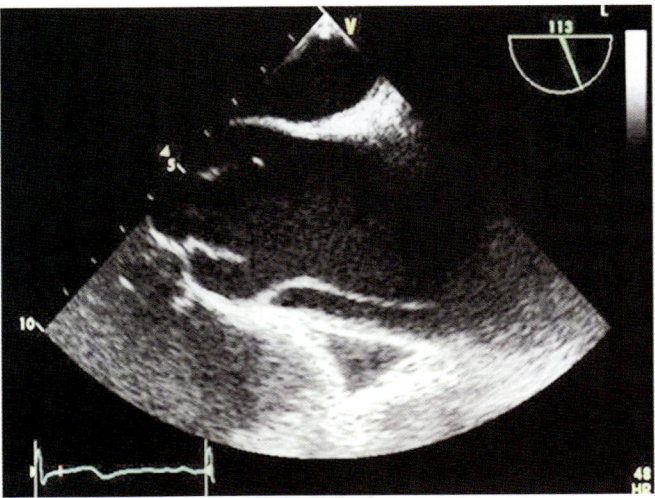

**Fig. 7.26:** Modified ME view, ascending aorta

blood flow moving slightly earlier. The false lumen is typically larger than the true lumen's diameter, involving half to two-thirds of the circumference, and expands in diastole. Sometimes, clots or venous stasis (spontaneous echo contrast) can be seen inside this channel. The false lumen can rupture into the pericardium, the pleural space, or the abdomen. TEE is therefore helpful in differentiating the true lumen from the false lumen-which is crucial, especially during procedures such as endovascular aortic stenting. If the image were a normal aorta and an artifact, the lower image would mirror the upper and there would not be a difference in the direction of flow during the cardiac cycle.

## TRANSESOPHAGEAL ECHOCARDIOGRAPHY TO KNOW ENTRY AND EXIT POINT OF THE DISSECTION

The intimal tear creates one or several entry and re-entry points through which blood may enter and exit the false lumen. The intimal tear frequently occurs in the thoracic aorta. Blood can be seen entering the false lumen in systole. The aortic cannula has a completely different appearance on TEE and is usually seen in the ascending aorta. Aortic debris, another term for mobile or complex atheromas, does not have the linear appearance shown in the examples. Aortic rupture would involve extra-luminal blood collection.

TEE is a powerful diagnostic tool when aortic dissection is suspected. A complete TEE examination of the aorta should be done in order to assess and identify the intimal tear, the aortic true lumen, the extension of dissection, and potential complications as they all will have an impact on management.

## OTHER MONITORING

### Somatosensory Evoked Potentials

Somatosensory evoked potentials (SEPs) have been promoted as a means of assessing functional status of the spinal cord during periods of possible ischemia. Briefly, SEPs monitor spinal cord function by stimulating a peripheral nerve and monitoring the response in the brainstem and cerebral cortex. Normal SEPs seem to ensure the integrity of the posterior (sensory) columns. However, SEPs have several shortcomings. First, during aortic surgery, it is the anterior (motor) horns that are more at risk. Perhaps for this reason, there have been reports of patients who had normal SEPs during cross-clamping and who subsequently were found to have paraplegia. Second, it must be remembered that many anesthetics, including all of the halogenated drugs, nitrous oxide, and several

IV drugs (e.g. thiopental and propofol) will alter the amplitude and latency of the evoked potential. In addition, if simple cross-clamping is used, ischemia of the peripheral nerves will interfere with SEP interpretation.

Other than being used as an intraoperative tool to help identify intercostal arteries that should be reimplanted to preserve spinal cord perfusion, SEP monitoring has not been shown to decrease the incidence of paraplegia.

## Motor Evoked Potentials

Because of the limitations of SEPs, motor evoked potentials (MEPs) have been introduced to monitor the integrity of the anterior spinal cord. The motor cortex is stimulated transcranially with the use of electromagnetic or electrical energy, and the myogenic MEPs are recorded from the lower paravertebral muscles. Peripheral nerve ischemia does not appear to affect such measurement, as it does with SEPs. Complete muscle relaxation cannot be used during MEP recording. However, MEPs can be monitored in the presence of a stable degree of partial neuromuscular blockade. MEP monitoring has been shown to be highly sensitive and specific for the detection of significant motor tract injury in numerous experimental studies. Furthermore,

changes in MEP have been shown to reliably predict neurologic outcome and paraplegia after ischemia or mechanical injury. Monitoring of spinal cord evoked potentials is another electrophysiologic modality that has been used for the early detection of spinal cord ischemia. The use of MEP monitoring alone or in conjunction with SEP monitoring in patients undergoing aortic dissection.

### Pre-anesthetic Assessment of Aortic Dissections

A pre-anesthetic checkup is essential to decision for type of sternotomy to detect the following Urgency of operation, Pathology and extent of disease, Median sternotomy/thoracotomy/endovascular approach, Mediastinal mass effect and any Airway compromise/deviation.

Diagram of the assessment of cardiovascular risk (Fig. 7.27).

## ANESTHETIC CONSIDERATIONS

Anesthetists are involved in protective evaluation resuscitation and stabilization, pain relief, sedation for transesophageal echocardiography (TEE), transfer, anesthesia, and perioperative and postoperative care of aortic dissection patients. The anesthetist's role may also

| Table 7.5: Assessment of cardiovascular risk | |
|---|---|
| ECG: | Baseline, Prior MI: Risk stratification, dysrhythmias: Other than sinus: Risk, lacks sensitivity |
| Exercise ECG: | 30–70% cannot reach target HR, poor functional capacity, β blocker, etc. If 85% of predicted maximal HR achieved: Low risk, arm exercise: Fatigue precedes increase |
| Myocardial perfusion imaging: | DTI: Most common, non-invasive, steal phenomenon, 3 outcomes: Normal, myocardium at risk, fixed perfusion defect, Eagle, et al, and L'italien et al: No additional stratification for pts classified as low or high risk. Classified 80% of intermediate risk into low or high risk. |
| Ambulatory ECG monitoring: | Detect dysrythmias, sensitivity: In pts with high pretest probability, 80–90% MI silent: Periop morbidity, low cost, not in LBBB, pacemaker dependency, LVH, significant strain or digitalis |
| Echocardiography: | With 5 or > abnormal segments: 4–6 fold ↑ risk of cardiac Cx |
| Stress echocardiography: | TEE superior to transthoracic, DSE: Sensitivity: and specificity 80–90%, stratifies pts only with risk factors, pericardiac events unlikely if result –ve, best predictor: |
| Radionuclide ventriculography: | LVF at rest or exercise, independent predictor of periop cardiac morbidity, EF < 35%: 75–85% MI risk or >35% : 19–20%, however limited use |

| Table 7.6: Assessment of aortic dissections | |
|---|---|
| Assessment of pulmonary risk: | Rule out COPD, smoking, chronic bronchitis, ABG: baseline PACO$_2$ >45=higher risk, PFT: FEV1<1lit/ MBC<50%, steroids short course: Helpful in copd/asthma, may benefit from epidural analgesia and anesthesia |
| Assessment of renal function: | HTN, atherosclerosis, diabetic nephropathy, renal artery stenosis, Pre and intraoperative dye loads: Nephrotoxic, aortic cross clamping: ↓ blood flow, embolic plaque, Fluctuations in CO and intravascular vol, ARF: about 7%, preoperative ARF most imp predictor of postoperative ARF, pathogenesis: ATN, Clamp, distal to subclavian A: 85–94% ↓ in blood flow, infrarenal: >30% ↓, S. creat >2 mg% : High risk |

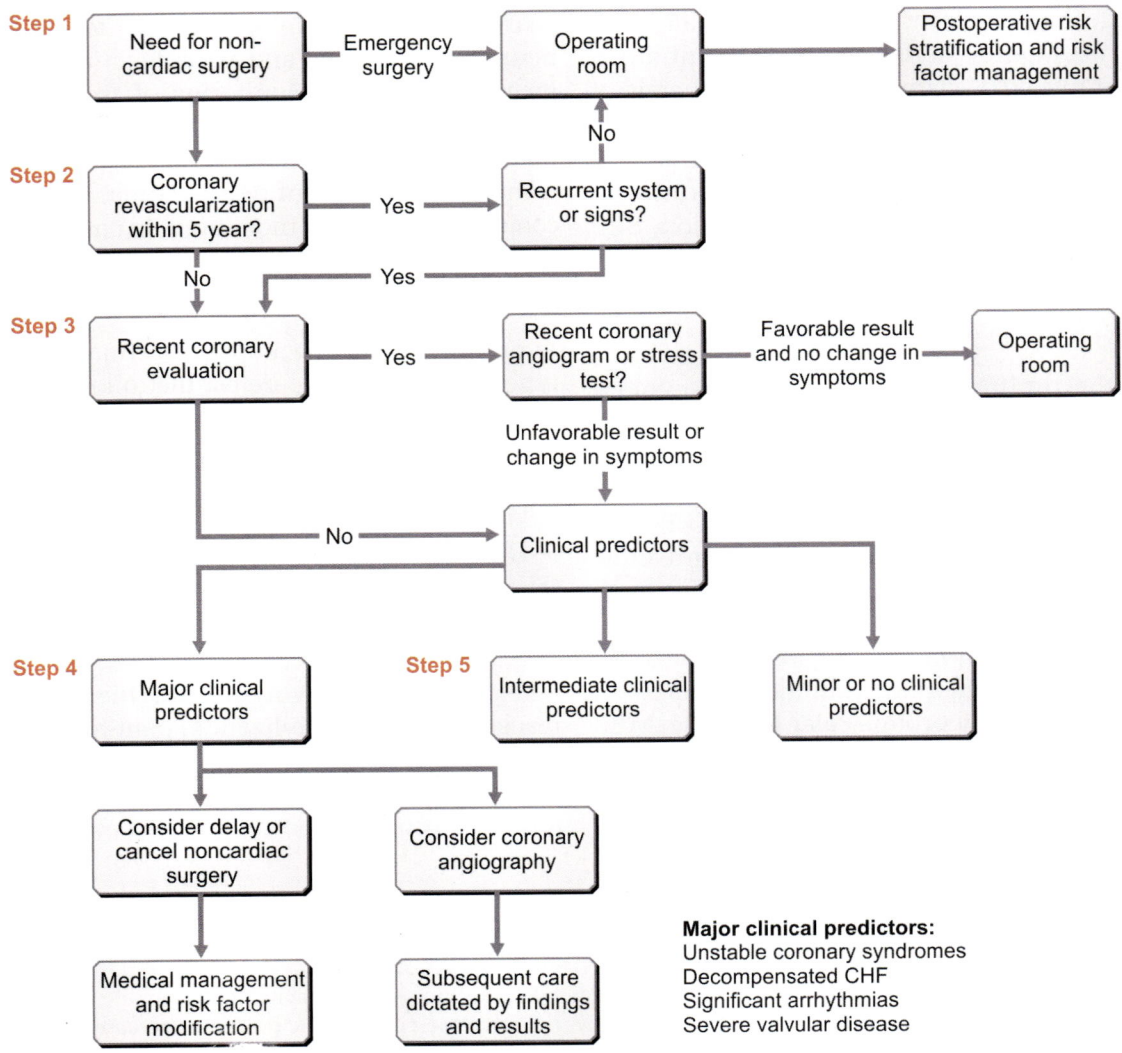

**Major clinical predictors:**
Unstable coronary syndromes
Decompensated CHF
Significant arrhythmias
Severe valvular disease

**Fig. 7.27:** Assessment of cardiovascular risk

include diagnostic perioperative TEE to aid surgical decision making. These will be discussed in detail under the following headings (Table 7.7).

In addition to the routine monitoring required for all anesthetized patients, these patients will require hourly urine output measurement, and central venous access,

**Table 7.7:** General anesthetic management under the following headings

- Hemodynamic monitoring
- Neurophysiologic monitoring
- OLV for thoracotomy
- Bleeding potential
- Antibiotic prophylaxis
- Temperature monitoring
- Blood sugar monitoring
- Aaesthetic depth monitoring
- Renal protective strategies

both for the administration of vasoactive drugs and for pressure monitoring. A pulmonary artery catheter (PAC) should also be inserted. Arterial pressure should be measured via a right radial arterial line; the left radial pressure wave may be lost if the origin of the left subclavian artery is clamped. This is also useful for blood sampling. Femoral or dorsalis pedis arterial access is required to monitor distal vascular bed perfusion in the event of shunt malfunction, if a shunt or bypass is used. Body temperature monitoring is advisable, and is essential if the patient is to be passively cooled (Fig. 7.28).

## ASCENDING AORTIC DISSECTION

Anesthetic management of these patients usually starts in the intensive care unit during the diagnostic evaluation. Large-bore intravenous lines and an intra-arterial line should be inserted as soon as the diagnosis of acute dissection is suspected (Fig. 7.29) .

**Table 7.8.** Preoperative general anesthesia consideration

| | |
|---|---|
| Neurophysiologic monitoring: | To monitor for intraoperative spinal ischemia: SSEP, MEP, EEG, Jugular venous oxygen saturation, lumbar CSF pressure, body temperature |
| Hemodynamic monitoring: | • ECG, IBP for proximal aortic pressure, R radial—Innominate A |
| | • BP: Repair of arch/proximal, L radial, |
| | • A: ACP, B/L, femoral: Distal aortic pressure, avoided in PVD |
| | • CVP: RAP, vasoactive drugs |
| | • PAC: PAP, CO, mixed $Svo_2$, (CPB, DHCA, partial LSHB, aortic-cross clamping), TEE: Ventricular ft |
| Temperature monitoring: | **Core:** Urinary catheter with temp probe, PAC probe, nasopharyngeal probe, rectal probe |
| SSEP: | Electrical stimuli to peripheral nerves and record evoked potential at peripheral nerves, spinal cord, brainstem, thalamus, cerebral cortex; ↓/ disappearance of amplitude in LL v/s UL, balanced anesthesia technique, MAC <0.5, Monitors only posterior column not motor |
| MEP: | Paired stimuli to scalp and record evoked potential in anterior tibialis muscle ; ↓/ disappearance of amplitude in LL v/s UL, TIVA without N-M blockade |
| OLV | Left thoracotomy or Left thoracoabdominal approach of TAAA. It improves surgical exposure to decrease lung contusion or torsion and protects R lung in bleeding, DLT/BB, advantages and disadvantages of each, If DLT- exchange to angle lumen tube at the end of Sx |

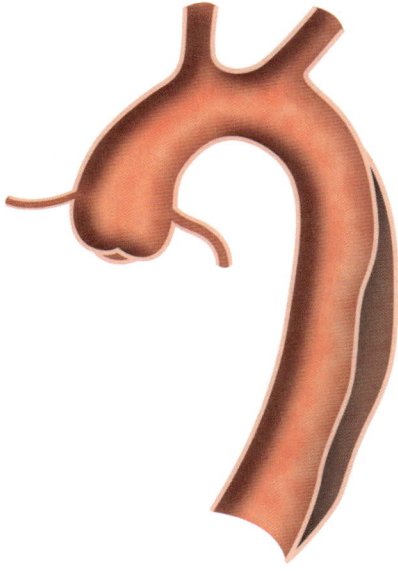

Fig. 7.28: The descending thoracic aorta

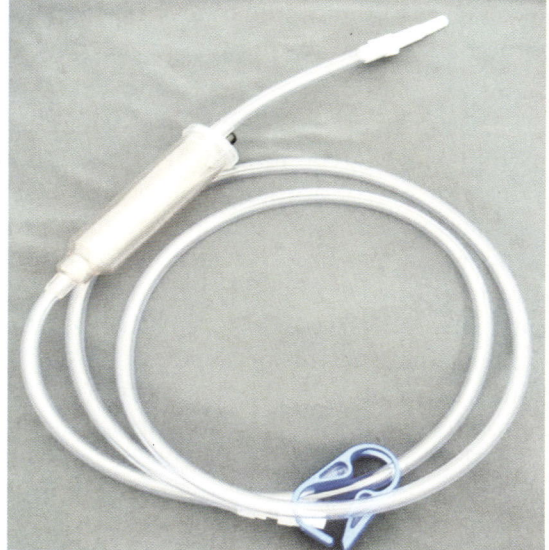

Fig. 7.29: Large bore intravenous (IV) Set

Titration of fluid infusions is paramount as overzealous fluid administration may lead to progression of dissection and rupture. Left radial arterial pressure monitoring is preferred as the innominate artery may be involved in the dissection and therefore affect right radial artery Pressures. Anatomy should be verified prior to insertion of the arterial line. However, some recommend also placing a right radial arterial catheter to detect the presence of a malperfusion state after the initiation of cardiopulmonary bypass (CPB).

A femoral artery is acceptable for monitoring; however, one side is likely to be used for CPB arterial inflow (Fig. 7.30). Central venous and pulmonary artery (PA) catheters are inserted to monitor filling pressures and CO and to administer vasoactive drugs.

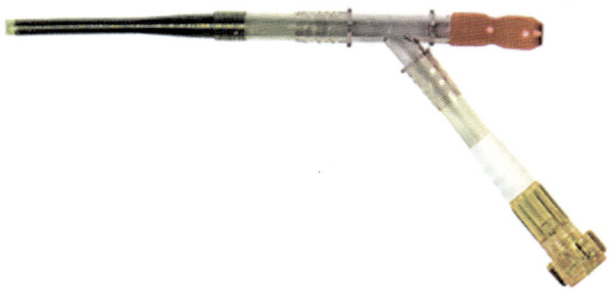

Fig. 7.30: Femoral arterial cannulation

ECG gives basic information on heart rate and rhythm, ECG monitoring with ST segment analysis may also allow for diagnosis of coronary malperfusion in the perioperative phase and after the operation is completed give important information with regard to the adequacy of coronary perfusion if root replacement with coronary reimplantation is required.

## PERIOPERATIVE TEE IN ASCENDING AORTIC ANEURYSMS

In addition to its preoperative diagnostic importance, TEE is a useful adjunct in the intraoperative management of these patients. The diagnosis of hypovolemia, hypocontractility, myocardial ischemia, intracardiac air, and valvular dysfunction can be made with TEE. Caution should be exercised when placing this probe in the presence of a large aortic aneurysm. For evaluating brain function, either raw or processed electro-encephalographic data may be helpful for judging the adequacy of cerebral perfusion during CPB. Newer monitors such as the bispectral index may help to assess the depth of anesthesia during these procedures.

## MANAGEMENT OF BLOOD PRESSURE

Special emphasis is given to control of blood pressure and the rate of rise of aortic pressure (dP/dT), using β-blockers and vasodilators, which are maintained into the postoperative period. The anesthetic implications of the presence of aortic valve incompetence should be appreciated. Anesthesia concerns for patients with aortic insufficiency include the presence of impaired left ventricular function and the necessity for afterload reduction and avoidance of bradycardia. Inadequate myocardial protection may occur because of the presence of hypertrophied left ventricle and may contribute to the post by pass ventricular dysfunction. Intramyocardial catecholamines are depleted in patients with chronic aortic regurgitation.

## INOTROPIC SUPPORT

Inotropic support may be needed to successfully wean the patient from CPB. Because regurgitation occurs during diastole, a slower heart rate provides more opportunity for backward flow. Faster heart rates are therefore preferred to decrease the regurgitation time. Bradycardia and afterload increase the regurgitant fraction in the presence of significant aortic insufficiency. Intramyocardial catecholamines are also depleted in patients with chronic aortic incompetence, which may predispose to post-bypass left ventricular dysfunction. Because of advances in surgical and anesthetic management, the operative mortality rate for ascending aortic surgery has decreased from 5 to 10%. Predictors of poor outcome include emergency surgery, advanced patient age, preoperative functional status, and cross-clamping time and duration of circulatory arrest.

## BLOOD LOSS AND ITS MANAGEMENT

Surgery for acute dissection is usually complicated by more blood loss in comparison to other cardiac surgical procedures. Difficulties with hemostasis result from friability of the aortic tissues, suture line bleeding, long CPB and DHCA durations, and activation of the coagulation antifibrinolytic cascades by the dissection process, resulting in disseminated intravascular coagulopathy. Intraoperative red blood cell (RBC) salvage techniques should be employed. Antifibrinolytic drugs (aprotinin, ε-aminocaproic acid [EACA], and tranexamic acid) were shown to significantly reduce bleeding. Because of concerns about thrombosis and renal dysfunction, aprotinin is better deferred until after circulatory arrest. Platelets, fresh-frozen plasma, and cryoprecipitate should be available. Advances in surgical technique, including the widespread use of Teflon felt and both fibrin and gelatin resorcinol fibrin biologic glue, collagen, or gelatin-impregnated graft have significantly decreased the incidence of excessive hemorrhage and operative mortality. Major causes of morbidity and mortality include hemorrhage, renal failure, myocardial infarction, left ventricular failure, and stroke. Ventricular dysrhythmias are reported to occur in 20 to 30% of patients. Excessive antihypertensive and anti-impulse therapy are continued after separation from CPB and in the intensive care unit.

Hypothermic CPB is used in most cases of ascending aneurysms. Deep hypothermic circulatory arrest (DHCA) is needed if the proximal arch is involved. If femoral cannulation is used and the femoral artery is small, a smaller cannula may be needed. This probably will delay cooling and rewarming, because lower blood flows are used to avoid excessive arterial line pressures. Extra time for cooling and rewarming must be allowed in this setting.

## AORTIC ARCH SURGERY

In most cases the patient is supine and the surgery is performed through a median sternotomy. In some cases the procedure is done with the patient in the left lateral thoracotomy position. CPB is established via the femoral artery with venous drainage achieved through right atrial, bicaval, or femoral venous cannulation.

Electroencephalography can be useful not only for ensuring that adequate cooling has been achieved but also for titration of the thiopental dose for brain protection. Nasal temperature will verify adequate brain cooling. TEE provides useful information similar to that for ascending aortic surgery, but care should be taken when placing the probe.

Management of hypothermic circulatory arrest—the technique involves core cooling to 15° to 20°C, packing the head in ice, using other cerebral protective agents, avoiding glucose-containing solutions, and using proper monitoring.

Complications related to anesthesia for this procedure are uncommon. One is myocardial depression secondary to the use of thiopental for cerebral protection, and inotropic agents may be needed to wean the patient from CPB.

In the presence of aortic dissection, the $dP/dt_{max}$ must be minimized to that amount that is just sufficient to permit adequate tissue perfusion. β-Adrenergic receptor blocking agents, supplemented with vasodilators, are excellent for this purpose. The use of inotropic drugs in the presence of aortic dissection could be hazardous because of the increase in $dP/dt_{max}$. The anesthetic technique should allow for complete neurologic assessment within a few hours after surgery.

## CONDUCT OF ANESTHESIA BEFORE AND DURING CROSS-CLAMPING

Before the aorta is cross-clamped, mannitol (0.5 g/kg) should be infused to provide some renal protection during clamping. Even though a shunting procedure will be used, changes in the distribution of renal blood flow make mannitol administration prudent.

After the clamp is applied, it is important to closely monitor acid–base status with serial arterial blood gas measurements. It is common for metabolic acidosis to develop due to hypoperfusion of critical organ beds, and this should be treated aggressively if the patient is normothermic. If simple cross-clamping without adjuncts is used, proximal hypertension should be controlled, again with the realization that distal organ flow may be diminished. In treating proximal hypertension, regional blood flow studies have shown that nitroprusside infusion may decrease renal and spinal cord blood flow in a dose-related fashion. Ideally, cross-clamp time (regardless of technique) should be less than 30 minutes, because the incidence of complications, especially paraplegia, begins to increase above this limit.

If a heparinized shunt has been placed and proximal hypertension cannot be treated without producing subsequent distal hypotension (less than 60 mm Hg), the surgeon should be made aware that there might be a technical problem with shunt placement. If partial bypass (ECC) is used, the pump speed or venous return can be adjusted so that control of proximal hypertension can be maintained by adequate unloading while the lower body is simultaneously perfused. Usually little or no pharmacologic intervention is necessary in this case because the pump speed and manipulation of venous return provide rapid control of proximal and distal pressures. Before removal of the cross-clamp, a vasopressor should be available. The anesthesiologist must be constantly aware of the stage of operation so that major events such as clamping and declamping may be anticipated.

| Comparison between ascending and descending TAA aneurysm | |
|---|---|
| *Ascending TAA* | *Descending TAA* |
| ■ Mortality: 3–5% | ■ Mortality: 4% |
| ■ Median sternotomy | ■ Lateral thoracotomy/thoraco-abdominal incision |
| ■ TEE: valve sparing Sx, diameter, AR post repair | ■ Cross clamping/ partial L heart bypass/DHCA |
| ■ CPB | ■ Spinal cord, mesenteric, LL protection Endovascular stent grafts |
| ■ Wheat procedure: AVR + tube graft | |
| ■ Bentall procedure: AVR | |
| ■ Ross procedure: PV ≥ AV | |
| ■ Carbol technique: coronary reimplantation | |

## DECLAMPING SHOCK

The most consistent observation on release of the cross-clamp is an acute fall in systemic blood pressure. This is caused mostly by a decrease in systemic vascular resistance (SVR) and a reactive hyperemia in the previously ischemic vascular beds. Whereas the release of an infrarenal aortic cross-clamp usually produces a modest decrease in blood pressure, the release of a supraceliac cross-clamp can result in profound hypotension. Before unclamping, vasodilators should be discontinued and intravascular volume should be increased. Transient vasopressor support is frequently required. Pulmonary capillary wedge pressure should be increased to about 2 to 4 mm Hg above the baseline value.

Acidosis may contribute to hypotension by producing myocardial depression and systemic vasodilation. The level of vasoactive intestinal peptide measured in mixed venous blood doubles with reperfusion of the splanchnic organs after supraceliac cross-clamp release and could contribute to hypotension by causing peripheral arterial vasodilation.

Total-body oxygen consumption increases with unclamping as tissues return to aerobic metabolism.

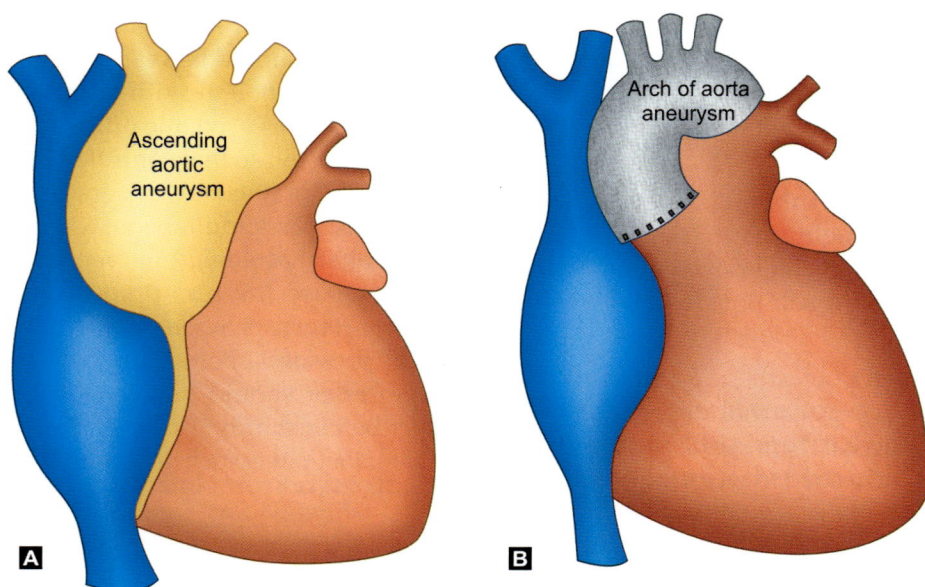

**Figs 7.31A and B:** Ascending aortic aneurysms and aortic arch aneurysms

Mixed venous oxygen saturation shows an abrupt decrease within minutes after unclamping but rapidly returns to control values. Carbon dioxide is elevated in arterial and venous blood within moments of unclamping. This rapid increase is caused by the buffering of lactic acid and other organic acids that are washed out from the distal circulation after reperfusion. Ventilation should be increased before unclamping to eliminate the excess $CO_2$ load. Bolus administration of sodium bicarbonate at this stage can produce further increase in $PaCO_2$ and worsening of intracellular acidosis. That is why it is preferable to administer bicarbonate gradually by an infusion during the entire period of cross-clamping rather than as a bolus injection after unclamping (Fig. 7.32). Unclamping of the descending thoracic aorta after 45 minutes of occlusion results in a 4 mmol/L increase in serum lactate concentration that usually returns rapidly to normal after complete restoration of hepatic and renal blood flow. It is uncommon for significant lactate elevations to persist into the postoperative period unless hepatic and intestinal ischemic injury has occurred. Partial bypass and shunt techniques maintain near-adequate perfusion of most tissues below the cross-clamp and significantly reduce lactic acid production and accumulation.

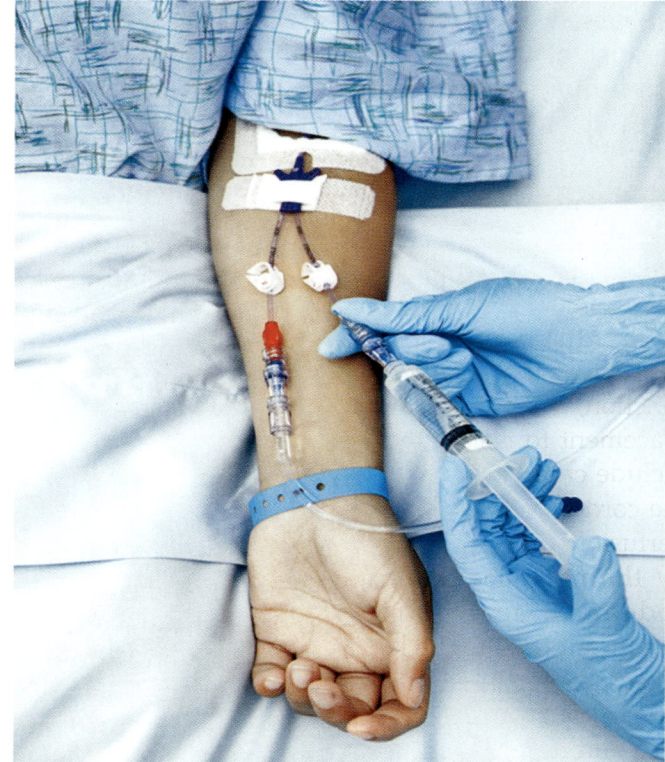

**Fig. 7.32:** The administer bicarbonate is gradually administered by an infusion during the entire period of cross-clamping rather than as a bolus injection after unclamping

## FLUID THERAPY AND TRANSFUSION

Even patients undergoing elective repair of a descending aneurysm may be relatively hypovolemic, and fluid therapy should have the following aims: correct this fluid deficit, provide maintenance fluids, compensate for evaporative and "third space" losses, decrease red cell loss by mild hemodilution, and replace blood loss as needed.

Despite proximal and distal control of the aorta, blood loss can be considerable in these cases due to back-bleeding from the intercostal arteries. These collateral vessels often are ligated on opening the aorta. Use of cell-scavenging devices has become common and has reduced the need for banked blood, but because massive losses may occur, banked blood may still be needed. As long as liver perfusion is adequate, even with a large blood loss, citrate toxicity usually is not a problem because of rapid first-pass metabolism in the liver. Repair of a thoracic aneurysm with simple clamping, however, presents a unique situation—the liver is not perfused. In this circumstance, transfusion of large amounts of banked blood may rapidly produce citrate toxicity, resulting in myocardial depression that requires calcium chloride infusion.

## SPINAL CORD PROTECTION

Several methods have been espoused to provide protection of the spinal cord during cross-clamping in addition to ECC, shunts, and expeditious surgery.

### Maintaining Perfusion Pressure

Some groups prefer to maintain perfusion pressure of the distal aorta in the range of 40 to 60 mm Hg to increase blood flow to the middle and lower spinal cord. This practice should be regarded as controversial because at present there are few data on outcome supporting this position. No method used to maintain blood flow to the distal aorta (i.e., shunt or partial bypass) guarantees that spinal cord blood flow, and therefore function, will be maintained. Proximal and distal clamp placement to isolate the diseased aortic segment may include critical intercostal vessels that provide flow to the cord and whose loss is not compensated by distal perfusion. In addition, distal perfusion may be hindered by the presence of atherosclerotic disease in the abdominal aorta, a condition that may prevent significant flow to the kidneys and spinal cord. Lastly, these crucial vessels may be disrupted in gaining surgical exposure. One should never assume that the cord and kidneys are absolutely "protected" because a shunt or partial bypass has been used. The largest studies have shown no difference in the incidence of paraplegia regardless of the surgical adjunct used.

## HYPOTHERMIA

Allowing the core temperature to be reduced to approximately 33° to 34°C will lower the metabolic rate of the spinal cord tissue and may provide some protection from reduced or interrupted blood flow. Adequate temperature reduction usually can be accomplished with topical cooling agents (cooling blankets, bags of crushed ice). Iced saline gastric lavage also may be used. Administration of even 1 or 2 units of cool banked blood (only if indicated) will lower the core temperature. Precise control of temperature is difficult. At temperatures below 32°C, the myocardium may become more irritable and prone to ventricular arrhythmias. These facts, plus the lack of improved outcome data, have resulted in sparse use of this technique.

## SPINAL DRAINS

Experimental data show that spinal cord damage may be mediated through the increase in cerebrospinal fluid (CSF) pressure that accompanies the reduction in spinal cord blood flow during cross-clamping. CSF pressure may be increased to as high as the mean distal arterial pressure. Because spinal cord blood flow is proportional to the mean arterial pressure minus the higher of the CSF or venous pressure, perfusion in this circumstance may be reduced to zero.

A spinal drain would allow not only for measurement of the intraspinal pressure but also for therapeutic reduction of CSF pressure by its removal and an increase in spinal cord blood flow. As a note of caution, removal of CSF in the presence of an elevated intraspinal pressure may provide a gradient for herniation of cerebral structures. In addition, placement of a spinal drain followed by systemic heparinization may lead to the formation of an epidural hematoma as a rare complication (Fig. 7.33). The use of spinal drains has increased because of the associated low morbidity and

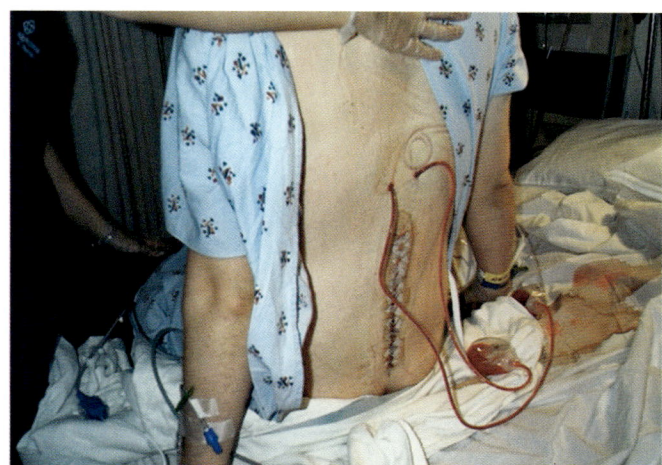

Fig. 7.33: The spinal drain followed by systemic heparinization may lead to the formation of an epidural hematoma as a rare complication

possible significant benefits. To date, no controlled study has demonstrated a reduction in morbidity associated with the use of spinal drains.

## OTHER

Additional "protective" measures, such as IV steroids, pharmacologic suppression of spinal cord function through IV or intrathecal drug administration, local hypothermia, and free radical scavengers, are not widely used or are considered experimental.

## PREVENTION OF RENAL FAILURE AND RENAL PROTECTION

The etiologic cause of renal failure is thought to be ischemia from interruption of blood flow by clamping, although embolism remains another possibility. Use of CPB or a shunt may be protective, but superior outcome data are lacking, and renal failure still occurs despite these surgical adjuncts (Fig. 7.34).

Adequate volume loading should be used and probably is most important in renal protection. Mannitol may help, and because its use is innocuous in most patients, it is recommended.

Adequate hydration and renal perfusion pressure are important factor for renal protection. The changes in renal blood flow are significantly attenuated if adequate intravascular volume and cardiac output are maintained.[25] There are so many methods[17] like minimizing aortic cross clamp time, maintaining

adequate renal perfusion (adequate intravascular volume, ventricular function and cardiac output), decreasing renal metabolic rate (cold perfusion to renal artery, frusemide, systemic hypothermia), decreasing reperfusion injury (mannitol, calcium channel blocker, superoxide dismutase), using pharmacological manipulation of renal blood flow (low dose dopamine, mannitol, frusemide, fenoldopam, PGE), are there to protect renal function.

Endovascular stent graft repair for isolated descending thoracic aortic aneurysms with a proximal landing zone that involves the left subclavian artery can be accomplished using a two-stage procedure. The most critical phase of the surgical procedure is device deployment. Tachycardia and hypertension should be avoided. Older devices are predisposed to distal migration as a result of forward aortic blood flow. Device malposition secondary to inadvertent migration may result either in occlusion of major arterial branches or incomplete aneurysm exclusion. Induced hypotension may be needed to reduce device migration. Other methods include the administration of high-dose adenosine or the induction of ventricular fibrillation to temporarily induce asystole and hence a "still" field. Newer-generation endografts are either thermally or mechanically activated ("self-deploying" stents), which do not require those maneuvers.

## COMPLICATIONS OF AORTIC DISSECTION

- Hemopericardium
- Acute severe AR
- Coronary malperfusion
- Aortic arch branch vessel malperfusion
- Cardiac tamponade
- Pleural effusion
- Hemopericardium
- Circumferential pericardial effusion
- Chamber compression
- Diastolic chamber collapse

TEE is useful for detecting complications like aortic regurgitation, coronary artery malperfusion, hemo-pericardium, etc. Hemopericardium is usually best seen on echocardiogram (Fig. 7.35A and B). Multiple echo-cardiographic views can help in evaluation of aortic regurgitation associated with aortic dissection (Fig. 7.36A and B). If the aortic dissection extends beyond the sinotubular junction, enlargement of the aortic root can result in aortic regurgitation. If the dissection causes coronary artery malperfusion then ventricular dysfunction should be evaluated on TEE (Fig. 7.36C). TEE also plays a useful role for evaluating traumatic aortic injury (Fig. 7.36D).

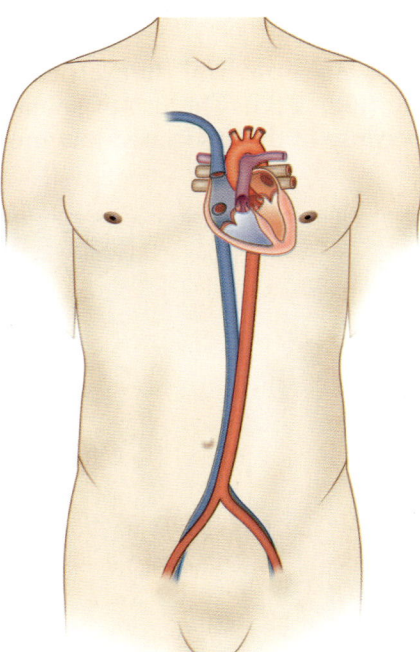

**Fig. 7.34:** The CPB or a shunt may be protective, but superior outcome data are lacking, and renal failure still occurs despite these surgical adjuncts

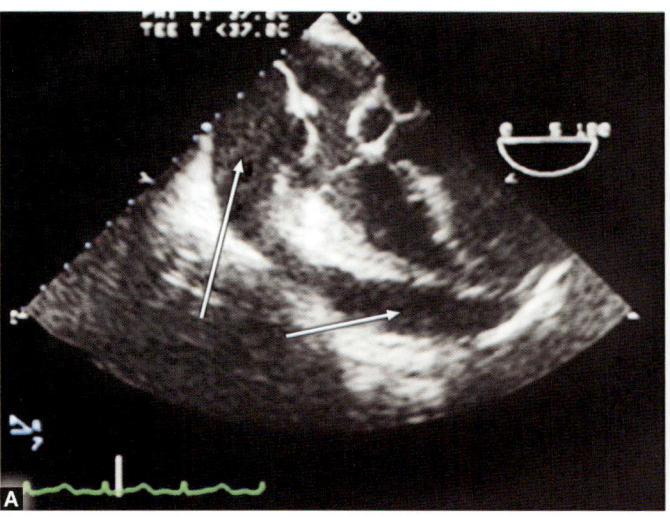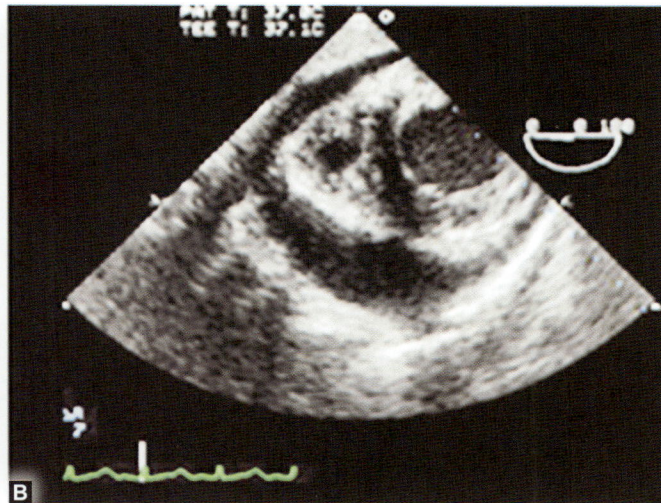

**Figs 7.35A and B:** The complications of aortic dissection

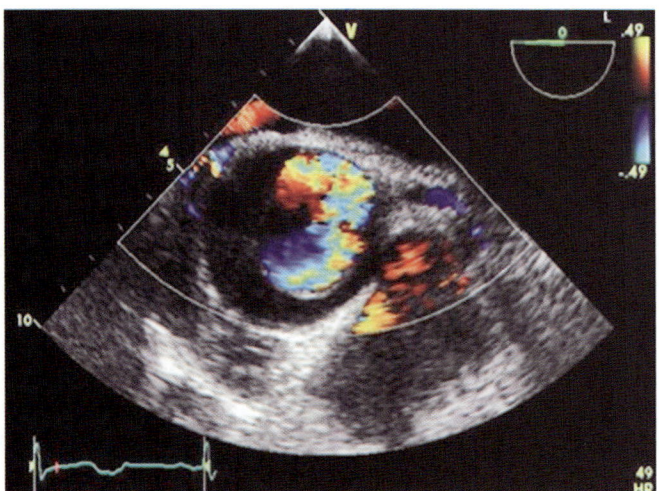

**Fig. 7.36A:** Modified ME AV LAX, color Doppler

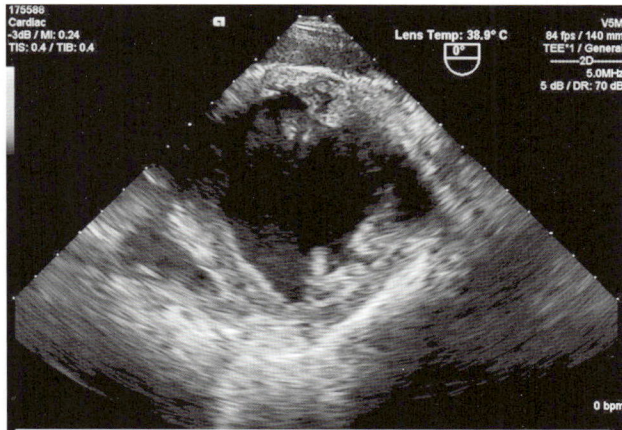

**Fig. 7.36C:** Coronary artery malperfusion on TEE demonstrates:
- Right ventricular dysfunction
- Left ventricular inferior wall hypokinesis

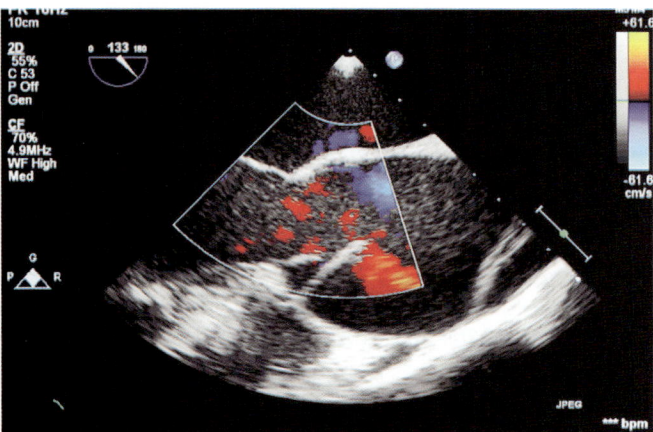

**Fig. 7.36B:** Aortic regurgitation best seen on TEE:
- Dilation of the aortic root
- Dissection into the aortic root
- Malsuspension of the aortic valve cusps
- Prolapse of the intimal flap through the aortic valve

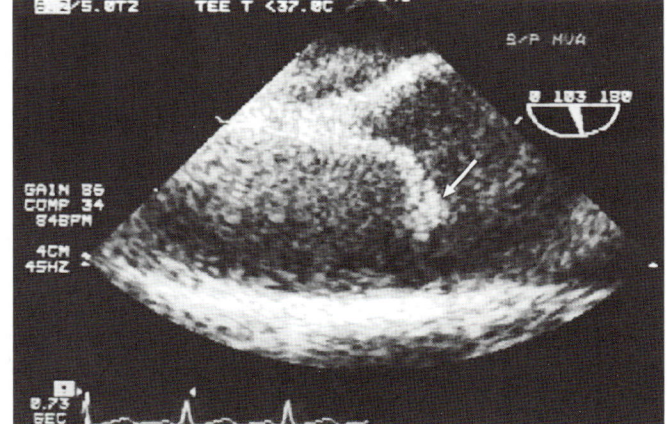

**Fig. 7.36D:** Traumatic aortic injury on TEE, shows site of:
- Intimal tear
- Intimal flap
- Pseudoaneurysm
- Aortic rupture

## ROLE OF ENDOVASCULAR THERAPY IN AORTIC DISSECTIONS

The endovascular stent-grafts were custom-designed for each patient according to measurements obtained from the diagnostic imaging studies (Fig. 7.37). Since it is difficult to know the original diameter of the aorta in cases of aortic dissection, the diameter of the nondissected portion of the aorta proximal to the entry tear (as measured by CT, MRI, or quantitative aortography with a calibrated catheter) was used to plan the diameter of the stent-graft. In this way, the residual radial force of the stent could provide an effective frictional seal against the aortic wall and dissection flap.

The anesthetist's role here is in doing TEE which shows the following:

- Type B aortic dissection
- Additional information to angiography/fluoroscopy
- Guiding correct stent-graft placement
- Detect peristent leaks and/or small re-entry tears
- Guidewire repositioning from the false to the true lumen
- Correct guidewire entrance into elephant trunk prostheses

## CONCLUSION

Acute aortic dissection is uncommon, but complication develops rapidly and the outcome is often fatal. The typical presentation is characterized by acute onset of severe pain. However, clinical manifestations are diverse, and what were previously considered to be classic symptoms and signs are often absent. Therefore, a high clinical index of suspicion is nece-ssary.

Despite significant advances in diagnostic and therapeutic techniques, morbidity and mortality rates remain high. Although it is clear that during the past 2 centuries much progress has been made, these data support the need for continued improvements in our ability to understand, diagnose and manage this devastating condition.

Echocardiography particularly TEE is an invaluable tool in the evaluation of Aorta. Its role in acute aortic syndrome is well proved and comparable to other modalities. TEE with epiaortic scanning has become a gold standard for detection of aortic atherosclerosis. Its role in endovascular therapy is also expanding to guide placement of stent and detection of leaks.

## REFERENCES

1. Braverman AC, Thompson RW, Sanchez LA. Diseases of the aorta. In: Bonow RO, Mann DL, Zipes DR, Libby P (Eds). Braunwald's Heart Disease, 9th edn. Philadelphia, PA: Saunders, 2012, p. 1309–37.
2. Hagan PG, Nienaber CA, Isselbacher EM, et al. The International Registry of Acute Aortic Dissection (lRAD): new insights into an old disease. JAMA 2000;283(7):897–903.
3. Apostolakis E, Akinosoglou K. What's new in the bio-chemical diagnosis of acute aortic dissection: problems and perspectives. Med Sci Monit 2007;13(8):RA 154–8.
4. Kouchoukos NT, Dougenis D, surgery of the thoracic aorta. N Engl J Med 1997;336:1876–1888.
5. Kamp TJ, Goldschmidt-Clermont PJ, Brinker JA, Resar JR. Myocardial infarction, aortic dissection, and thrombolytic therapy. Am Heart J 1994;128:1234–7.
6. Hartnell GG. Imaging of aortic aneurysms and dissection: CT MRI. J Thorac Imaging 2001;16:35–46.
7. Mehta RH, Suzuki T, Hagan PG, et al. Predicting death in patients with acute type A aortic dissection. Circulation 2002; 105:200.
8. Abbott OA. Clinical experiences with application of polythene cellophane upon the aneurysms of the thoracic vessels. J Thorac Surg 1949;18(4):435–61.
9. De Bakey ME, Cooley 0, Creech 0 Jr, et al. Surgical considerations of dissecting aneurysm of the aorta. Ann Surg. 1955;142(4):586–610.
10. Ince H, Nienaber CA. The concept of interventional therapy in acute aortic syndrome. J Card Surg. 2002;17(2):135–42.
11. Nienaber CA, Fattori R, Lund G, et al. Nonsurgical recons-truction of thoracic aortic dissection by stent graft placement. N Engl J Med 1999;340(20):1539–45.
12. Dake MD, Kato N, Mitchell RS, et al. Endovascular stent-graft placement for the treatment of acute aortic dissection. N Engl J Med 1999;340(20):1546–52. 7

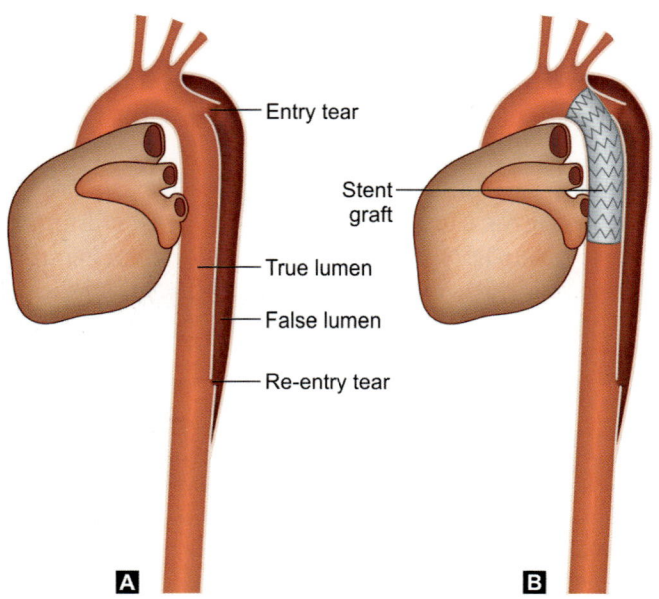

**Figs 7.37A and B:** Endovascular treatment of aortic dissection

13. Walkers PJ, Miller DC. Aneurysmal and ischemic complications of type B (type III) aortic dissections. Semin Vasc Surg 1992;5:198–214.

14. Knott AW, Kalra M, Duncan AA, et al. Open repair of juxta renal aortic aneurysms (jAAA) remains a safe option in a the era of fenestrated endografts. J Vasc Surg 2008;47: 695–701.

15. Novick AC. Renal hypothermia: invivo and exvivo. Urol Clin North Am 1983;10:637–44.

16. Erbel R, Alfonso F, Boileau C, et al. Task Force on Aortic Dissection Diagnosis and Management of aortic dissection. Eur Heart J 2001;22:1642–81.

17. Willens HJ, Kessler KM. Transesophageal echocardiography in the diagnosis of diseases of the thoracic aorta: Part 1. Aortic dissection, aortic intramural hematoma, and penetrating atherosclerotic ulcer of the aorta. Chest 1999; 116:1772.

18. Keren A, Kim CB, Hu BS, et al. Accuracy of biplane and multiplane transesophageal echocardiography in diagnosis of typical acute aortic dissection and intramural hematoma. J Am Coll Cardiol 1996;28:627.

19. Anju Sarupria, Poonam Malhotra Kapoor, Usha Kiran, Milind Hote, et al. Multiple ruptured aneurysm of left sinus of valsalva: A rare entity. Annals of Cardiac Anaesthesia 2011;14(1):48–50.

20. Sawyers JL, Adams JE, Scott HW Jr. Surgical treatment for aneurysm of the aortic sinuses with aorticoatrial fistula. Surgery 1957;41:26.

21. Blaivas M, Sierzenski PR. Dissection of the proximal thoracic aorta: A new ultrasonographic sign in the subxiphoid view. Am J Emerg Med 2002;20:344.

22. Navin C Nanda, Ming Chon Hsiung, Andrew P Miller, Fadi G Hage, et al. Aortic valve and aorta. Live/Real Time 3D Echocardiography, 1st edn. 2010.

23. Xu Q, Peng Z, Rahko PS. Doppler echocardiographic characteristics of sinus of Valsalva aneurysms. Am Heart J 1995;130:1265–9.

24. Chiang CW, Lin FC, Fang BR, Kuo CT, Lee YS, Chang CH. Doppler and two dimensional echocardiographic features of sinus of Valsalva aneurysm. Am Heart J 1988;116:1283–8.

25. Cronenwett JL, Lindenaauer SM. Distribution of blood flow following aortic clamping and declamping.J Surg Res 1977; 22:469–82.

26. O' Conner CJ, Rothenber DM. Anaesthetic consideration for thoracic aortic surgery. Cardiothoracic Vasc Anaesth 1995;9:734.

# CHAPTER 8

# Ruptured Aortic Aneurysm

Vishwas Malik, Arun Subramaniam

## INTRODUCTION

Aortic aneurysms may leak or burst. The term ruptured or leaking aneurysm applies to the situation in which blood has escaped through the wall of the aortic aneurysm. Sometimes leaking aneurysm is ascribed to the condition when the blood escapes from the aneurysm but hemodynamics are still stable and rupture is referred to a situation when the blood pressure is low and patient presents in shock due to the leakage of blood from the aneurysm resulting in major blood loss.

The risk of an aneurysm rupturing varies with the aneurysm size. The larger the aortic aneurysm the more risk of rupture (Fig. 8.1). Small aneurysms less than 5.5 cm in diameter have an annual risk of rupture of less than 1% (1 in 100). This means that a patient, with an aortic aneurysm less than 5.5 cm in diameter, has approximately 1 in 100 chance of it bursting over the next 12 months.

### Presentation

Rupture of thoracic aneurysm can be associated with excruciating chest pain or back pain. Patient might have difficulty in breathing or can lose consciousness as a result of decreased cerebral perfusion because of

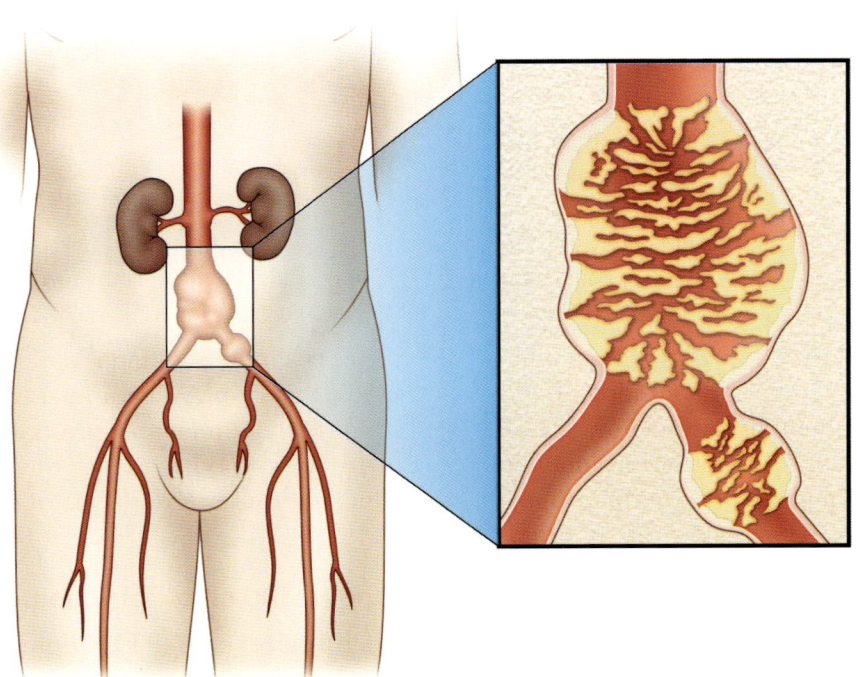

**Fig. 8.1:** Pictorial representation of large aneurysm

exsanguination. Thoracic aortic aneurysm most commonly ruptures in pleural space or mediastinum resulting in hypotension. Less commonly it can rupture in adjacent structures resulting in aortoesophageal or aortobronchial fistula presenting as hematemesis or hemoptysis respectively (Fig. 8.2).

A ruptured aneurysm of abdominal aorta usually occurs in patients older than 60 years and in men more commonly than women (because men are more likely to have an aneurysm). The classic presentation of a ruptured abdominal aortic aneurysm AAA is the sudden onset of abdominal or back pain in association with an episode of syncope or hypotension and a pulsatile abdominal mass. However, this combination of symptoms and signs is not always present and misdiagnosis or delayed diagnosis is common. Pain may have been present for days or weeks before presentation or may not be apparent, particularly in patients presenting with confusion or an impaired conscious level. Blood pressure may be normal on admission and palpation of the aneurysm may be difficult if the patient is obese. Other symptoms such as vomiting and dizziness may be present. On the other hand, a patient with a AAA which has not ruptured who has another cause of abdominal or back pain or shock such as cholecystitis or a myocardial infarction may mistakenly be thought to have a ruptured aneurysm.

Occasionally abdominal aortic aneurysm rupture into the inferior vena cava to produce an aortocaval fistula or into the bowel, resulting in an aortoenteric fistula.

An aortocaval fistula may be diagnosed before surgery from clinical signs of venous engorgement, high output cardiac failure and a continuous 'machinery' abdominal murmur or thrill, or on CT scan or it may be a surprise finding during surgery. A primary aortoenteric fistula occurs when the aneurysm erodes into bowel, usually into adherent duodenum. A secondary aortoenteric fistula is a complication of previous aortic surgery and usually there is erosion of the proximal aortic suture line into the duodenum. In both types, minor episodes of gastrointestinal hemorrhage may occur initially followed by massive exsanguinating hemorrhage hours to weeks later.

A portable ultrasound examination in the emergency department can confirm the presence of an aneurysm but is not a reliable guide as to whether an aneurysm has ruptured. In the past it was considered inappropriate to undertake a CT scan of the abdomen if there was a high suspicion of a ruptured AAA because the delay caused by the investigation may result in the patient's condition deteriorating and death occurring before surgery. However, now that many emergency departments have CT scanners in or immediately beside the department, a CT scan can often be undertaken very quickly and if endovascular repair of a ruptured AAA is contemplated, a preoperative CT scan is usually required to decide if that approach is possible and to plan the procedure. Specific signs on CT include 'high attenuating crescent' sign and (Fig. 8.3A) 'draped aorta' sign (Fig. 8.3B).

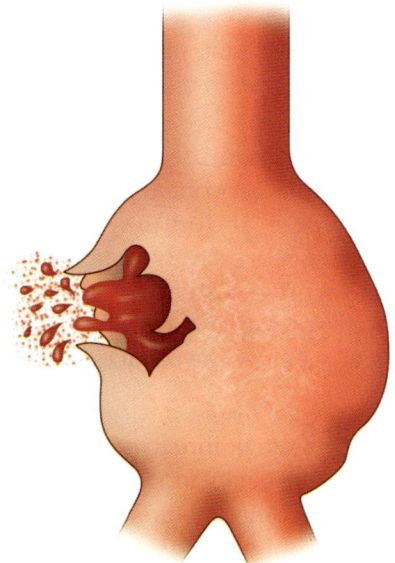

**Fig. 8.2:** Pictorial representation of ruptured aneurysm

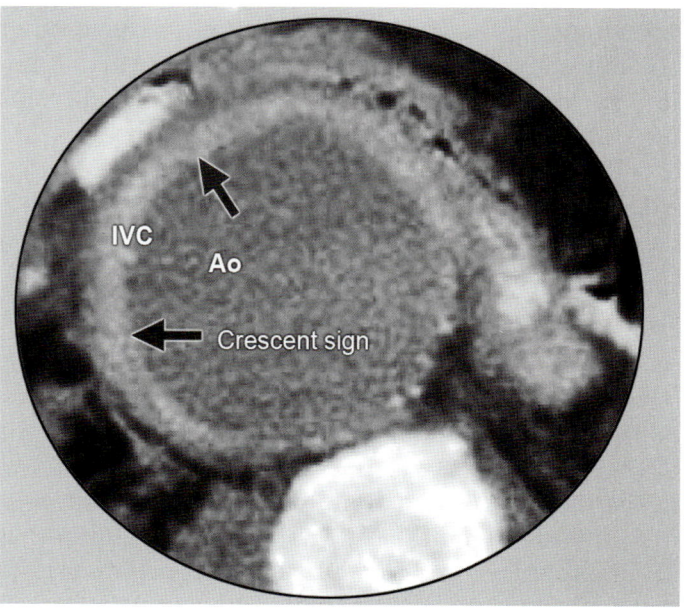

**Fig. 8.3A:** Crescent sign

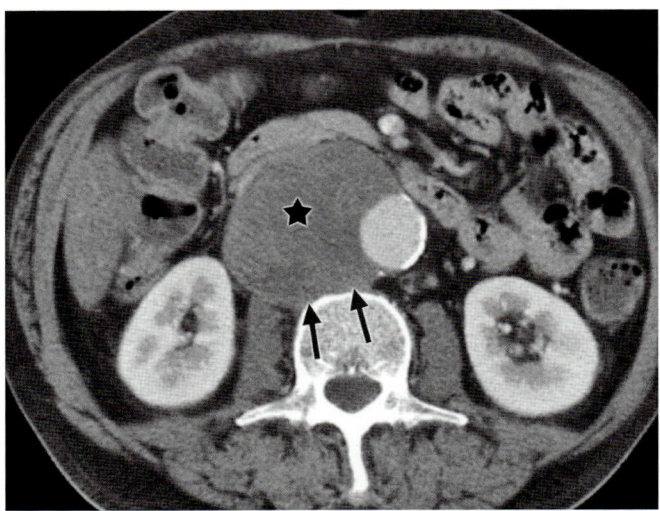

**Fig. 8.3B:** Draped aorta sign

## Management

Planning for anesthesia and repair of ruptured aortic aneurysm is one of the most challenging situations faced by an anesthesiologist. Anesthesia and surgery are very urgent. The patient is usually elderly and often has cardiac, respiratory or renal disease but the information available is frequently incomplete and the time for assessment and investigations is very limited.

When an aneurysm reaches 5.5 cm most surgeons would consider offering surgical intervention. This is because, at this size, the aneurysm has a greater risk of rupture. It then becomes as safe to have an operation to repair the aneurysm, as it is to leave the aneurysm alone. Surgery may also be considered if aneurysm is rapidly growing on regular scans or it starts to cause other complications. Rapid expansion means more than 7 mm in 6 months or 10 mm in one year. Aortic aneurysms are painless but become tender before rupture.

## MANAGEMENT OPTIONS

There are three options for management of a ruptured aortic aneurysm:
1. Open surgical repair
2. Endovascular repair
3. Conservative management, i.e. palliative care.

The patient may have been previously assessed for elective repair of an asymptomatic aneurysm and the decision made at that time that the risks of surgery exceeded the benefits. It does not necessarily follow that an attempt to repair the aneurysm is inappropriate now that it has ruptured. Rupture of an aneurysm is almost always fatal if repair is not undertaken so the balance of risk and benefit may now be very different.

However, repair of ruptured aneurysm is associated with a high rate of death and complications and may be considered inappropriate in some patients for example:
- Patients with underlying medical conditions that preclude any significant long-term survival (e.g. terminal cancer)
- Patients with underlying conditions that already result in poor quality of life (e.g. demented elderly patients)
- Patients in whom a combination of age, comorbidity, clinical presentation and, when known, aneurysm extent (i.e. suprarenal or thoracoabdominal aneurysm) makes survival with a reasonable quality of life appear unlikely.

Various scoring systems have been used as an aid to predicting the outcome of ruptured abdominal aortic aneurysm (AAA) repair.[1] Those that rely on the results of laboratory investigations such as serum creatinine have the disadvantage that the required information may not be available at the time, the decision as to whether or not to attempt to repair the aneurysm is made. Incorporating preoperative hemoglobin into a score is less of a problem because point of care measurement of hemoglobin is commonly available in the emergency department. An example of such a scoring system, the Edinburgh Ruptured Aneurysm (ERA) score, is shown in Table 8.1.

In a prospective study of several scoring systems, 27 of 111 patients with a diagnosis of ruptured AAA did not undergo attempted operative repair.[1] In 13 of these cases the reason for not attempting repair was refractory cardiac arrest/loss of consciousness. The remaining 84 patients underwent open surgery. The 30-day or in-hospital mortality was 26% in patients with an ERA score of 1, 59% in patients with a score of 2 and 82% in patients with a score of 3.

The commonest operation for a ruptured AAA is open surgery with a transperitoneal approach through a midline or transverse abdominal incision to an aneurysm that has ruptured retroperitoneally. The posterior peritoneum, often distended with hematoma, is exposed before dissecting and clamping the neck of the aneurysm–usually below the renal arteries. There is

**Table 8.1:** Edinburgh ruptured aneurysm (ERA) score.[1] One point is allocated for each preoperative variable that fulfils the criterion resulting in a score of between 0 and 3 points

| Preoperative variable | Score |
| --- | --- |
| Hemoglobin <9 g/dl | 1 |
| Best recorded in-hospital Glasgow Coma Scale of <15 | 1 |
| Recorded in-hospital blood pressure of <90 mm Hg | 1 |

a risk of tearing the left renal vein or its tributaries during the dissection and the resulting venous bleeding can be difficult or impossible to control. Sometimes the aorta is clamped above the renal arteries or above the coeliac axis. After clamping the neck of the aneurysm, both common iliac arteries are clamped, the aneurysm is opened and its contents evacuated. Bleeding occurs from the orifices of lumbar arteries in the posterior wall of the aneurysm and these are oversewn. The inferior mesenteric artery, if patent, is usually tied off. A prosthetic tube or Y-shaped graft is sutured end-to-end to the neck of the aneurysm to form the top anastomosis, then a clamp is applied to the graft and the upper aortic clamp is removed to test the anastomosis. The lower end of the graft is then sutured to the aortic bifurcation in the case of a tube graft, or in the case of a Y-graft to the bifurcation of each common iliac artery. The graft is thoroughly flushed to remove any clot before the lower anastomosis is completed and the clamps on the iliac arteries are released one side at a time.

*Endovascular repair* of ruptured AAAs has become a common technique in some centers in recent years. A contrast-enhanced CT scan is usually undertaken to determine if endovascular repair is possible and the size of the stent-graft(s) required. At the start of the procedure a balloon may be inserted via the femoral artery into the supracoeliac aorta and inflated to produce temporary control of bleeding until the stent-graft is deployed. Two types of stent-graft are available for this procedure (Fig. 8.4).

Modular bifurcated stent-grafts may be used, as are commonly used for elective endovascular repair. A main aortic body with ipsilateral iliac leg is inserted through one femoral artery. The other iliac leg is inserted through the contralateral femoral artery and attached to the main body to form a Y-shaped graft. It is necessary to have a large variety of sizes of the modular stent-graft components in stock to ensure that suitable sizes are immediately available. Alternatively, an aorto-uni-iliac stent-graft can be inserted through one femoral artery to exclude the aneurysm from the circulation. This may be inserted more quickly than a bifurcated stent-graft and a smaller selection of graft sizes needs to be stocked. However, after insertion of an aorto-uni-iliac stent it is necessary to occlude the contralateral iliac artery to prevent retrograde flow into the aneurysm sac and then an open surgical femoro-femoral bypass graft is required to restore the circulation to the contralateral leg.

*Conventional open surgery* is typically associated with an operative (30-day or in-hospital) mortality rate of

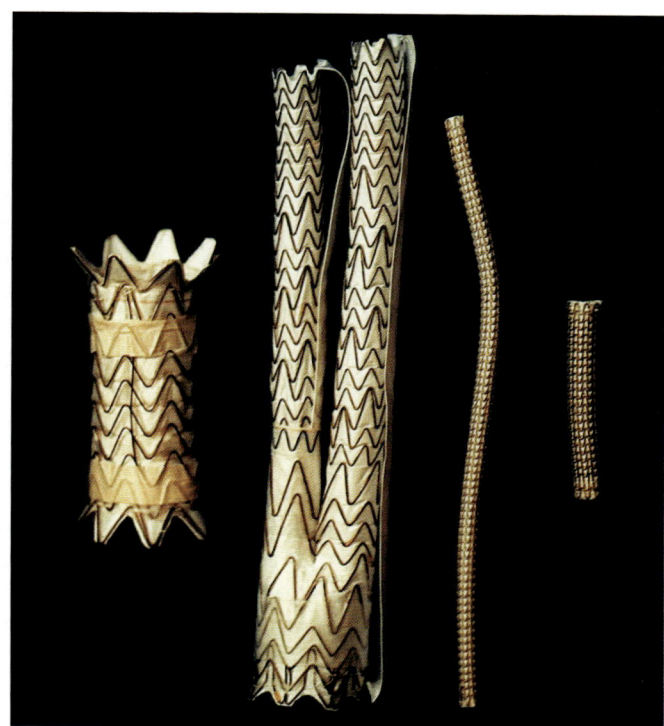

**Fig. 8.4:** Types of endovascular grafts

around 40–50%. This figure is affected by a hospital's policy on the selection of patients for surgery and tends to be higher in units that operate on almost all patients with ruptured aneurysms than in those that elect not to operate on moribund patients. A number of case series of endovascular repair of ruptured AAA report lower mortality rates than this. However, patients selected for endovascular repair were typically hemodynamically stable and had 'favourable anatomy' for endovascular repair, i.e. with an infrarenal neck of the aneurysm long enough for the top of the stent-graft to obtain a seal and without severe iliac artery disease. These factors would also tend to result in a lower mortality rate for open surgical repair. Some centers have reported reduced overall mortality rates after adopting a policy of endovascular repair for suitable patients with ruptured AAA.[2,3] However, there may be publication bias with hospitals whose results improve being more likely to publish than those whose results remain unchanged or get worse.

## PREOPERATIVE ASSESSMENT

When it has been decided that surgery should be undertaken to repair a suspected ruptured aortic aneurysm, the patient should be transferred to the operating room as quickly as possible because their condition may rapidly deteriorate at any moment leading to cardiorespiratory arrest. Investigations should not delay transfer to theatre except when it has been decided that an emergency CT scan is appropriate. Preparation should include arterial cannula or central venous catheter insertion. Oxygen should be given by face-mask and at least one large peripheral intravenous cannula inserted if possible in the emergency department. Blood samples should be taken when the cannula is inserted for a full blood count, coagulation screen, urea and electrolytes and glucose and for blood transfusion but there is no need to wait for the results of blood tests before surgery. If point of care testing is available, rapid results of, for example, the hemoglobin concentration may be obtained. Blood components, e.g. 10 units of red cells, 4 units of fresh frozen plasma (FFP) and 2 standard adult doses of platelets, should be requested for issue as soon as possible. An ECG and portable chest X-ray and insertion of a urethral catheter can be performed very quickly in most emergency departments and may well already have been done by the time, the decision is made that the patient should have surgery.

If not, they *should not be allowed to delay transfer to operation room.* A brief assessment of the patient should be undertaken before or during transfer to theatre. A history of the previous state of health and any drugs being taken (e.g. oral anticoagulants or dual antiplatelet therapy) may be obtained from the patient, relatives or any case notes that are available. A brief clinical examination should include assessment of the heart rate and rhythm, blood pressure, peripheral perfusion, conscious level, whether dentures are present and whether there is likely to be any difficulty with tracheal intubation. Vascular surgery patients may have a significant difference in blood pressure between the two arms, usually because of a subclavian artery stenosis, and if this is the case the higher reading should be regarded as being correct.[4] The results of any investigations that are available should be reviewed. A chest X-ray may reveal that the aneurysm extends to involve the thoracic aorta. Analgesia may be required if the patient is in severe pain and small doses of intravenous fentanyl are appropriate in this situation. However, shocked elderly patients may be very sensitive to the effects of opioids which may decrease blood pressure, depress conscious level and result in airway obstruction. Therefore, the aim should be to relieve severe pain while getting the patient to theatre as quickly as possible, rather than making the patient completely comfortable, unless it has been decided that surgery is inappropriate.

**Patients with ruptured aortic aneurysm presenting for aortic surgery may be very unstable hemodynamically because of ongoing hemorrhage, cardiac tamponade, myocardial ischemia, or congestive heart failure.** Organ malperfusion is also a major problem. It is therefore recommended that patients who present for emergency aortic surgery is intensively monitored to control blood pressure and resuscitate appropriately.

Emergency operations are independent risk factors for major complications, and therefore these remain high-risk procedures even with an optimal preoperative evaluation.

**When surgery is required on an urgent basis, and thus preoperative optimization of the patient is not always feasible.** Large-bore intravenous access is extremely important in aortic surgery. Aortic rupture may always occur, and the ability to rapidly infuse intravenous fluids, blood or blood products is necessary. One or 2 large-bore peripheral intravenous lines are recommended along with some form of central venous access. Because the left innominate vein may be injured or intentionally divided during aortic arch surgery, left-side intravenous access should be avoided if aortic arch repair is anticipated. A rapid infusion system with a heat exchanger should be immediately available. Blood should also be immediately available and possibly even primed through the rapid infusion system.

**Coagulopathy** commonly occurs during and after descending thoracic aortic aneurysm repair. The causes include dilutional coagulopathy, qualitative platelet dysfunction, heparin effects, and fibrinolysis. The extensive product and fluid requirements of descending thoracic aortic aneurysm repairs may approach several blood volumes. Qualitative and quantitative platelet deficiencies are the most common cause of perioperative bleeding, most likely attributable to extracorporeal circulation and hypothermia.

**Antifibrinolytic agents** should be considered during the perioperative period. Compared with placebo, tranexamic acid use during thoracic aortic surgery decreases perioperative bleeding with subsequent reduction erythrocyte and total amount of allogeneic transfusion. No increased risk of thrombotic complications has been observed. Aprotinin is a nonspecific serine protease activity and inhibits plasmin, thrombin, trypsin, and tissue and plasma kallikrein. In addition, aprotinin prevents activation of platelet thrombin receptors (PAR-1,3,4,) and the platelet glycoprotein receptors (GPIb,IIa and GPIIbIIIa).

## PREOPERATIVE FLUID RESUSCITATION

It is common practice to avoid or restrict giving intravenous fluids to a patient with a ruptured aortic aneurysm until anesthesia is induced and surgery is about to start even if the patient is hypotensive. The rationale for this **'permissive hypotension' or 'hypotensive resuscitation'** is that after initial bleeding from the aortic aneurysm, clot formation, retroperitoneal tamponade and hypotension may be important in limiting further hemorrhage.

Fluid resuscitation to restore blood pressure before the aorta is clamped may dislodge clot and overcome tamponade. It may result in further hemorrhage and in dilutional anemia and coagulopathy. There have been no randomised trials of preoperative fluid resuscitation (nor of anesthetic techniques) in ruptured aortic aneurysm patients. However, a randomised trial in hypotensive patients with penetrating torso injuries found that mortality and complication rates were reduced by not giving intravenous fluid until the patients reached the operating room.[5] Animal models of aortic hemorrhage have also provided support for a policy of hypotensive resuscitation.[6] In practice, hypotensive resuscitation may involve either maintaining an arbitrary minimum value of blood pressure, e.g. a systolic of 70 mm Hg, or not giving any intravenous fluids unless hypotension is producing cerebral or myocardial ischemia. It is essential that any delay before surgery is minimized to avoid a prolonged period of preoperative hypotension. If intravenous fluids are given before surgery red cells may need to be given as well as clear fluids to avoid a severe dilutional anemia.

## MANAGEMENT IN THE OPERATING THEATRE: OPEN REPAIR

General anesthesia is required for open repair of a ruptured aneurysm and the insertion of an epidural catheter before surgery is not appropriate. The patient should be transferred directly into the operating room as rapidly as possible and not into an anesthetic induction room. Anesthesia is usually induced after the surgeons have disinfected and draped the parts so that the operation can start as soon as the patient is asleep. Occasionally tracheal intubation is required before this for airway protection or to assist ventilation in the unconscious moribund patient and if surgery is considered appropriate in this situation little anesthesia may be required before aortic clamping.

### Preparation

Two experienced anesthesiologists are required for satisfactory management of the patient (Table 8.2). Red cells should be in the operating theatre ready to transfuse before anesthesia is induced, but surgery should not be delayed by waiting for blood grouping, antibody screens or cross-matching. In emergency group O blood should be used if group-specific blood is not yet available. Invasive blood pressure monitoring at the time of induction is useful because severe hypotension may occur at this stage and progress to cardiac arrest. If an arterial cannula is in place before induction a sample may be withdrawn for point-of-care testing of hemoglobin.

The arterial cannula should be inserted in an upper limb artery, usually radial or brachial. However, if the blood pressure is low, it may be difficult to insert an arterial cannula and prolonged attempts should not be allowed to significantly delay surgery. It is desirable to position one or both of the upper limbs on arm boards perpendicular to the body so that there is access during surgery to existing intravenous and arterial cannulae or for the insertion of new ones. If a urethral catheter is not already in place it may be inserted before induction. A central venous catheter is not required before surgery unless, it has proved impossible to insert a large peripheral venous cannula, in which case a large central venous catheter is useful. Depth of anesthesia monitoring of both induction and maintenance of anesthesia is a useful aid to avoiding awareness while not giving unnecessarily large doses of anesthetic agents. A shocked elderly patient may require much lower doses of anesthetic than are typically used.

### Induction

A rapid sequence induction should be performed. Etomidate or ketamine are appropriate for induction if the patient is hypotensive; thiopentone may be considered if the blood pressure is normal. The use of propofol for induction is not appropriate. Unless the patient has already received opioid analgesia or is profoundly hypotensive, intravenous opioid should be

**Table 8.2:** Minimum requirements for satisfactory management of the start of anesthesia for ruptured aortic aneurysm

Two anesthesiologists

At least one, preferably two, large intravenous cannulae

Rapid fluid infuser and warmer

Red cell concentrate in theatre

Anesthetic drugs for rapid sequence induction

Monitoring: five-lead ECG and ST segments, blood pressure, pulse oximetry

Vasoconstrictor/inotrope drugs, e.g. syringes of ephedrine, phenylephrine, and epinephrine 1 in 100 000 given before induction to reduce the risk of a hypertensive response to laryngoscopy causing further bleeding. Fentanyl is appropriate but morphine should be avoided because renal failure may occur, impairing the excretion of the active metabolite morphine-6-glucuronide. A large fall in blood pressure may occur on induction because of vasodilation, reduction in sympathetic tone and circulating catecholamine levels, reduced venous return secondary to positive pressure ventilation and abdominal muscle relaxation reducing tamponade and allowing further bleeding. The anesthetist should aim to maintain the blood pressure around the preinduction level (unless the pre induction blood pressure was considered to be unacceptably low), avoiding or correcting large falls in pressure but not raising the blood pressure of a patient who was hypotensive before induction to normal until the aorta is clamped. Rapid infusion of fluids and sometimes also the administration of vasoconstrictor or inotrope drugs may be required to maintain the blood pressure at an acceptable level. If the hypotension is severe the operating table should be tilted head down and only gentle positive pressure ventilation given. If continuous invasive blood pressure monitoring is not possible at induction, palpation of the carotid pulse and observation of the capnography trace may give an early indication of a profound fall in blood pressure and cardiac output. Rapid infusion of clear fluids can very quickly result in a severe dilutional anemia. Therefore, unless the hemoglobin concentration is known to be high, red cells should also be given.

## Maintenance

Surgery may commence as soon as the patient is unconscious. If suxamethonium was given for muscle relaxation during induction, a non-depolarising relaxant should be given as soon as the tracheal tube is in place. Maintenance of anesthesia may be either with a volatile anesthetic or a propofol infusion. A low concentration of volatile anesthetic/low target concentration or infusion rate of propofol will be appropriate initially if the blood pressure is low and depth of anesthesia monitoring is very useful for guiding appropriate adjustment. Once the surgeon has clamped the aorta, blood pressure usually rises and the aim should now be to maintain a blood pressure around normal. Severe hypertension and/or signs of myocardial ischemia may require treatment during aortic clamping. Further opioid analgesia and an increase in the depth of anesthesia may be given as may specific treatment with an intravenous beta-blocker or an infusion of glyceryl trinitrate (GTN). Intravenous beta-blocker may be given if tachycardia is associated with ECG signs of ischemia.

## Monitoring

Additional monitoring that is recommended during emergency aortic surgery is shown in Table 8.2. If not already in place an arterial cannula, central venous catheter, nasogastric tube and nasopharyngeal temperature probe should now be inserted. Central venous pressure (CVP) monitoring is of limited value in determining how much intravenous fluid is required.[7] While a low CVP during surgery suggests hypovolemia, CVP may also be normal or high in this situation. Other monitors of cardiac output or filling or aortic flow are more useful as a guide to intravenous fluid administration. Examples include pulse contour analysis of the arterial pressure waveform, transoesophageal echocardiography and esophageal Doppler. Pulse contour analysis has the advantage of being quick to set up and not requiring any additional probe to be inserted. The displayed absolute values of stroke volume and cardiac output are unlikely to be accurate in the presence of the marked hemodynamic changes that occur during aneurysm repair. However, the percentage increase in stroke volume in response to an intravenous fluid challenge may give a useful indication of whether hypovolemia is present, as may the pulse pressure variation or stroke volume variation over the respiratory cycle. Temperature should be monitored and attempts made to maintain or restore normothermia by raising the temperature in the operating room, warming intravenous fluids, forced-air warming of the upper body and under-body warming of the upper body, and ensuring the head is wrapped or covered. Warming of the lower limbs, which will be ischemic during the period of aortic clamping, should be avoided. Point-of-care monitoring of hemoglobin, coagulation, arterial gases and acid–base status, electrolytes and glucose is extremely useful in guiding the appropriate administration of blood components and the correction of acid–base and electrolyte abnormalities during surgery.

## Transfusion and Correction of Coagulopathy

Sufficient red cells should be transfused to avoid the development of severe anemia, e.g. the hemoglobin should be maintained above 8.0 g/dl. The use of intraoperative red cell salvage reduces the need for allogeneic blood transfusion. Patients having surgery for a suspected ruptured aortic aneurysm may have massive hemorrhage and severe coagulopathy, or a small contained rupture with little blood outside the aorta or indeed be found to have an aneurysm which hasn't in fact ruptured. There is, therefore, great variation in the presence and severity of abnormalities of hemostasis between patients and there may also be rapid changes during surgery. For example, a patient with a ruptured aortic aneurysm may have relatively normal coagulation at the start of surgery but develop a severe coagulopathy during the operation.

In general, the greater the blood loss and the greater the degree of shock, the more severely coagulation is impaired. It is not uncommon for elderly patients presenting with a ruptured AAA, particularly patients with atrial fibrillation, to be taking warfarin and this should be reversed with prothrombin complex concentrate.

Dual antiplatelet therapy, for example, with aspirin and clopidogrel, is another cause of excessive bleeding. Once the aorta is clamped, the surgeon may be able to assess whether or not there is diffuse microvascular bleeding. Point-of-care testing of coagulation with thromboelastometry/thromboelastography is extremely useful and permits the rapid identification and treatment of abnormalities such as a low fibrinogen concentration, thrombocytopenia or excessive fibrinolysis. If there are clinical signs of severe coagulopathy with diffuse bleeding and point-of-care testing is not available, it is preferable to treat the problem empirically, e.g. with transfusions of FFP and platelets, rather than waiting for laboratory results. Heparin is not usually given to patients with a ruptured aortic aneurysm if the clinical picture is of significant bleeding and impaired coagulation or if point-of-care testing indicates a coagulopathy. However, if there has been little blood loss and there is no evidence of impaired coagulation clinically or on point-of-care testing, intravenous heparin may be given before aortic clamping.

## Renal Function

Renal dysfunction is common after ruptured AAA repair. In addition to the causes of renal dysfunction after elective aneurysm repair, there may also have been a period of preoperative renal ischemia as a result of hemorrhagic shock. Measures that reduce the incidence or severity of renal dysfunction are avoiding or minimising the duration of suprarenal aortic clamping, maintaining an adequate blood pressure and cardiac output (after any initial period of permissive hypotension) by giving sufficient intravenous fluid, and the avoidance of nephrotoxic drugs. No specific pharmacological measures have been shown to be of benefit.

## CLAMP RELEASE

A large fall in blood pressure may occur when the iliac clamps are released, reperfusing the ischemic pelvis and lower limbs. Cardiac arrest may occur at this stage. The hypotension results from a combination of hypovolemia as the vasodilated vessels of the lower body are refilled with blood (and bleeding from anastomoses may also occur), and the effects of ischemic metabolites returning from the lower body causing pulmonary hypertension and reduced myocardial contractility (Fig. 8.5). Intravenous fluid loading before clamp release reduces the fall in blood pressure. It is important that the surgeon gives the anesthetist advance warning of clamp release to permit fluid loading and so that the anaesthetist is ready to treat marked hypotension with further rapid intravenous fluid infusion and/or the intravenous injection of a vasoconstrictor/inotrope such as ephedrine. The clamps should be released slowly, reperfusing one leg at a time, and if the fall in blood pressure is excessive clamps may be reapplied or the iliac arteries temporarily compressed by the surgeon. Other changes that occur on clamp release include a temporary fall in oxygen saturation, an increase in arterial and end-tidal carbon dioxide concentration and a worsening of the metabolic acidemia that is usually already present. Minute ventilation should be increased provided that there is not severe hypotension. If there is little or no fall in blood pressure or rise in carbon dioxide when the circulation to a leg is restored, the possibility that blood flow to the limb is obstructed by thrombus or emboli should be considered. If the leg appears ischemic the surgeon may pass an embolectomy catheter into the femoral artery.

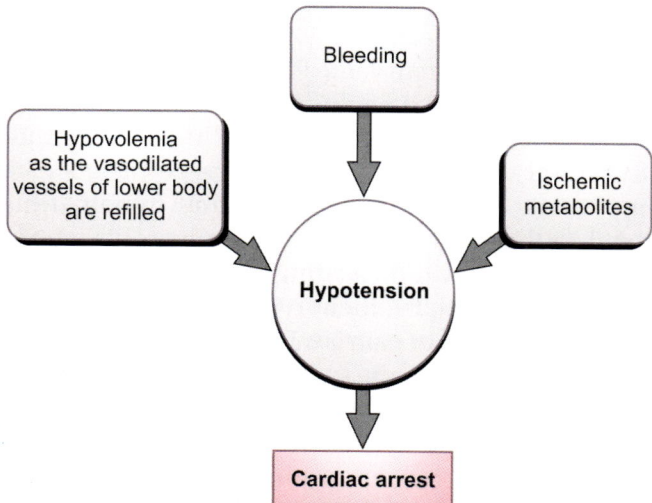

**Fig. 8.5:** Pathophysiology of clamp release

## ANESTHESIA FOR ENDOVASCULAR REPAIR OF RUPTURED ABDOMINAL AORTIC ANEURYSM

Endovascular repair of a ruptured abdominal aortic aneurysm may be undertaken under local (infiltration) anesthesia or general anesthesia. A combined technique may be used—the initial part of the procedure is performed under local anesthesia and then, after the stent-graft has been deployed and the patient is hemodynamically stable, general anesthesia is induced. If an aorto-uni-iliac stent-graft is deployed followed by a surgical femoro-femoral cross-over graft, the latter procedure is likely to be poorly tolerated by a patient under local anesthetic because of ischemic leg pain. The use of spinal or epidural anesthesia has been described but has the disadvantages that coagulopathy may increase the risk of an epidural hematoma and that the sympathetic block may worsen hypotension before surgery, resulting in intravenous fluid administration and in uncertainty about whether the fall in blood pressure is the result of the anesthetic or further bleeding from the aneurysm. Much of the discussion above about management of open AAA repair applies to management of endovascular repair. Permissive hypotension is commonly employed before deployment of the stent and any delay before repair of the aneurysm must be minimised. The assessment of blood loss and clinical assessment of coagulopathy is made more difficult when the abdomen has not been opened. Intravenous heparin is given in some centres and avoided in others. Whether the overall mortality and complication rate is reduced by endovascular repair of ruptured AAA is uncertain.

## POSTOPERATIVE COMPLICATIONS

### Cardiac Complications

Postoperative myocardial infarction (MI) is the most common cause of death following surgery for repair of ruptured aortic aneurysm. Predisposing factors for myocardial ischemia include pre-existing coronary artery disease, pain, mobilization of third-space fluid into central circulation, stress and hypermetabolism, sympathetic overactivity, anemia, and hypothermia. Added to the hemodynamic stress is hypofibrinolysis and thrombin activation leading to prothrombotic state and myocardial injury. Identifying perioperative MI is difficult because chest pain is infrequent (fewer than 50% of ischemic episodes are symptomatic) and disguised by analgesics. ECG is the mainstay of the diagnosis, but the changes may be subtle and transient. Most of the postoperative MIs are of the non-Q wave variety. Moderate elevations of creatinine kinase myocardial band fraction can occur in aortic surgical patients.

Cardiac troponin (TnI) elevation may be more specific. Elevated TnI has been demonstrated in 46% of the patients who survived ruptured aortic aneurysm repair and was associated with increased cardiac dysfunction and death.[1] In doubtful cases of perioperative MI, echocardiography and nuclear scans may help in diagnosis. Therapy of non-ST elevation MI includes oxygen, analgesics, nitrates, beta-blockers, angiotensin converting enzyme inhibitors, and anticoagulation with aspirin and heparin, when approved by the surgeon. An increased bleeding risk precludes the use of thrombolytics in the immediate postoperative period. Cardiology consultation is initiated immediately for percutaneous interventions, such as cardiac catheterization, angioplasty, stenting, or surgery in patients who still have ischemia despite maximal medical therapy. Intervention is required in all cases of ST elevation MI. Treatment of cardiogenic shock require invasive monitoring, such as a PAC with continuous cardiac output and mixed venous saturation monitoring and inotropic support.

### Pulmonary Complications

Various perioperative factors influence the development of respiratory failure after AAA repair (Box 8.1).

---

**Box 8.1**

**Preoperative factors**
1. Advanced age
2. Cigarette smoking
3. History of COPD
4. Morbid obesity
5. Abnormal pulmonary function tests (FEVI or FVC <70% predicted, Expiratory flow rate less than 200 ml/min)
6. Arterial blood gas ($PCO_2$ >45 mmHg on room air)

**Intraoperative factors**
1. Prolonged surgery
2. Large volume infusion
3. Large midline vertical incision
4. Transperitoneal approach

**Postoperative factors**
1. Abdominal distension from ileus
2. Inadequate analgesia
3. Large doses of parenteral narcotic administration
4. Hypothermia
5. Bed rest in supine position
6. Impaired cough and mucociliary clearance
7. Pneumonia

Pneumonia is usually caused by *Pseudomonas aeruginosa* and *Staphylococcus aureus* and associated with mortality of 21%. Pulmonary complications can be minimized by:

- Aggressive perioperative pulmonary toilet
- Lung expansion maneuvers, such as deep breathing exercises and incentive spirometry
- Antibiotics for pneumonia
- Epidural or paravertebral analgesia, which allow for early extubation and mobilization.[9]

## Renal Insufficiency

Pre-existing renal dysfunction with creatinine levels higher than 2 mg/dl is associated with operative mortality of 19% *versus* 4.2% mortality if the creatinine was less than 2 mg/dl.[10] Patients with creatinine levels more than 4 mg/dl require preoperative initiation of hemodialysis.[11] AAA may be associated with renal artery stenosis or ureteric obstruction, which should be evaluated preoperatively by renal ultrasound and excretory urography, respectively. The incidence of new onset of renal failure after infrarenal clamping is 3% and the rates for suprarenal occlusion are five times greater. Transient renal insufficiency is more common and patients who develop renal insufficiency have longer periods of intubation, ICU, and hospital length of stay. Aortic cross-clamping increases renal vascular resistance and decreases renal cortical blood flow and increases renin–angiotensin secretion and decreases glomerular filtration rate (GFR). Suprarenal clamping decreases blood flow by 80% and infrarenal clamping decreases by 38%. The incidence of renal failure following ruptured AAA repair ranges from 8 to 46% and is associated with a mortality of 57–97%.[12] Additional perioperative factors that contribute to the development of renal insufficiency are given below.

- Pre-existing cardiac disease
- Advanced age
- Contrast studies without proper hydration
- Suprarenal clamping
- Ischemic time >30 min
- Hypovolemia (due to fasting, bowel preparation, and blood loss)
- Hypotension
- Large volume transfusion
- Rhabdomyolysis
- Early reoperation
- Atheromatous plaque embolization.

Urine output does not correlate with GFR and oliguria does not predict postoperative renal insufficiency.

The incidence of postoperative renal insufficiency may be decreased by preventing hypovolemia, maintaining cardiac output, and by diagnosing and treating oliguria early.

## Neurologic Complications

The two major neurologic complications include spinal cord ischemia and postoperative cognitive dysfunction. Ruptured aneurysms produce significant hypotension, require supraceliac cross-clamping, and usually heparin is not used; all these factors predispose to Spinal Cord injury (SCI). SCI can occur with infrarenal and supra-renal aortic cross-clamps and with both surgery for AAA and aorto-iliac occlusive disease.[13] The low incidence of paraplegia after elective AAA surgery may be explained by the low level of clamping relative to the origin of arteria radicularis magna and the presence of adequate pelvic collaterals. In general, when the greater radicular artery is open and of normal size, the pelvic blood supply is of minor importance. When greater radicular artery is compromised, the pelvic blood supply becomes critically important. Interference of pelvic blood supply has to be avoided preventing significant hypotension, revascularization of internal iliac artery with a separate graft, and gentle surgical techniques to avoid embolization.[14] SCI after infrarenal AAA and iliac surgery has a poor prognosis and may be reversed by spinal fluid drainage.

## Gastrointestinal Complications

Paralytic ileus is the most common complication which is due to bowel manipulation and fluid sequestration. The return of GI function depends on the technique employed and the level of the clamp. GI function returns more rapidly with the retroperitoneal technique and infrarenal crossclamping. Infrarenal cross-clamping produces little effect on splanchnic blood flow compared to suprarenal or supraceliac cross-clamping. A rare (0.6–1%) but more devastating complication is ischemic colitis, which is associated with a higher mortality rate (50–75%). Ruptured AAA repair, ligation of a patent inferior mesenteric artery, marginal collateral circulation, and perioperative low flow state are risk factors. Inferior mesenteric stump pressure less than 40 mmHg and loss of mesenteric Doppler signals are predictors of the development of colonic ischemia. The risk is reduced by inferior mesenteric artery revascularization and ensuring the circulation is preserved through at least one internal iliac artery. Signs and symptoms of ischemic colitis include excessive fluid requirement, abdominal pain, fever, leukocytosis, diarrhea, and bloody stools. Nonsurgical treatment includes bowel rest, aggressive fluid resuscitation, and antibiotics. Surgical treatment is indicated for full thickness bowel necrosis.

## Hemorrhage

Hemorrhage is the second most common postoperative complication and is almost always the result of technical error. Continued hemorrhage increases transfusion requirements and mortality.

If the administration of platelets and clotting factors fail to improve the bleeding or if the TEG and coagulation studies are normal, the patient may require a reoperation to search for a surgical bleeding (Box 8.2). Patients undergoing repair of a ruptured AAA have a higher incidence of postoperative bleeding and hence re-explorations.

### Symptomatic Abdominal Aortic Aneurysm

A symptomatic AAA is one which is causing abdominal or back pain, is tender and is thought to be at a high risk of rupturing soon. Mortality rates from repair of symptomatic aneurysms are substantially higher than from elective aneurysm repair. The term, however, covers a spectrum of different presentations from the patient with a slightly tender aneurysm when seen at the outpatient clinic who the surgeon decides it is wise to admit with a view to repair on the next available elective operating list to a patient whose symptoms and signs may in fact be the result of a contained rupture. The appropriate anesthetic management will also vary, therefore, from management similar to that of an elective AAA repair to management similar to that of a ruptured aneurysm. The urgency with which surgery is planned may be a guide as to the likelihood that a contained rupture has already occurred or is imminent but may be influenced by factors other than the patient's condition—for example, by the surgeon's schedule and when the next available space on an elective list is available.

A CT scan will usually have been undertaken before repair of a symptomatic aneurysm but a contained rupture can sometimes be difficult to identify. An

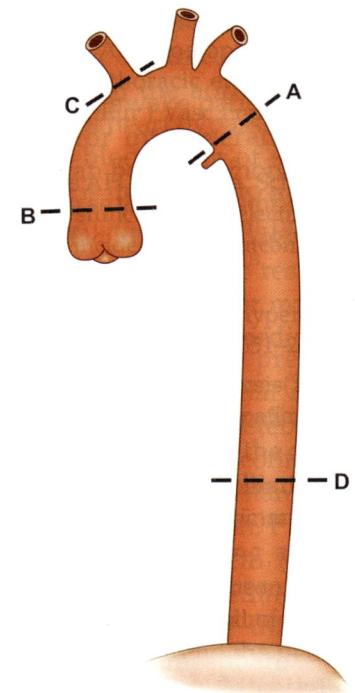

**Fig. 8.6:** Commonest site of aortic disruption—(A) Most common site adjacent to the ligamentum arteriosum. (B) Ascending aorta. (C) Avulson of the innominate artery from the aortic arch. (D) Lower descending aorta (*From Stene JK, Grande CM, Bernhard WN, et al. Perioperative anesthetic management of the trauma patient: thoracoabdominal and orthopaedic injuries. In: Stene JK, Grande CM, eds. Trauma anesthesia. Baltimore: Williams & Wilkins, 1991:218, with permission*)

important decision that the anesthsiologist managing a patient who is to have repair of a symptomatic aneurysm may have to make is whether or not to insert an epidural catheter before surgery. **If immediate surgery is planned, insertion of an epidural catheter may cause some delay and if local anesthetic (even a 'test dose') is injected through the catheter there is potential for confusion and misdiagnosis if hypotension then occurs because it may be the result of vasodilation from the epidural or of rupture of the aneurysm. Insertion of an epidural catheter is best avoided if the patient has had an episode of severe pain, syncope or hypotension and there is concern that this might have been the result of aneurysm rupture.** On the other hand, if there is no history of these events, the CT scan suggests that it is unlikely the aneurysm has ruptured and coagulation is normal, then insertion of an epidural catheter is reasonable.

## TRAUMATIC AORTIC DISRUPTION

During blunt chest trauma, abrupt deceleration of the thorax applies a shearing force to the aortic wall that is greatest at the origin of the subclavian artery and, in

| Box 8.2 | Surgical and nonsurgical causes of hemorrhage |

**Surgical causes of hemorrhage:**
1. Persistent retroperitoneal bleeding
2. Anastomotic disruption
3. Injury to adjacent venous structures

**Nonsurgical causes of hemorrhage:**
1. Dilutional coagulopathy
2. Disseminated intravenous coagulation
3. Preoperative anticoagulants, such as antiplatelet agents.

the ascending aorta, at the level of the coronary ostia. Traumatic disruption of the aorta is immediately fatal in approximately 85% of cases. A minority of patients survive because of containment and tamponade of the hemorrhage by adjacent mediastinal structures. Often the adventitia remains intact and prevents immediate exsanguination, but sudden aortic rupture may develop later. Alternatively, an intimal tear may be produced, with subsequent formation of a dissecting aneurysm. Occasionally patients are asymptomatic and remain undiscovered after injury, only to present with chronic traumatic aneurysm formation several years later. The causes and mechanism include steering wheel impact during a motor vehicle accident, penetrating trauma, crush injuries, and falls from great heights. The most common sites of traumatic aortic rupture are (a) just distal to the origin of the left subclavian artery at the ligamentum arteriosum (80 to 90%), (b) at the root of the aorta (with possible dissection back to the coronary ostia, (c) at the innominate artery (avulsion from the aortic arch), and (d) at the aortic hiatus at the level of the diaphragm.

Clinical findings of aortic rupture include the following diagnostic triad, which is seen in more than 50% of cases: (a) increased arterial blood pressure and pulse amplitude in the upper extremities, (b) decreased pressure and pulse amplitude in the lower extremities, and (c) a widened superior mediastinum on the chest radiograph (Table 8.3). Additional symptoms in the conscious patient include retrosternal or interscapular pain, dysphagia due to esophageal compression, ischemic extremity pain, dyspnea, and hoarseness due to recurrent laryngeal nerve dysfunction. Associated injuries may include the steering wheel imprint on the chest wall, massive hemothorax, cardiac contusion, rib fractures, and tension pneumothorax. Diagnosis should be suspected in trauma victims when the chest radiograph shows a widened superior mediastinum.

After confirming the diagnosis by *CT angiography*, surgical repair should be accomplished as soon as possible.

### Anesthetic Management

The usual anesthetic concerns of patients with multiple trauma needs to be applied for those with acute traumatic aortic rupture. These include the need for full-stomach precautions; the concern of associated injuries, the need for large-bore intravenous access; the need for massive transfusions of blood and coagulation factors; and the susceptibility to intraoperative hypothermia. The possibility of acute alcohol intoxication should also be kept in mind. In addition to the usual routine monitors, intraoperative invasive hemodynamic monitoring should include a right radial arterial line in case of descending traumatic aortic rupture and a left radial arterial line in case of ascending traumatic aortic rupture. In all, but the most emergent cases, PA catheterization is also desirable because proximal aortic occlusion imposes a severe afterload stress on the left ventricle and may precipitate left ventricular failure. In addition, monitoring of cardiac filling pressures guides intraoperative fluid management. Descending thoracic aortic tears are usually approached via a left thoracotomy. A DLT double lumen endotracheal tube is highly desirable to facilitate surgical exposure and to isolate the dependent right lung from the parenchymal hemorrhage that frequently occurs in the left lung as a result of surgical retraction. This can be a particularly serious problem in patients who are heparinized for femorofemoral bypass.

Surgical technique may consist of a simple clamp-and-sew technique, the use of a Gott shunt, partial CPB, or the use of an atriofemoral left heart centrifugal pump bypass. When methods that provide distal perfusion are to be employed, an additional arterial line in the femoral artery is helpful to monitor distal aortic perfusion pressure. The prevention of renal, spinal cord, and

| Table 8.3: Traumatic rupture of aorta | |
|---|---|
| *Clinical features* | *Radiographic features* |
| Increased arterial pressure and pulse amplitude of upper extremities | Widened mediastinum |
| | Unsharp aortic contours |
| | Opacified pulmonary window |
| Decreased arterial pressure and pulse amplitude of lower extremities | Broadened paratracheal stripe |
| Retrosternal or interscapular pain | Displacement of the left main stem bronchus |
| Hoarsesness | |
| Systolic flow murmur over the precordium or medial to the left scapula | Rightward deviation of the esophagus |
| Neurologic deficits in the lower extremities | Sternal and/or upper rib fractures |
| | Left hemothorax |

mesenteric ischemia follows similar guidelines as discussed earlier. The use of full CPB and DHCA for spinal cord protection has been described. The induction of anesthesia depends on the patient's mental status and the degree of hemodynamic instability as well as other associated injuries. Useful induction agents include etomidate or ketamine together with succinylcholine and rapid intubation of the trachea. Hypertension should be prevented during induction and intubation in order to avoid the free rupture of a previously contained aortic tear. Maintenance of anesthesia is usually with a narcotic-oxygen-relaxant technique supplemented with low-dose volatile agents or benzodiazepines as tolerated by the patient's hemodynamic status. The patient remains intubated and ventilated postoperatively in the intensive care unit.

Injury is confined to the ascending aorta in fewer than 10% of patients with traumatic aortic rupture. These patients usually present with cardiac tamponade and may have concurrent involvement of the coronary arteries or the aortic valve. Repair of these lesions require median sternotomy, CPB, and cardioplegia for myocardial preservation. Frequently, when aortic cross-clamping is not possible, DHCA is used.

Survival after traumatic avulsion of the arch vessels is extremely rare, but successful repairs have been reported. Total CPB is initiated using femoral artery cannulation. Profound hypothermia is achieved, and repair of the arch is completed during a period of DHCA. The mortality rate may be as high as 30%, especially in patients with multiple associated injuries. Mortality is directly related to the injury severity score, the number of injured organ systems and the time from the accident to arrival at the emergency department, but it does not correlate directly with the time taken in the hospital to make a definitive diagnosis or to reach the operating room. Advanced age and preoperative hypotension are risk factors for intraoperative death.

## Points to Remember

- Ruptured abdominal aneurysm is an emergency necessitating utmost priority on hospital admission.
- A majority of patients are elderly with a multitude of comorbid conditions.
- Sudden onset abdominal pain with hypotension is the commonest presentation.
- Modern day CT scanners can aid in a rapid diagnosis of a ruptured aneurysm.
- The presence of more than one experienced anesthetist is mandatory during such procedure.
- All patients are considered full stomach, so a rapid sequence/modified rapid sequence induction is mandatory.
- Hypotensive resuscitation has a place in limiting further hemorrhage prior to laparotomy.
- Sufficient blood and blood products must be available at the time of surgery.
- Traumatic aortic disruption commonly occurs at the origin of subclavian artery in ascending aorta and is fatal in 85% of cases.
- Postoperatively, myocardial infarction is the commonest complication followed by hemorrhage.

## REFERENCES

1. Tambyraja AL, Lee AJ, Murie JA, Chalmers RT. Prognostic scoring in ruptured abdominal aortic aneurysm: A prospective evaluation. J Vasc Surg 2008;47:282–6.
2. Moore R, Nutley M, Cina CS, et al. Improved survival after introduction of an emergency endovascular therapy protocol for ruptured abdominal aortic aneurysms. J Vasc Surg 2007;45:443–50.
3. Wibmer A, Schoder M, Wolff KS, et al. Improved survival after abdominal aortic aneurysm rupture by offering both open and endovascular repair. Arch Surg 2008;143:544–9.
4. Frank SM, Norris EJ, Christopherson R, Beattie C. Right- and left-arm blood pressure discrepancies in vascular surgery patients. Anesthesiology 1991;75:457–63.
5. Bickell WH, Wall MJ, Jr, Pepe PE, et al. Immediate versus delayed fluid resuscitation for hypotensive patients with penetrating torso injuries. N Engl J Med 1994;331:1105–9.
6. Roberts K, Revell M, Youssef H, Bradbury AW, Adam DJ. Hypotensive resuscitation in patients with ruptured abdominal aortic aneurysm. Eur J Vasc Endovasc Surg 2006; 31:339–44.
7. Gelman S. Venous function and central venous pressure: a physiologic story. Anesthesiology 2008;108:735–48.
8. Djavani Gidlund K, Wanhainen A, Björck M. Intra-abdominal hypertension and abdominal compartment syndrome after endovascular repair of ruptured abdominal aortic aneurysm. Eur J Vasc Endovasc Surg 2011;41:747.
9. Ghansah JN, Murphy JT. Complications of major aortic and lower extremity vascular surgery. Semin Cardiothorac Vasc Anesth 2004;8:335–61.
10. Sladen RN, Endo E, Harrison T. Two hour versus 22-hour creatinine clearance in critically ill patients. Anesthesiology 1987;67:1013–1016.
11. Luft FC, Hamburger RJ, Dyer JK, Szwed JJ, Kleit SA. Acute renal failure following operation for aortic aneurysm. Surg Gynecol Obstet 1975;141:374–8.
12. Sakalihasan N, Limet R, Defawe OD. Abdominal aortic aneurysm. Lancet 2005;365:1577–89.
13. Rosenthal D. Risk factors for spinal cord ischemia after abdominal aortic operations. Is it preventable? J Vasc Surg 1999;30:391–399.
14. Cambria RP, Brewster DC, Abbott WM, et al. Transperitoneal versus retroperitoneal approach for aortic reconstruction: A randomized prospective study. J Vasc Surg 1990;11: 314–324.

# CHAPTER 9

# Anesthesia for Peripheral Vascular Revascularization

Suruchi Hasija, Palleti Rajashekar

## PERIPHERAL VASCULAR DISEASE

The problem of peripheral vascular disease (PVD) is considerable. Up to 5% men and 2.5% women older than 60 years have symptoms of PVD.[1] It is usually accompanied by severe multi-system atherosclerosis. The anesthetic management of patients presenting for lower limb revascularization is challenging as they are invariably elderly with limited physical reserve and coexisting medical issues such as hypertension, diabetes mellitus, coronary artery disease (CAD), cerebrovascular disease, renal vascular disease and chronic obstructive pulmonary disease.

## ACUTE ISCHEMIA OF THE LOWER EXTREMITIES

Acute ischemia of the lower extremities may be caused by embolism, thrombosis, trauma, vasospasm or iatrogenic (e.g. after percutaneous vascular interventions). Thrombosis is more commonly implicated in acute arterial occlusion than embolism. The origin of the embolus may be cardiac (85%) or extracardiac (5%). It may arise from an atrial thrombus (associated with atrial fibrillation and mitral stenosis), ventricular thrombus [associated with myocardial infarction (MI), left ventricular aneurysm or dilated cardiomyopathy], prosthetic heart valve, infective endocarditis, left atrial myxoma, tumour, aortic/peripheral aneurysm, aortic mural thrombus, migrated atherosclerotic plaque, paradoxical venous embolus or iatrogenic during angiography, angioplasty, placement of stent, endograft or intra-aortic balloon pump. The constellation of clinical findings in acute lower limb ischemia includes pain, paresthesia, pallor, pulselessness, paralysis and poikilothermia.

The clinical categories of acute limb ischemia have been classified by the Society of Vascular Surgeons (Table 9.1).[2] These patients do not allow enough time for extensive preoperative evaluation. Nevertheless, their medical condition must be optimized within the available time. In striking contrast to chronic limb ischemia, blood flow must be restored within 4 to 6 hours to salvage the limb. Hematocrit, platelet count, serum electrolytes, prothrombin time, activated partial thromboplastin time (PTT) and electrocardiogram must be sought whenever possible. If time permits, an echocardiogram must be obtained to rule out cardiac source of the embolus. The localization of obstruction is aided by ultrasound Doppler, angiography, contrast computed tomography and magnetic resonance angiography.

Anticoagulation with heparin, intra-arterial thrombolysis, surgical embolectomy, angioplasty, stenting or bypass grafting comprise the therapeutic options available for acute limb ischemia. Systemic heparinization (100 U/kg followed by 1000 U/hr infusion) is initiated immediately with the target PTT maintained between 60 and 80 seconds in order to prevent propagation of thrombus and further embolization. The sites of occlusion by an arterial embolus are aortoiliac, popliteal and superficial femoral in decreasing order of frequency. Proximal emboli are amenable to catheter embolectomy whereas distal emboli require thrombolysis. An attempt must be made to achieve catheter-directed thrombolysis (with streptokinase/antistreplase/urokinase/tissue plasminogen activator/alteplase/reteplase/tenecteplase) or percutaneous mechanical thrombectomy unless the situation is immediately limb threatening, where surgical intervention is indicated. In this regard, patients in

**Table 9.1:** Clinical categories of acute limb ischemia[2]

| Category | Description/Prognosis | Findings | | Doppler signals | |
|---|---|---|---|---|---|
| | | Sensory loss | Muscle weakness | Arterial | Venous |
| I. Viable | Not immediately threatened | None | None | Audible | Audible |
| II. Threatened; | | | | | |
|   a. Marginally | Salvageable if promptly treated | Minimal (toes) or none | None | (Often) inaudible | Audible |
|   b. Immediately | Salvageable with immediate revascularization | More than toes, associated with rest pain | Mild, moderate | (Usually) inaudible | Audible |
| III. Irreversible | Major tissue loss or permanent nerve damage inevitable | Profound, anesthetic | Profound, paralysis | Inaudible | Inaudible |

category I and caterogy IIa are managed by thrombolytic therapy. Patients in category IIb require an urgent operative intervention and those in category III require amputation of the affected limb.

Thrombolysis is performed under local anesthesia and monitored anesthesia care. The contraindications of thrombolysis are listed in Table 9.2. Its complications include intractable local hemorrhage necessitating surgical re-exploration, intracerebral hemorrhage, stroke, retroperitoneal hemorrhage, pseudoaneurysm, renal failure and gastrointestinal bleeding. Thrombolysis is successful in 50–80% cases.[3] Fasciotomy is performed in case of prolonged ischemia or development of compartment syndrome. Amputation becomes necessary in some patients with prolonged ischemia and non-viable extremity.

Embolectomy is usually performed under local anesthesia, and parentral sedation and analgesia. However, since these patients invariably have underlying medical disease, it is prudent to provide monitored anesthesia care. More invasive procedures are performed under general anesthesia. As this procedure is done on emergency basis, rapid sequence induction of anesthesia is preferred. Regional anesthesia is contraindicated in fully heparinized patients.

Once the artery is isolated, a Fogarty catheter is passed proximally and distally in the artery and the thrombus is extracted (Figs 9.1 and 9.2). Distal patency of the artery can be evidenced on the operating table by observing good back flow or by performing an arteriogram if available. In very small vessels in the lower limb one can perform direct popliteal cut down to gain access and then repair it using a patch from a homologous vein graft/polytetrafluoroethylene (PTFE) graft or performing bypass grafting of the affected segment. In cases where acute limb ischemia is due to

**Table 9.2:** Contrindications to thrombolysis[2]

**Absolute contrindications**
- Established cerebrovascular event (excluding transient ischemic attack within previous 2 months)
- Active bleeding diathesis
- Recent gastrointestinal bleeding (within previous 10 days)
- Neurosurgery (intracranial, spinal) within previous 3 months
- Intracranial trauma within previous 3 months

**Relative contrindications**
- Cardiopulmonary resuscitation within previous 10 days
- Major nonvascular surgery or trauma within previous 10 days
- Uncontrolled hypertension (systolic >180 mmHg or diastolic >110 mmHg)
- Puncture of noncompressible vessel
- Intracranial tumour
- Recent eye surgery

**Minor contraindications**
- Hepatic failure, particularly those with coagulopathy
- Bacterial endocarditis
- Pregnancy
- Diabetic hemorrhagic retinopathy

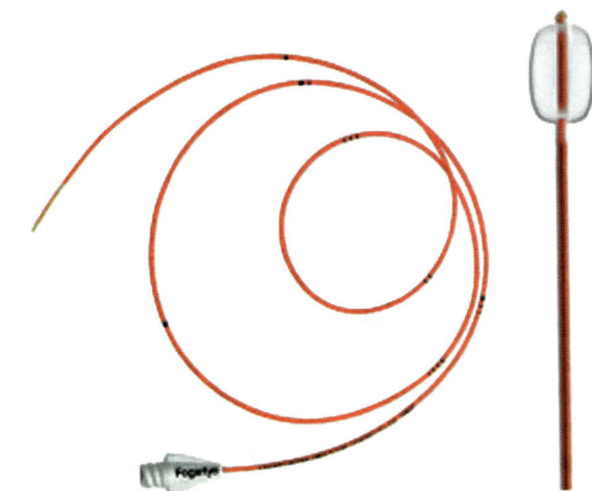

**Fig. 9.1:** Fogarty catheter

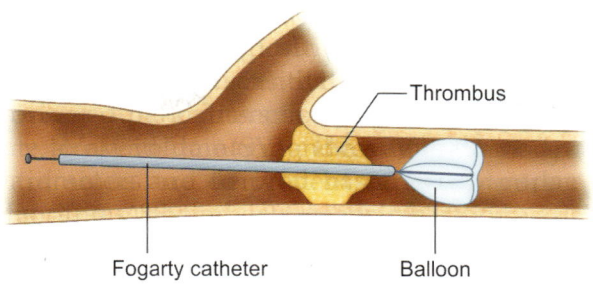

**Fig. 9.2:** Extraction of thrombus with a Fogarty catheter

**Table 9.3:** Clinical classification of peripheral arterial disease

| Fontaine classification | | Rutherford classification | |
|---|---|---|---|
| Stage | Clinical | Grade | Clinical |
| I | Asymptomatic | 0 | Asymptomatic |
| IIa | Mild claudication | 1 | Mild claudication |
| IIb | Moderate to severe | 2 | Moderate claudication |
| | claudication | 3 | Severe claudication |
| III | Ischemic rest pain | 4 | Ischemic rest pain |
| IV | Ulceration or | 5 | Minor tissue loss |
| | Gangrene | 6 | Major tissue loss |

trauma, it is most important to get adequate proximal and distal control of the injured artery prior to exploring the wound site. An end-to-end anastamosis is preferable whenever possible in such cases.

Restoration of the arterial circulation may cause severe reperfusion injury secondary to hyperkalaemia and acidosis manifesting as myocardial depression, cardiac arrhythmias, cardiac arrest, myoglobinemia and acute renal failure. This can be dealt with hydration, diuresis, hyperventilation, and administration of sodium bicarbonate and glucose-insulin. If the indicators of rhabdomyolysis (CPK, myoglobin, potassium, lactate, base deficit) are elevated, good urine output must be ensured with the use of furosemide and mannitol to prevent acute renal injury.

The operative mortality in patients with acute lower limb ischemia is 10–15%, limb loss occurs in 10% and late mortality is around 40%. Prognosis is worse in the elderly, those with CAD, congestive heart failure, aortoiliac occlusion and respiratory compromise.

## CHRONIC ISCHEMIA OF THE LOWER EXTREMITIES

Pathophysiologic processes that necessitate surgical intervention of the lower limb arteries include atherosclerosis, aneurysm, fibromuscular disease, embolism and trauma. The risk factors for developing peripheral atherosclerosis and CAD are similar: Diabetes mellitus, hypertension, dyslipidemia, tobacco abuse, hyperhomocysteinemia, male gender and family history. The clinical history and physical examination often identify the location and relative severity of the patient's vascular disease. The clinical classification of peripheral arterial disease is given in Table 9.3. The principal symptoms of peripheral atherosclerosis are intermittent claudication characterized by pain, cramping or fatigue in muscles induced by exercise and relieved at rest. Characterizing the pain—location, precipitating, aggravating and relieving factors, frequency, duration, and evolution—can allow one to diagnose or exclude most arterial and venous diseases with a high degree of

sensitivity, even before examining the patient. Infra-inguinal atherosclerosis most commonly involves the superficial femoral artery followed by the popliteal and infrapopliteal arteries. Therefore, the usual location of pain is in the calf. Claudication may also involve the thigh in case of aorto-iliac obstruction. The arterial system affected is usually one level above the symptomatic muscle group. The obstruction in the arterial system to particular limb compromises its perfusion and leads to pain which worsens progressively to rest pain and sometimes awakens the patient from sleep.

The findings include absent arterial pulses, bruit, subcutaneous atrophy, hair loss, muscle wasting, coolness, pallor and cyanosis. Audible bruits indicate the anatomic site of arterial stenosis. Patients with critical limb ischemia suffer skin breakdown (ulcers or gangrene) and pain at rest. Confirmation of diagnosis is aided by Doppler ultrasound derived ankle brachial index (ABI: ratio of ankle systolic blood pressure to brachial systolic blood pressure), transcutaneous oximetry, magnetic resonance imaging and contrast angiography. The normal ABI is >1, with claudication it is between 0.3 and 0.9, with critical limb ischemia it is <0.5 and with gangrenous extremities it is <0.2. The differential diagnosis of intermittent claudication is given in Table 9.4.

Almost 28% patients also have CAD,[1] but cardiac symptoms may be masked owing to limitation of exercise by claudication, arthritis, previous amputation or general debility.[4] Perioperative cardiac complications majorly contribute to the morbidity and mortality. The combined incidence of cardiac death and non-fatal MI has been reported to be >5% and the reported 30 day mortality after elective lower limb revascularization is 5–8%.[5] Medical and behavioral therapy is targeted towards modification of risk factors for PVD such as cessation of smoking, moderation in alcohol intake, control of hypercholesterolemia, blood pressure and diabetes (Table 9.5). Anticoagulant and antiplatelet medications are started to halt disease progression, decrease thromboembolic events and prevent graft occlusion.

**Table 9.4:** Differential diagnosis of intermittent claudication[2]

| Condition | Location of pain or discomfort | Characteristic discomfort | Onset relative to exercise | Effect of rest | Effect of body position | Other characteristics |
|---|---|---|---|---|---|---|
| Intermittent claudication | Buttock, thigh, or calf muscles and rarely the foot | Cramping, aching, fatigue, weakness, or frank pain | After some degree of exercise | Quickly relieved | None | Reproducible |
| Nerve root compression (e.g. herniated disc) | Radiates down leg, usually posteriorly | Sharp lancinating pain | Soon, if not immediately after onset | Not quickly relieved (also often present at rest) | Relief may be aided by adjusting back position | History of back problems |
| Spinal stenosis | Hip, thigh, buttocks (follows dermatome) | Motor weakness more prominent than pain | After walking or standing for variable lengths of time | Relieved by stopping only if position changed | Relief by lumbar spine flexion (sitting or stooping forward) | Frequent history of back problems, provoked by intra-abdominal pressure |
| Arthritic, inflammatory process | Foot, arch | Aching pain | After variable degree of exercise | Not quickly relieved (and may be present at rest) | May be relieved by not bearing weight | Variable, may relate to activity level |
| Hip arthritis | Hip, thigh, buttocks | Aching discomfort, usually localized to hip and gluteal region | After variable degree of exercise | Not quickly relieved (and may be present at rest) | More comfortable sitting, weight taken off legs | Variable, may relate to activity level, weather changes |
| Symptomatic Baker's cyst | Behind knee, down calf | Swelling, soreness, tenderness | With exercise | Present at rest | None | Not intermittent |
| Venous claudication | Entire leg, but usually worse in thigh and groin | Tight, bursting pain | After walking | Subsides slowly | Relief speeded by elevation | History of iliofemoral deep vein thrombosis, signs of venous congestion, edema |
| Chronic compartment syndrome | Calf muscles | Tight bursting pain | After much exercise (e.g. jogging) | Subsides very slowly | Relief speeded by elevation | Typically heavy muscled athletes |

**Table 9.5:** Treatment modalities for peripheral vascular disease

Stop smoking

Moderation of alcohol intake

Exercise

Cholesterol lowering drugs, e.g. statin

Antiplatelet drugs, e.g. aspirin or clopidogrel

Diabetes control

Blood pressure control

Non-surgical interventions—angioplasty/stenting

Surgical revascularization

Whenever possible, such as for single, short, segmental stenoses, minimally invasive procedures like angioplasty and endovascular stent placement are considered as the first line treatment for PVD. It is usually performed by radiologists under local anesthesia with or without sedation. Other advantages of angioplasty include low treatment cost, rapid recovery and decreased hospital stay. Complications arise in up to 10% cases and include technical difficulty in negotiating the catheter through the stenoses, hemorrhage, dissection, distal embolization, formation of pseudoaneurysm or arteriovenous fistula.[6] When angioplasty is unsuccessful or inappropriate, surgical arterial bypass is performed using either synthetic (Dacron or PTFE) graft, human umbilical vein or autologous saphenous vein graft. Upper extremity cephalic and basilic veins may also be used as a graft. In patients with unilateral iliac artery obstruction, femorofemoral bypass is performed. Other infrainguinal bypass procedures include femoropopliteal and tibioperoneal reconstruction. According to the recent American College of Cardiology and American Heart Association (ACC/AHA) guidelines, peripheral vascular revascularization is considered as a high risk surgery.[5] Lumbar sympathectomy is rarely used to treat ischemic (and dilated) vessels. Amputation is performed in cases of advanced limb ischemia or in cases of impossible or failed revascularization. The approach to a patient with PVD is summarized in Fig. 9.3.

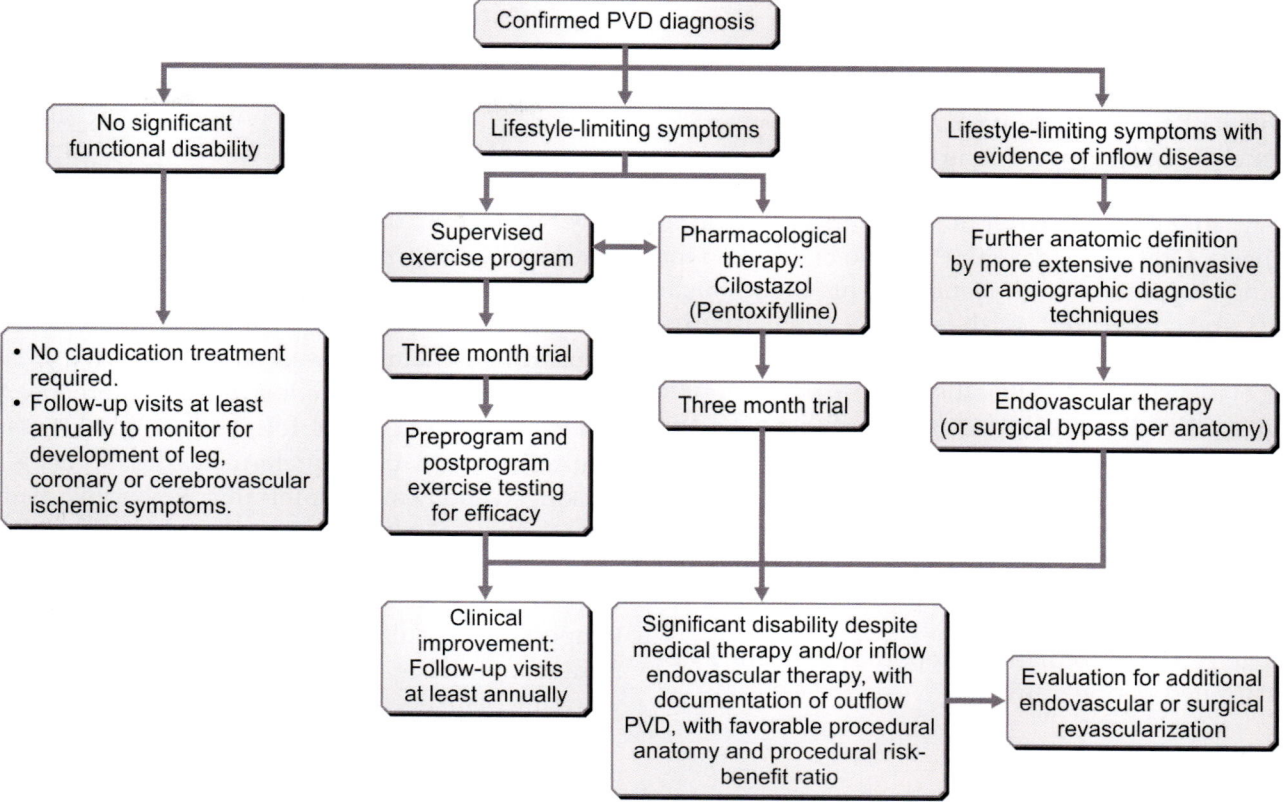

**Fig. 9.3:** Approach to a patient with peripheral vascular disease

## Preoperative Assessment

The important preoperative risk factors are known cardiovascular conditions, comorbidities and functional capacity (Table 9.6). The minimum investigations ordered include complete blood count, blood urea, serum creatinine, electrolytes, blood glucose, electro-cardiogram and chest X-ray. An echocardiogram may also be required in indicated cases. According to ACC/ AHA guidelines patients with intermediate and major clinical risk factors should undergo non-invasive cardiac testing with exercise or pharmacological stress testing, or myocardial perfusion scanning.[5,7] It is noteworthy that many patients with PVD are unable to exercise owing to claudication. In these cases, dobutamine stress echocardiography or myocardial perfusion scanning become applicable. Patients in heart failure need evaluation of left ventricular function. If the underlying cause is CAD, they should be considered for coronary angiography and revascularization. However, in patients who have undergone coronary revasculariza-tion in the preceding 5 years and do not exhibit cardiac symptoms, further testing is not mandated. Coronary evaluation is recommended in case symptoms are manifest or revascularization was performed over 5 years ago. Peripheral vascular revascularization should be delayed for at least 4–6 weeks after balloon angioplasty, coronary stenting or bypass grafting.[5]

| Table 9.6: ACC/AHA clinical predictors of preoperative risk[5] |
| --- |
| **Major** |
| • Unstable coronary syndromes (unstable angina/MI within 30 days) |
| • Decompensated congestive cardiac failure |
| • Significant arrhythmias |
| • Severe valvular disease |
| **Intermediate** |
| • Mild angina pectoris |
| • Previous MI (>30 days earlier) |
| • Compensated or previous congestive cardiac failure |
| • Diabetes mellitus |
| • Renal insufficiency |
| **Minor** |
| • Advanced age (>70 years) |
| • Abnormal electrocardiogram |
| • Non-sinus rhythm |
| • Low functional capacity |
| • History of stroke |
| • Uncontrolled systemic hypertension |

## Preoperative Management

The treatment of associated diseases should be optimized before surgery. Most cardiac medications are continued till the day of surgery. Angiotensin converting enzyme inhibitors and angiotensin II receptor antagonists may be discontinued on the morning of surgery, for they cause hypotension on induction of anesthesia. Oral hypoglycemics are also omitted on the morning of surgery. In diabetic patients blood sugar levels are controlled with sliding scale insulin perioperatively. It is prudent to start β-blockers since recent evidence suggests that they reduce perioperative ischemia, MI and mortality in high risk patients.[8] Statin therapy has also been shown to improve long-term outcome in patients with vascular disease.[9] Aspirin is usually continued till the surgery as it reduces cardiovascular morbidity and mortality.[10] However, clopidogrel and ticlopidine should be witheld for 7 days prior to surgery. Pentoxifylline and cilostazol, drugs having antiplatelet and vasodilating properties used for PVD, are continued perioperatively.

## Intraoperative Management

No specific anaesthetic technique has been recommended as there are no reported differences in graft function, cardiac morbidity or mortality between regional and general anesthesia.[11,12] The procedure can be performed under local anesthesia with sedation, regional anesthesia or general anesthesia. Regional anesthesia with combined spinal-epidural or continuous epidural infusion is frequently employed. Regional anesthesia can also be used to supplement general anesthesia. Sensory and motor blockade up to T10 level is adequate for performing lower limb revascularization. The advantages of regional anesthesia over general anesthesia include reduced blood loss, attenuation of the stress response to surgery, less increase in systemic vascular resistance with aortic cross-clamping, improved postoperative respiratory function, postoperative analgesia and attenuation of the hypercoagulable state induced by surgery.[13] Peripheral nerve blocks (and continuous catheter techniques) such as sciatic, femoral, popliteal and ankle, may be performed given the risk associated with neuraxial anesthesia in these anticoagulated patients. These procedures are preferably done under ultrasound and peripheral nerve stimulation guidance. The concerns of bleeding cannot be altogether avoided in patients who have received anticoagulants. There is the additional concern of local anesthetic toxicity as large volumes are required for performing these nerve blocks.

The main aims of anesthesia for peripheral vascular revascularization are to maintain hemodynamic stability, adequate hydration, oxygenation, adequate analgesia, and prevent hypothermia, acidosis and anemia. Prolonged vascular clamping can induce ischemia reperfusion injury. As mentioned earlier, hyperventilation, administration of intravenous sodium bicarbonate and treatment of hyperkalemia help abate the phenomenon. Hemodynamic perturbations such as tachycardia, hypertension and hypotension induce myocardial ischemia. Based on the underlying cardiorespiratory status, induction of and emergence from general anesthesia are performed in a smooth manner. Controlled ventilation is preferred as the surgery is often prolonged and hemodynamically demanding. Pain and hypothermia also increase oxygen demand and cause myocardial ischemia. Necessary steps should be taken to mitigate heat loss including control of ambient temperature, insulation of exposed areas, warming of intravenous fluids, use of a thermal mattress and topical warming blankets. Analgesia is provided with regional blocks, opioids and non-steroidal anti-inflammatory drugs. Volume status should be optimized to ensure adequate graft perfusion. Unfractionated heparin (1 mg/kg intravenous) is routinely administered before application of the arterial clamp in order to achieve an activated clotting time of >250s. Its effect can be reversed with protamine. Dextran may be administered intraoperatively and continued into the postoperative period to improve graft patency.

The timing of regional anesthesia is tailored according to heparin administration. Neuraxial block is performed at least 1 hr before or 4 hr after the administration of unfractionated heparin, and 4 hr before or 12 hr after the administration of low molecular weight heparin.

## Monitoring

The essential monitoring for peripheral vascular revascularization includes multi-lead ECG (including lead $V_5$ and II, with ST-segment analysis), pulse oximetry, capnography, invasive blood pressure, central venous pressure, temperature and urine output. Transesophageal echocardiography or pulmonary artery catheterization are useful to assess ventricular function, guide fluid management and detect myocardial ischemia in high-risk patients. In cases of profoundly ischemic limbs with metabolic derangements, such as hyperkalemia, metabolic acidosis, myoglobinuria, rhabdomyolysis and azotemia, attention must also be paid to the acid–base and electrolyte status.

## Surgical Technique

### Aorto Iliac Diseases

Aortobifemoral bypass with a prosthetic graft via the transabdominal or retroperitoneal approach is performed when the diseased segment involves common femoral arteries. Preoperative imaging delineates the target vessels, usually the common femoral or profunda femoris arteries. Proximal anastomoses can be performed in end-to-end or end-to-side configuration. For patients with occlusive disease, the end-to-side configuration is more commonly used because it may preserve perfusion to the pelvis via the diseased but patent iliacs and lumbar collaterals. End-to-end anastomosis (Fig. 9.4) improves flow dynamics and has the potential for decreased friction between the overlying bowel and graft. Alternative sources include the thoracic aorta, axillary artery and contralateral femoral artery if disease is unilateral.

### Lower Extremity Occlusive Disease

The classification of lower extremity occlusive disease is shown in Fig. 9.5. Vascular control is achieved with minimal traction with vascular loops. End-to-end or end-to-side anastomoses are done with evenly placed bites to include all layers of the vessel wall. Lesions involving the common femoral artery and origin of the profunda artery are approached by open groin exploration, to perform common femoral artery endarterectomy, and

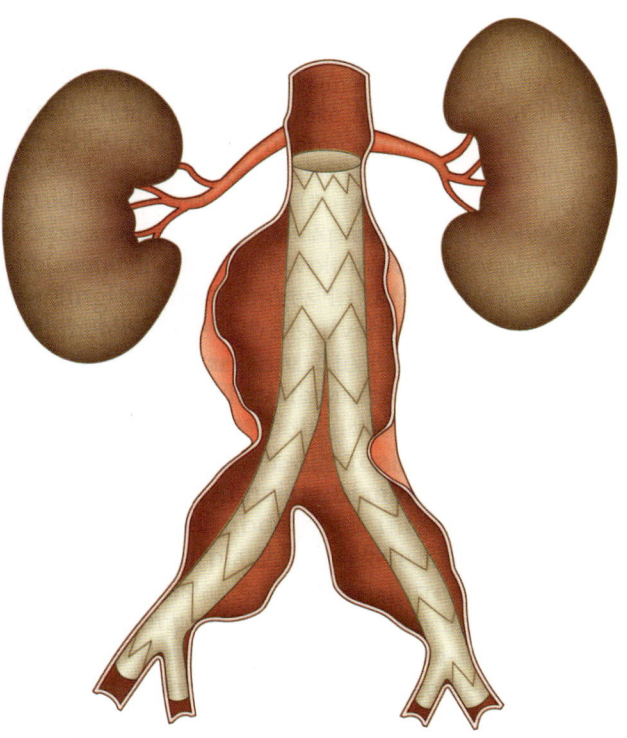

Fig. 9.4: End-to-end aortobifemoral bypass graft

profundaplasty or ileofemoral bypass. If concomitant iliac artery or superficial femoral artery disease is present, patients may undergo hybrid procedures with iliac stent placement via open femoral access if facilities are available or by femoropopliteal bypass or stenting of superficial femoral artery.

## Surgical Technique and Choice of Conduits

The two main graft types used for lower extremity bypasses are the great saphenous veins and PTFE grafts with heparin coating. The greater saphenous veins should be used preferentially in all bypasses because of inherent anti-thrombotic properties, especially in below-knee popliteal and small tibial arteries as the distal target vessels. PTFE grafts can be used for bypasses to above-knee popliteal arterial segments with satisfactory patency rates.

The great saphenous vein can be placed in situ or reversed because of the presence of valves. For the in situ vein graft, there is better size match—larger thigh vein for the common femoral artery and smaller leg vein for the tibial artery. Other choices when great saphenous vein is not available are small saphenous vein of the leg, the cephalic and basilic veins from the upper extremities, but these veins have thinner walls. Several veins can be joined to form a composite graft to achieve adequate length, but risk of thrombogenicity increases. Alternative conduits include cryopreserved arteries and veins, which have been shown to be more resistant to infection.

For endarterectomy patch angioplasty, vein patch or prosthetic patches of PTFE or Dacron can be used. Bovine pericardial patches are also available.

The femoropopliteal bypass is used in patients with superficial femoral and popliteal arterial occlusion with a popliteal artery segment distal to the occlusion that is patent, with luminal continuity with any of the tibial arterial branches (Fig. 9.6). Bypass can be performed even if one or more tibial arterial branches are occluded in the leg. Infrapopliteal bypass is performed on arteries beyond the popliteal artery when there is arterial disease that involves the popliteal or proximal tibial artery and there is no obstruction in the distal tibial artery. With femoropopliteal and infrapopliteal bypasses, a tibial artery with stenosis of less than 50% distal to the distal anastomosis is acceptable. But the contraindications are the absence of a complete plantar arch or the presence of vascular calcification. The common femoral artery is generally used as the inflow for these bypasses and shorter bypass grafts are preferred because of improved patency.

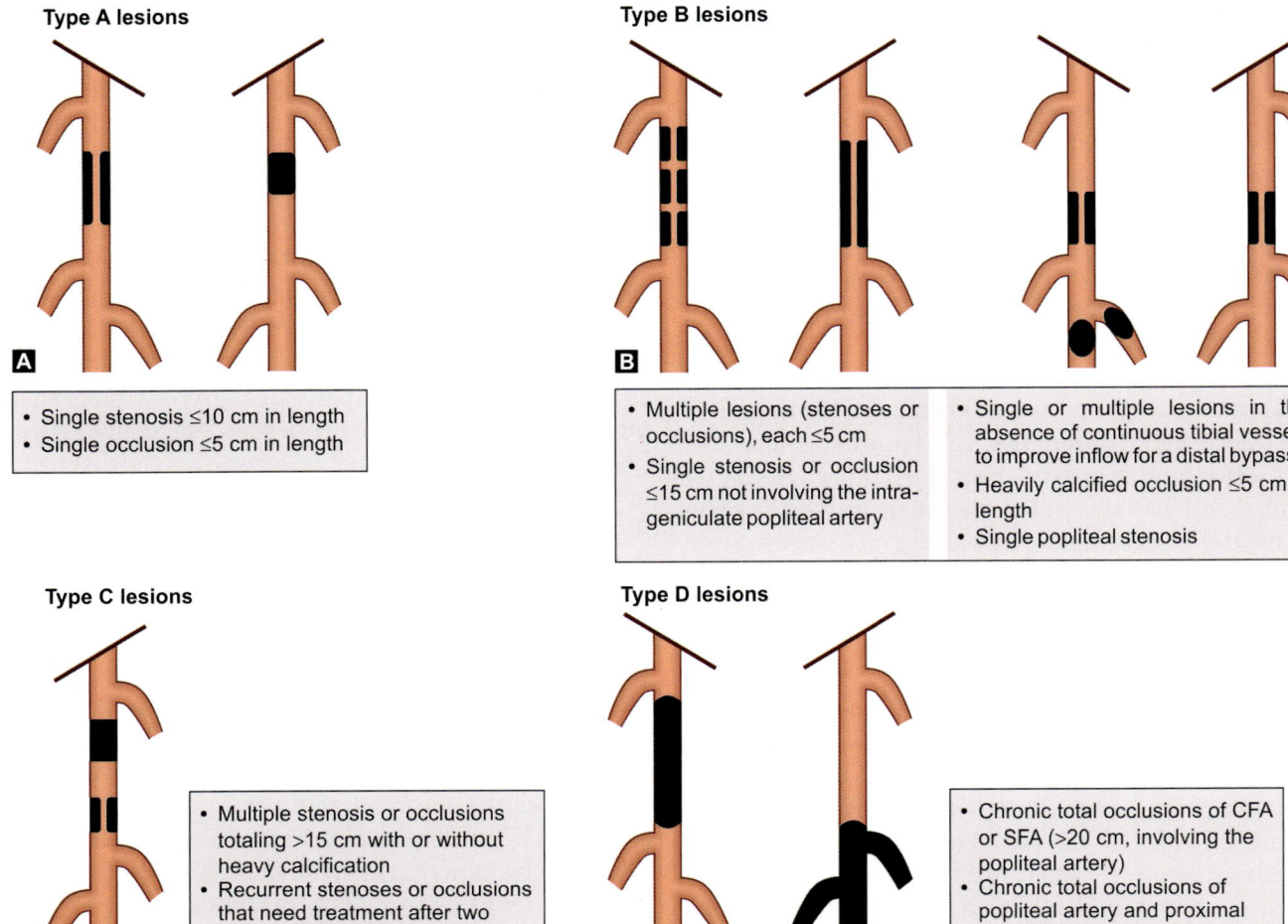

**Type A lesions**

A

- Single stenosis ≤10 cm in length
- Single occlusion ≤5 cm in length

**Type B lesions**

B

- Multiple lesions (stenoses or occlusions), each ≤5 cm
- Single stenosis or occlusion ≤15 cm not involving the intra-geniculate popliteal artery

- Single or multiple lesions in the absence of continuous tibial vessels to improve inflow for a distal bypass
- Heavily calcified occlusion ≤5 cm in length
- Single popliteal stenosis

**Type C lesions**

C

- Multiple stenosis or occlusions totaling >15 cm with or without heavy calcification
- Recurrent stenoses or occlusions that need treatment after two endovascular interventions

**Type D lesions**

D

- Chronic total occlusions of CFA or SFA (>20 cm, involving the popliteal artery)
- Chronic total occlusions of popliteal artery and proximal bifurcation vessels

**Figs 9.5A to D:** Trans-Atlantic Inter-Society Consensus (TASC) classification of femoropopliteal lesions

## Complications

As with any other surgery, infection of the wound (superficial and deep) is the most common complication. Sometimes the graft itself may get infected. The most dreadful complication of aortic bypass is aortoduodenal fistula. The treatment is extra-anatomic bypass and graft removal, with debridement of the retroperitoneal tissues.

Other complications include groin hematoma, lymphatic leak or lymphocele, femoral nerve entrapment, limb swelling and knee contracture.

## Postoperative Management

Pain, temperature, fluid and electrolyte management, and oxygenation require attention after surgery. Analgesia is provided with epidural infusion of local anesthetic and opioid, intravenous opioid and/or non-steroidal anti-inflammatory drugs. Normothermia is maintained by active warming methods. Oxygen is supplemented to prevent postoperative myocardial ischemia. Heart rate and blood pressure need to be carefully controlled. ECG must be continuously checked for ST changes. Anemia (hemoglobin <9 g/dL) is treated with blood transfusion. Lower limb pulses are inspected to verify graft patency. High-risk patients are prescribed β-blockers and aspirin perioperatively. Warfarin may be administered postoperatively to maintain graft patency and prevent deep venous thrombosis.

## Mycotic Aneurysms in Drug Abusers

Mycotic aneurysms are most commonly found in intravenous drug abusers. These pseudoaneurysms are caused by microbes introduced during injection of infected material by non-sterile technique combined with trauma from inadvertent or deliberate arterial puncture. The patients present with a tender indurated inflammatory mass overlying the course of an artery such as the brachial or femoral artery (Figs 9.7A and B).

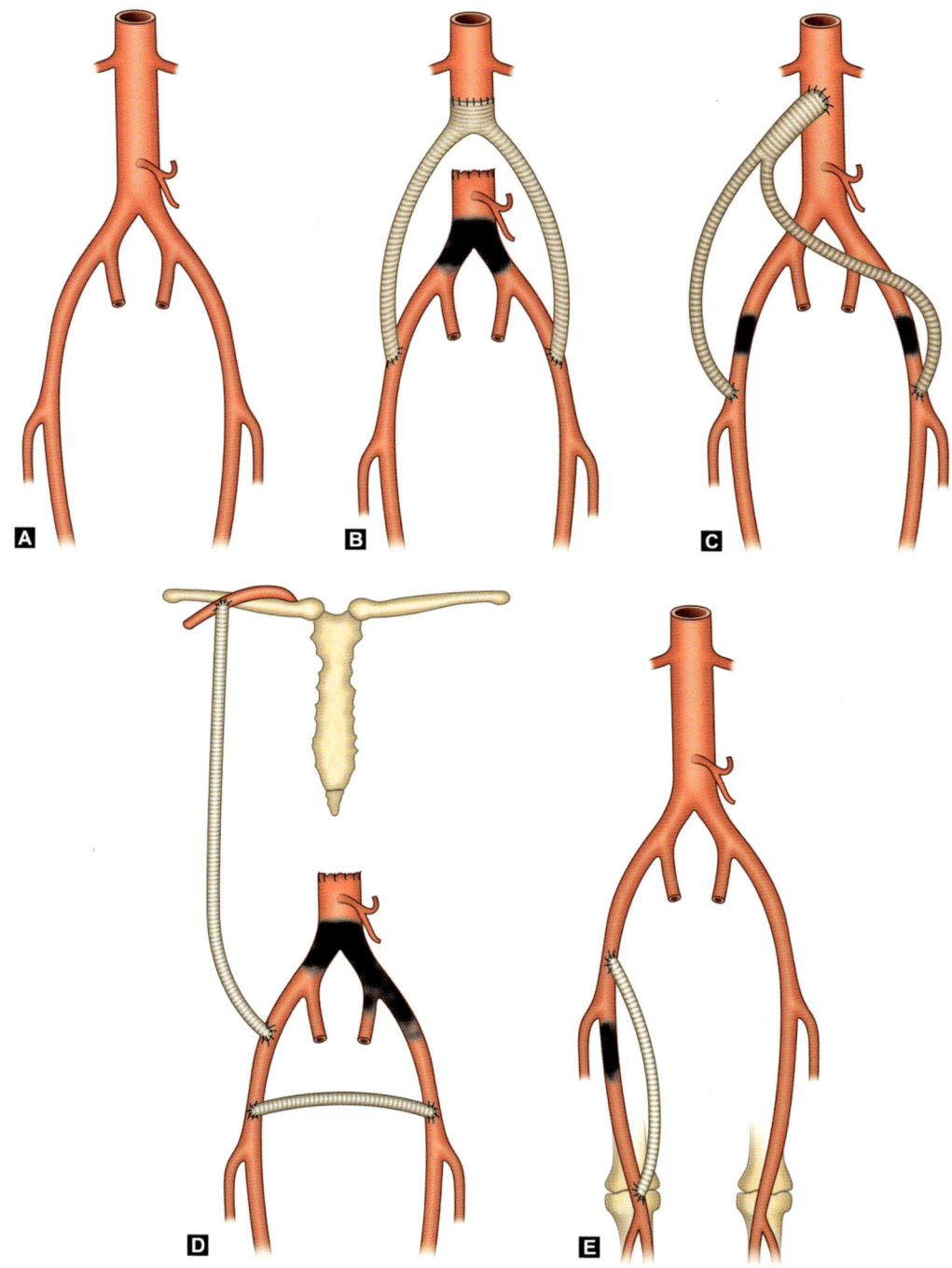

**Figs 9.6A to E:** Surgical technique of lower extremity arterial bypass: (A) normal arterial tree, (B) aortobifemoral bypass: end-to-end anastomosis, (C) aortobifemoral bypass: end-to-side anastomosis, (D) extra-anatomic axillofemoral and femorofemoral bypass, (E) femoropopliteal bypass

The patients are frequently also positive for human immunodeficiency virus and hepatitis B virus. The diagnosis is made on arteriogram. Its treatment includes debridement of infected and necrotic tissue, vascular repair and appropriate antibiotic coverage. Blood cultures are usually positive for *Staphylococcus aureus* although other organisms may be present. Although a limb may appear non-viable before operation because the presence of sepsis, hematoma, and aneurysm exaggerate the ischemia; viability should be reassessed following drainage of sepsis and debridement. Vascular reconstruction is carried out when the limb continues to remain non-viable. Autologous graft is not immune from the risk of infection. Synthetic grafts should be placed in an extra-anatomical plane avoiding the infected region. Whenever possible, late reconstruction

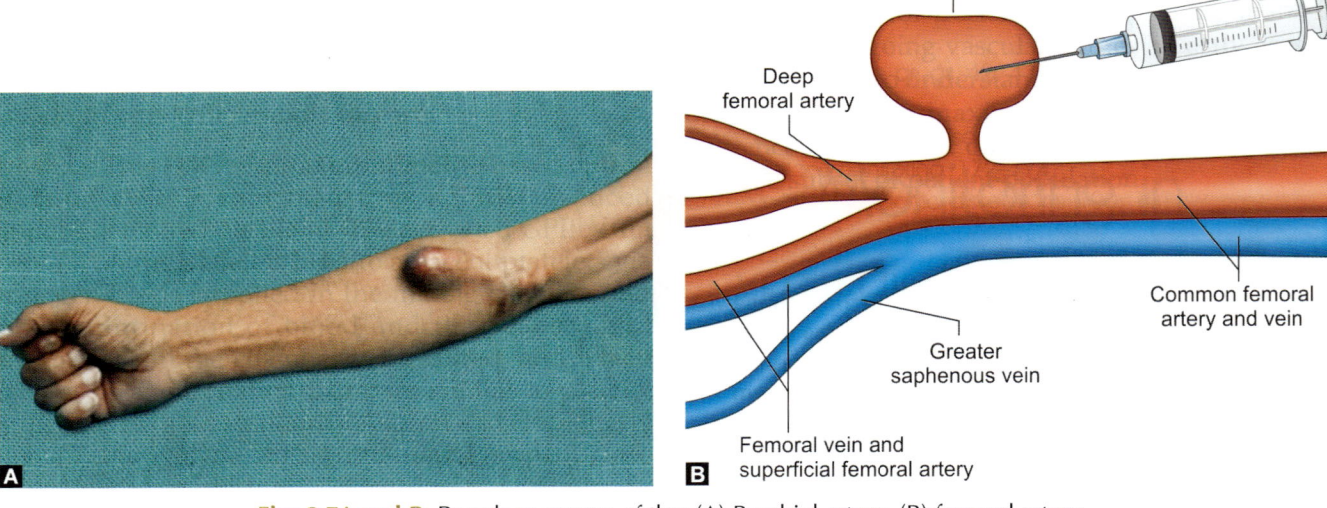

**Figs 8.7A and B:** Pseudoaneurysm of the: (A) Brachial artery, (B) femoral artery

should be performed after sepsis has been eradicated. Complications include hemorrhage and graft infection.

## Key Points

1. Surgery for lower limb revascularization carries high risk of cardiac morbidity and mortality because of associated comorbidities.
2. Preoperative cardiac risk assessment is important and steps should be initiated to reduce the risk expeditiously.
3. Acute limb ischemia presents as an emergency that may preclude extensive preoperative cardiac evaluation. Time is the most crucial factor and blood flow must be restored within 6 hr to salvage the limb.
4. The quality of anesthetic management and not any particular technique has an important influence on patient outcome.
5. Reperfusion injury occurs on establishing revascularization.
6. Although regional anesthesia has several advantages, the risk associated with anticoagulation raises concern.
7. The entire perioperative period carries high risk for myocardial ischemia. Necessary protective steps must be taken to mitigate this risk.
8. Perioperative β-blockade decreases the incidence of perioperative cardiac complications.

## REFERENCES

1. Weitz JI, Byrne J, Clagett GP, et al. Diagnosis and treatment of chronic arterial insufficiency of the lower extremities: A critical review. Circulation 1996;94:3026–49.
2. Trans-Atlantic Inter-Society Concensus. J Vasc Surg 2000; 31: Supplemental issue.
3. Golledge J. Lower-limb arterial disease. Lancet 1997; 350:1459–65.
4. Thompson JP, Smith G. Anesthesia for vascular surgery on the lower limb. In: Bannister J, Wildsmith JAW (Eds). Anaesthesia for Vascular Surgery. London: Arnold, 2000.
5. Eagle KA, Berger PB, Calkins H, et al. ACC/AHA guideline update for perioperative cardiovascular evaluation for noncardiac surgery: executive summary. A report of the American College of Cardiology/American Heart Association Task Force on Practice Guidelines (Committee to Update the 1996 Guidelines on Perioperative Cardiovascular Evaluation for Noncardiac Surgery). Circulation 2002;105:1257–67.
6. Matsi PJ, Manninen HI. Complications of lower-limb percutaneous transluminal angioplasty. A prospective analysis of 410 procedures on 295 consecutive patients. Cardiovasc Intervent Radiol 1998;21:361–66.
7. Chassot PG, Delabays A, Spahn DR. Preoperative evaluation of patients with, or at risk of, coronary artery disease undergoing non-cardiac surgery. Br J Anaesth 2002;89:747–59.
8. Poldermans D, Boersma E, Bax JJ, et al. Bisoprolol reduces cardiac death and myocardial infarction in high-risk patients as long as 2 years after successful major vascular surgery. Eur Heart J 2001;22:1353–8.
9. Poldermans D, Bax JJ, Kertai MD, et al. Statins are associated with a reduced incidence of perioperative mortality in patients undergoing major noncardiac vascular surgery. Circulation 2003;107:1848–51.
10. Jackson MR, Clagett GP. Antithrombotic therapy in peripheral arterial occlusive disease. Chest 2001;119:283S–299S.
11. Bode RH, Lewis KP, Zarich SW, et al. Cardiac outcome after peripheral vascular surgery: Comparison of general and regional anesthesia. Anesthesiology 1996;84:3–13.
12. Pierce ET, Pomposelli FB, Stanley GD, et al. Anesthesia type does not influence early graft patency or limb salvage rates of lower extremity arterial bypass. J Vasc Surg 1997; 25:226–32.
13. Christopherson R, Beattie C, Frank SM, et al. Perioperative morbidity in patients randomized to epidural or general anesthesia for lower extremity vascular-surgery. Anesthesiology 1993;79:422–34.

# CHAPTER 10

# Anesthesia for Carotid Artery Disease

Suruchi Ladha, Sandeep Chauhan, Akshay Kumar Bisoi, Ujjawal K Chwudhary

## INTRODUCTION

The word carotid is derived from the Greek word "karos", which means deep sleep. Around 400 BC Hippocrates was amongst the first to describe the symptoms of stroke. C. Miller Fisher first described the relationship between carotid artery disease, transient ischemic attacks (TIAs) and stroke.

Stroke is one of the leading causes of death and disability. Carotid artery disease is an important risk factor for stroke. There are above 8,00,000 strokes and 3,00,000 TIA each year in the USA[1]. Extracranial carotid atherosclerosis causes approximately 15–20% of ischemic stroke in adult population.[2] Large trials suggest that the incidence of stroke associated with ipsilateral carotid artery stenosis is 1–2% per year.[3] Carotid endarterectomy (CEA) is the most frequently performed noncardiac vascular procedure in the United States.[4] The first successful CEA was performed by DeBakey in 1953. The rate of carotid endarterectomies has fluctuated significantly since the early 1970s.

A marked increase in the number of carotid endarterectomies occurred after the results of two large-scale, prospective randomized trials namely the North American Symptomatic CEA Trial[5] and the European Carotid Surgery Trial[6] as both the trials demonstrated the benefit of CEA in symptomatic patients with high-grade carotid stenosis (70 to 99%).

## ANATOMY OF THE CAROTID ARTERIES

*Carotid artery:* The right common carotid artery (CCA) originates from the innominate artery and the left common carotid artery originates from the aortic arch. The CCA divides into the internal carotid artery (ICA) and external carotid artery (ECA) at the level of the superior border of the thyroid cartilage corresponding to the C3/C4 intervertebral disc space. The origin of the carotid arteries is shown in Fig. 10.1.

*External carotid artery:* The ECA supplies the face and scalp and provide collateral circulation to the brain. The branches of ECA include the superior thyroid, lingual, facial, ascending pharyngeal, occipital, posterior auricular, maxillary and superficial temporal arteries.

*Internal carotid artery:* The ICA has no branches in the neck. The cervical segment of the internal carotid extends from the carotid bifurcation until it enters the carotid canal of the petrous bone. The ICA runs within the carotid sheath with internal jugular vein and vagal nerve. It lies posterior and lateral to the ECA beneath the medial border of the sternocleidomastoid muscle.

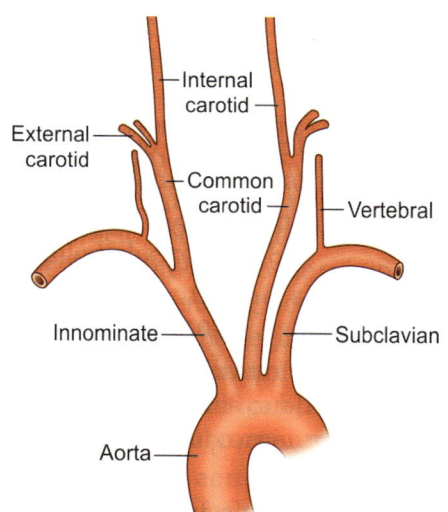

**Fig. 10.1:** Origin of the right common carotid from innominate artery and left common carotid from the aortic arch

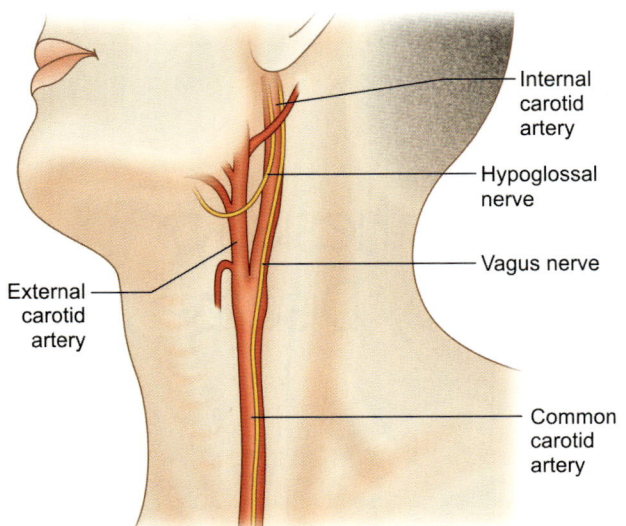

**Fig. 10.2:** The course of the carotid artery in the neck along with its relationship to vagus and hypoglossal nerve

The course of the carotid artery in the neck along with the relationship to the nerve is shown in Fig. 10.2.

However, there is considerable variation in the normal anatomy of the aortic arch and cervical arteries that supply the brain. Also, variations resulting from different factors like tortuosity, calcification, stenosis, presence of collateral vessels, aneurysms and arteriovenous malformations have important implications in the clinical management of the patient.

*Carotid baroreceptor:* Baroreceptors are stretch sensitive mechanoreceptors. The carotid sinus baroreceptors are located in the carotid sinus, which is a small dilatation of the internal carotid artery. It is innervated by the sinus nerve of hering, which is a branch of glossopharyngeal nerve. They respond both to sustained pressure and pulse pressure. In response to low blood pressure or low carotid pulse pressure, the nerve fibers decrease their discharge rates stimulating the sympathetic nervous system and inhibiting the parasympathetic nervous system resulting in a compensatory increase in blood pressure and cardiac output. In patients with carotid atherosclerosis the reactivity of carotid sinus may be affected.

## PHYSIOLOGY OF CEREBRAL BLOOD FLOW

Cerebral blood flow (CBF) is approximately 12 to 15% of cardiac output. CBF is provided by the internal carotid arteries (80%) and the vertebral arteries (20%) which usually anastomose at the base of the brain to form the circle of Willis. Patients having occlusive cerebrovascular disease may be dependent on other collateral channels between different intracranial and extracranial

vessels to obtain adequate CBF. Adequate cerebral blood flow is needed to provide a continuous supply of oxygen and glucose to brain cell as the brain cells do not have any reserve of glucose or oxygen.

CBF is related to cerebral perfusion pressure (CPP) and cerebrovascular resistance (CVR) according to the formula:

$$CBF = CPP/CVR$$

- CPP equals mean arterial blood pressure (MAP) minus intracranial pressure or central venous pressure, whichever is higher.
- CVR is related to blood viscosity and the diameter of the cerebral resistance vessels
- Thus, any factor affecting CPP and CVR would lead to changes in the CBF. Several factors like changes in cereals metabloc rate (CMR), $paCO_2$ and $paO_2$, cause changes in the cerebral biochemical environment that leads to change of CBF.

The normal ranges of cerebral physiologic values are as follows:

| | |
|---|---|
| CBF Global | 45–55 ml/100 g/min |
| CMRO₂ | 3–3.5 ml/100 g/min |
| CVR | 1.5–2.1 mm Hg/ml/100 g/min |
| Cerebral venous PO₂ | 32–44 mm Hg |
| Cerebral venous SO₂ | 55–70% |
| ICP (supine) | 8–12 mm Hg |

CBF: Cerebral blood flow, CMRO₂: Cerebral metabolic rate of oxygen consumption, CVR: Cerebral vascular resistance, ICP: Intracranial pressure

*paCO₂:* CBF varies directly with $paCO_2$. In the range of physiologic $paCO_2$, this effect is prominent. CBF usually changes 1 to 2 ml/100 g/min for each 1–mm Hg change in $PaCO_2$ in the range of 20–80 mm Hg. $CO_2$ is the most potent vasodilator of the cerebral vascular system. The effect of carbon dioxide on the cerebral arteries is most pronounced in smaller arteries (diameter 0.5–1.0 mm), whereas arteries with a diameter of 2.5 mm or more (e.g., the carotid artery) show no substantial change. An increase in $paCO_2$ can cause all arterioles to dilate maximally. This can "steal" blood flow from areas of higher metabolic demand that require extra oxygen. This is particularly important during focal ischemia due to a blocked vessel. Hypocapnia associated with hyperventilation causes constriction of cerebral blood vessels and decreases cerebral blood flow in areas of normal $CO_2$ responsive brain vessels and thereby increase the blood flow to ischemic areas (Robin Hood effect). Thus, shunting of blood from adequately perfused cerebral tissues to compromised, potentially ischemic areas, is referred as the Robin Hood effect.

Cerebral steal also known as luxury perfusion, can be triggered if the patient is given a vasodilator (nitroglycerin, nitroprusside or hydralazine) or if the patient is hypoventilated. Steal phenomenon is also reported with the use of inhalational anesthetic like sevoflurane. Hypercapnia associated with hypoventilation causes dilatation of cerebral blood vessels and an associated increase in global cerebral blood flow. However, if there is hypoventilation in ischemic areas, $paCO_2$ increases, pH decreases, arterioles in non-ischemic brain dilate, and blood flow to non-ischemic brain increases. This vasodilation in non-ischemic brain tissue could theoretically result in "steal" of blood flow from the ischemic areas that require oxygen. This is also referred to as Inverse Steal.

Alterations in cerebral vascular resistance occur when pH of the cerebrospinal fluid is altered (which occurs quickly with changes in $paCO_2$). Since ions including $H^+$ and $HCO_3^-$ do not cross the blood–brain barrier, neither acute metabolic acidosis nor acute metabolic alkalosis alters cerebral blood flow.

In the absence of demonstrated clinical benefit with either hypocapnia or hypercapnia, it is advised to maintain normocapnia during CEA. This would lead to balancing the optimum cerebral blood flow with avoidance of steal phenomenon. However, during carotid cross clamping the regional cerebral blood flow is not predictable as the autoregulation is lost.

$paO_2$: $paO_2$ from 60 mm Hg to greater than 300 mm Hg have little influence on CBF. Below a $paO_2$ of 60 mm Hg, CBF increases rapidly. The mechanisms mediating cerebral vasodilation during hypoxia include neurogenic effects initiated by peripheral and neuraxial chemoreceptors and local humoral influences. Hypoxia leads to hyperpolarization by the opening of ATP-dependent $K^+$ channels, which leads to vasodilation.

## Autoregulation of Cerebral Blood Flow

Autoregulation is the ability of the cerebral circulation to adjust its resistance to maintain CBF constant over a wide range of mean arterial pressure (MAP). Autoregulation occurs between MAP values of approximately 70 and 150 mm Hg. However, some authors quote the lower limit of autoregulation as an MAP of 50 mm Hg. This phenomenon includes myogenic responses of the arterioles due to their ability to constrict in response to an increased distending pressure. Patients who are hypertensive demonstrate a shift of autoregulation of both the upper and the lower limit to higher pressures. Autoregulation can be abolished by trauma, hypoxia, and certain anesthetic and adjuvant anesthetic drugs.

During CEA, cerebral blood flow is more dependent on CPP as autoregulation to $paCO_2$ may not be predictable. Some advocate to maintain a higher MAP as autoregulation will maintain normal CBF in areas of normal brain vessels and in diseased areas, higher MAP will lead to higher CBF. The adverse effects of such deliberate hypertension include cerebral hemorrhage and cerebral edema. Systemic vasoconstriction needed to maintain higher MAP also leads to imbalance in myocardial oxygen supply and demand ratio. Patients receiving phenylephrine infusion to maintain higher MAP have been reported to have higher incidence of myocardial adverse events. Thereby routine intraoperative increase in blood pressure during CEA is not recommended. However, spontaneous increase of systolic blood pressure in the range of about 20% above the baseline may be acceptable during carotid cross clamping.

In a normothermic person with a normal brain autoregulation regional CBF is proportional to regional CMR. Electrophysiological changes associated with decrease in cerebral blood flow are as follows:

| |
|---|
| Normal CBF ≈50 ml/100 gm/min (average) grey > white |
| EEG starts to change ≈20–25 ml/100 gm/min |
| Loss of function starts at ≈20 ml/100 gm/min (awake patient) |
| Evoked potentials change ≈15–20 ml /100 gm/min |
| EEG flat ≈15–20 ml/100 gm/min |
| Membrane failure ≈10 ml/100 gm/min |

## Ischemic Pellucida and Ischemic Penumbra

In the brain, the critical lower value for cerebral blood flow is around 25 ml/100 g/min, under which two types of ischemic areas can be defined: the pellucida ("almost light") type where cerebral function is abolished, without permanent cerebral lesion and the penumbra ("almost shadow") type where cerebral tissue recovers only if flow is rapidly restored. In the penumbra type of ischemia, the duration is very important.

The term 'Penumbra' was introduced by Branston and colleagues. When CBF is interrupted, because of vessel occlusion there is a spectrum of injured neurons. In the affected region, there is a core of irreversibly damaged neurons surrounded by an area of electrically silent but viable neurons known as the ischemic penumbra. CBF in the penumbra area is been determined to be between 10 and 20 ml/100 g per minute. The area between electrical failure and membrane failure is termed the ischemic penumbra and is important in the explanation of how TIAs and the occurrence of transient major EEG changes may fail to produce long-term neurological deficits.

## Carotid Artery Occlusive Disease

### Natural History

The pathophysiology of carotid artery atherosclerosis is similar in most respect to atherosclerosis affecting other arteries as the atherosclerosis develops in regions of low wall shear stress. Most commonly, atherosclerosis involves the bifurcation of the common carotid artery with extension into both the internal and external carotid arteries. Cerebrovascular symptoms of carotid atherosclerosis results from embolization of thrombus or atheromatous debris and from a reduction in flow (hypoperfusion) secondary to stenosis. The relationship between plaque growth, vessel stenosis and clinical symptoms like TIA or stroke is widely varied and complex. The extent of cerebral injury depends on various factors like plaque morphology, characteristics of the embolus, hypoperfusion duration, cerebrovascular vasoreactivity, the circle of Willis and extent of cerebral collateral circulation.

Patient with carotid disease may have a varied spectrum of presentation. Usually the patient presents to the clinician in one of the following ways:

1. Patient is asymptomatic and carotid lesion is found on noninvasive screening test, like carotid ultrasonography;
2. Carotid bruit is auscultated on clinical examination; or
3. Extracranial carotid disease is found in patients having symptoms like previous stroke or transient ischemic attack.

It should however be emphasized that some patients have no carotid bruit but have significant carotid disease, and not all patients with a carotid bruit have significant extracranial carotid disease.

The risk for stroke depends on the degree of carotid artery stenosis. There is an annual stroke risk of about 1% in patients who are having asymptomatic carotid artery stenosis of less than 75%.

If the stenosis is greater than 75%, then the combined 1-year risk for TIA or stroke is about 10%.[7] *A new, tissue-based definition of TIA: a transient episode of neurological dysfunction caused by focal brain, spinal cord, or retinal ischemia, without acute infarction.*[8]

### Symptoms of Carotid Artery Territory Transient Ischemic Attacks

- Ipsilateral monocular blindness (amaurosis fugax)
- Contralateral weakness or paralysis
- Contralateral paresthesias, numbness or sensory loss
- Dysphasia
- Dysarthria
- Contralateral homonymous hemianopia

The incidence of symptoms is higher in patients having high-risk factors for atherosclerosis, patients with coronary artery disease and peripheral vascular disease. Simultaneously patients with carotid artery disease are at increased risk of MI and death attributable to cardiac disease.

## MEDICAL MANAGEMENT

Medical management of carotid atherosclerotic disease focuses on secondary prevention rather than acute interventions. Risk factors for carotid artery atherosclerotic disease and their management is considered first, and then it is followed by various medical treatments which are used to prevent different complications of carotid artery occlusive disease like ischemic strokes.[9]

The different risk factors of extracranial carotid disease are as follows:

### Nonmodifiable risk factors

- Advancing age,
- Gender,
- Race, and
- Previous TIA or stroke.

### Modifiable risk factors

- Arterial hypertension,
- Diabetes mellitus,
- Tobacco smoking,
- Heavy alcohol use,
- Hyperlipidemia, etc.

Risk factor management plays an important role in the treatment of the disease. The following ACC/AHA guidelines are recommended for the management of the modifiable risk factors:

1. **Hypertension:** The risk of stroke is increased in patients with hypertension.[10] The relationship between blood pressure and stroke is parallel. *In the Framingham Heart Study, a 2-fold greater risk of 25% carotid artery stenosis for each 20 mm Hg increase in systolic blood pressure was found.*[10] For patients with hypertension and asymptomatic extracranial carotid artery disease, antihypertensive treatment is recommended to maintain blood pressure below 140/90 mm Hg (Class 1, Level of Evidence: A).[11] In patients with heart failure, renal insufficiency, diabetes or other evidence of target organ damage or clinical cardiovascular disease, drug therapy combined with lifestyle modifications should be considered when BP is high-normal (systolic BP-130 to 139 mm Hg or

diastolic BP-85 to 89 mm Hg). However, in symptomatic patients with severe carotid artery stenosis, antihypertensive therapy may have both beneficial and harmful effect as it may reduce the cerebral perfusion.

2. **Smoking:** Patients with extracranial carotid atherosclerosis who smoke cigarettes are advised to quit smoking. *In the Framingham Heart Study, correlation was found between carotid artery stenosis and the quantity of cigarettes smoked.* Smoking cessation interventions can reduce the risks of progression of atherosclerosis and stroke (Level of Evidence: B).

3. **Hyperlipidemia:** Statins are recommended for all patients with carotid artery disease. It is advised to reduce low-density lipoprotein (LDL) cholesterol below 100 mg/dL Class I (Level of Evidence: B)[12] and to a level near or below 70 mg/dL in those with a history of ischemic stroke (Class 2 Level of Evidence: B).[11] Different studies have shown that lovastatin or pravastatin can reduce the development or progression of carotid atherosclerosis as measured by the thickness of the vessel intima-media complex on carotid ultrasonography.

4. **Diabetes:** Among available options, the American Diabetes Association (ADA) emphasizes lifestyle intervention over drugs with no available evidence, supporting the conclusion that treatment of impaired glucose tolerance (IGT) prevents macrovascular events. Intensive glycemic control (i.e. HbA1c <6% or <6.5%) does not appear to reduce all-cause mortality or stroke risk, however, a goal of <6.5% HbA1c may be appropriate in selected, mainly younger individuals if it can be accomplished safely and without frequent hypoglycemia.[11]

## Medical Management and Antithrombotic Therapy

The medical management of carotid artery occlusive disease focus on platelet anti-aggregrating drugs, which is one of the mainstay in the prevention of stroke.[13]

The various antiplatelet agents used are:

1. **Aspirin:** Aspirin is irreversibe inhibitor of platelet cyclo-oxygenase enzyme, which prevents the formation of thromboxane A2.Other advantage of aspirin include its effect on reducing cardiovascular deaths and in reducing the mortality after CEA. An overview of randomized trials of platelet anti-aggregant therapy in patients with a history of TIA or stroke showed about a 25% reduction in the risk for nonfatal stroke, nonfatal myocardial infarction, and death from vascular causes. However there is controversy regarding the adequate dose of aspirin .

In aspirin in CEA (ACE) trial, 2804 patients who had a CEA were enrolled.[14] The study compared the benefits of low-dose aspirin (81 to 325 mg/day) with high-dose aspirin (650 to 1300 mg/day). Three months after surgery, the risk for stroke, myocardial infarction, or death was 6.2% in the low-dose aspirin group compared with 8.4% in the high-dose aspirin group A low dose (81 to 325 mg) appears at least as effective as higher doses, and higher doses may in fact be less effective. The US. Food and Drug Administration recommends dose of 50 to 325 mg/day of aspirin.

2. **Ticlopidine:** Ticlopidine inhibits the adenosine phosphate pathway of platelet aggregation. It has been shown to reduce the risk for stroke, myocardial infarction, or vascular death in patients with recent noncardioembolic stroke. When compared with aspirin it is shown to reduce the relative risk for death or nonfatal stroke by 12%. The dose of ticlopidine is 250 mg twice daily.

3. **Clopidogrel:** It is a platelet adenosine diphosphate receptor antagonist. In a study of 19,185 patients clopidogrel (75 mg/day) was found to be more effective than 325 mg of aspirin in reducing the combined risk for ischemic stroke, myocardial infarction, or vascular death.[15-17]

4. **Dipyridamole:** It is a phosphodiesterase inhibitor that increases the levels of cyclic adenosine monophosphate (cAMP). The combination of clopidogrel and aspirin did not reduce stroke risk compared with either treatment alone in the MATCH[16] (Management of Atherothrombosis with Clopidogrel in High-risk Patients) and CHARISMA[17] (Clopidogrel for High Atherothrombotic Risk and Ischemic Stabilization, Management, and Avoidance) trials. The European Stroke Prevention Study-2 (ESPS-2) randomized patients with prior TIA or stroke to treatment with aspirin alone (25 mg twice daily), modified-release dipyridamole (200 mg twice daily), the two agents in combination, or a placebo. ESPS-2 concluded that aspirin 25 mg twice daily and dipyridamole, in a modified-release form, at a dose of 200 mg twice daily was effective for the secondary prevention of ischemic stroke and TIA.[18] The stroke rate decreased in the combined treatment arm compared with either agent alone.

5. **Other drugs:** The benefit of platelet glycoprotein IIb-IIIa receptor inhibitors in preventing ischemic stroke still awaits randomized studies.

Warfarin has also been used in the primary and secondary prevention of stroke in patients with nonvalvular atrial fibrillation. Warfarin has been used in patients with high-grade intracranial stenosis and severe ICA stenosis, but randomized clinical data are not available to support its use. Low molecular weight heparinoids are not recommended for patients with extracranial cerebrovascular atherosclerosis who develop transient cerebral ischemia or acute ischemic stroke.

## SELECTING THE APPROPRIATE THERAPY: MEDICAL MANAGEMENT, CAS, OR CEA

After proper identification of a patient with a clinically significant carotid stenosis appropriate treatment must be selected. Treatment is primarily aimed at the reduction of stroke risk. The risks of an interventional treatment have to be analysed according to individual patient when treatment choices are made. In different clinical trials the rates of stroke, MI, and death have been used while comparing medical management, carotid artery stenting (CAS) or CEA.

Since 1990, many well-designed studies defining the effectiveness of CEA in preventing strokes in both neurologically symptomatic and asymptomatic patients have been published. Carotid endarterectomy (CEA) is now well established as the standard treatment for severe symptomatic internal carotid artery stenosis. Carotid angioplasty and stenting (CAS) has also been advocated for stroke prevention in patients with atherosclerotic carotid artery disease, especially in patients who are at high risk for complications with CEA. The role of CAS in the treatment of patients with carotid artery disease however is controversial. At present, there are no data to prove superiority of CAS over CEA in either asymptomatic or symptomatic disease, and some authors believe that there is serious doubt about whether CAS is an equivalent treatment, except for patients who are simply unable to undergo CEA because of medical comorbidities. However, the CREST results suggest that outcomes are not significantly different between CAS and CEA when they are performed at centers with experienced clinician and when an aggregate end point of MI and stroke is used.[19]

ACC AHA makes the following recommendations for:

### Patients with Extracranial Carotid Atherosclerotic Disease are not undergoing Revascularization[20]

1. Antiplatelet therapy with aspirin, 75 to 325 mg daily, is recommended for patients with obstructive or nonobstructive atherosclerosis that involves the extracranial carotid for prevention of MI and other ischemic cardiovascular events, although the benefit has not been established for prevention of stroke in asymptomatic patients (Class I Level of Evidence: A).

2. In patients with obstructive or nonobstructive extracranial carotid or vertebral atherosclerosis who have sustained ischemic stroke or TIA, antiplatelet therapy with aspirin alone (75 to 325 mg daily), clopidogrel alone (75 mg daily), or the combination of aspirin plus extended-release dipyridamole (25 and 200 mg twice daily, respectively) is recommended (Level of Evidence: B) and preferred over the combination of aspirin with clopidogrel.

### ACC/AHA Recommendations for Selection of Patients for Carotid Revascularization

#### Class I

1. Patients at average or low surgical risk who have nondisabling ischemic stroke or transient cerebral ischemic symptoms, within 6 months (symptomatic patients) should undergo CEA if the diameter of the lumen of the ipsilateral internal carotid artery is reduced more than 70% as documented by non-invasive imaging (Level of Evidence: A) or more than 50% as documented by catheter angiography (Level of Evidence: B) and the anticipated rate of peri-operative stroke or mortality is less than 6%.

2. CAS is indicated as an alternative to CEA for symptomatic patients at average or low risk of complications associated with endovascular intervention when the diameter of the lumen of internal carotid artery is reduced by more than 70% as documented by non-invasive imaging or more than 50% as documented by catheter angiography and the anticipated rate of periprocedural stroke or mortality is less than 6% (Level of Evidence: B).

3. Selection of asymptomatic patients for carotid revascularization should be guided by an assessment of comorbid conditions, life expectancy, and other individual factors and should include a thorough discussion of the risks and benefits of the procedure with an understanding of patient preferences (Level of Evidence: C).

#### Class III: No Benefit

1. Carotid revascularization by either CEA or CAS is not recommended when atherosclerosis narrows the lumen by less than 50% (Level of Evidence: A).

2. It is not recommended for patients with chronic total occlusion of the targeted carotid artery (Level of Evidence: C).

3. It is not recommended for patients with severe disability caused by cerebral infarction that precludes preservation of useful function (Level of Evidence: C).

## CAROTID ENDARTERECTOMY VERSUS CAROTID ARTERY STENTING

| | Advantages | Disadvantages |
|---|---|---|
| **CEA** | ■ Widely available<br>■ Excellent result for high volume surgeons/hospital in low risk patients | ■ Outcome influenced by comorbidities<br>■ Longer hospital stay<br>■ Frequently performed under general anesthesia<br>■ Neck incision/scar<br>■ Neck complications/cranial nerve palsies<br>■ Not suitable for high or low carotid lesions |
| **CAS** | ■ Outcome less influenced by comorbidities<br>■ Local anesthesia<br>■ No neck incision/scar, usually next day discharges | ■ Fewer experienced operators<br>■ Risk of the procedure may increase in patients with severe peripheral vascular disease; severely calcified , tortuous/steep aortic arch<br>■ Femoral access site complications<br>■ May not be performed if aspirin/clopidogrel interference |

### Randomized Trials of Carotid Endarterectomy

Randomized trials have played an important role in the evolution of management of patients with the carotid artery disease.

### SYMPTOMATIC PATIENTS

Two important multicentric trials, NASCET and ECST, have clearly demonstrated the efficacy of CEA in symptomatic patients.

### North American Symptomatic CEA Trial (NASCET)[5]

Between January 1988 and February 1991, NASCET enrolled 659 patients at 50 clinical centers in the United States and Canada with symptomatic carotid stenosis in whom symptoms occurred within 120 days before entry into the trial. Three hundred thirty-one patients were randomized to medical therapy and 328 to surgery. The study was stopped early because of a clear and highly significant benefit from CEA in patients with high-grade (70 to 99%) stenosis. Subsequently, the

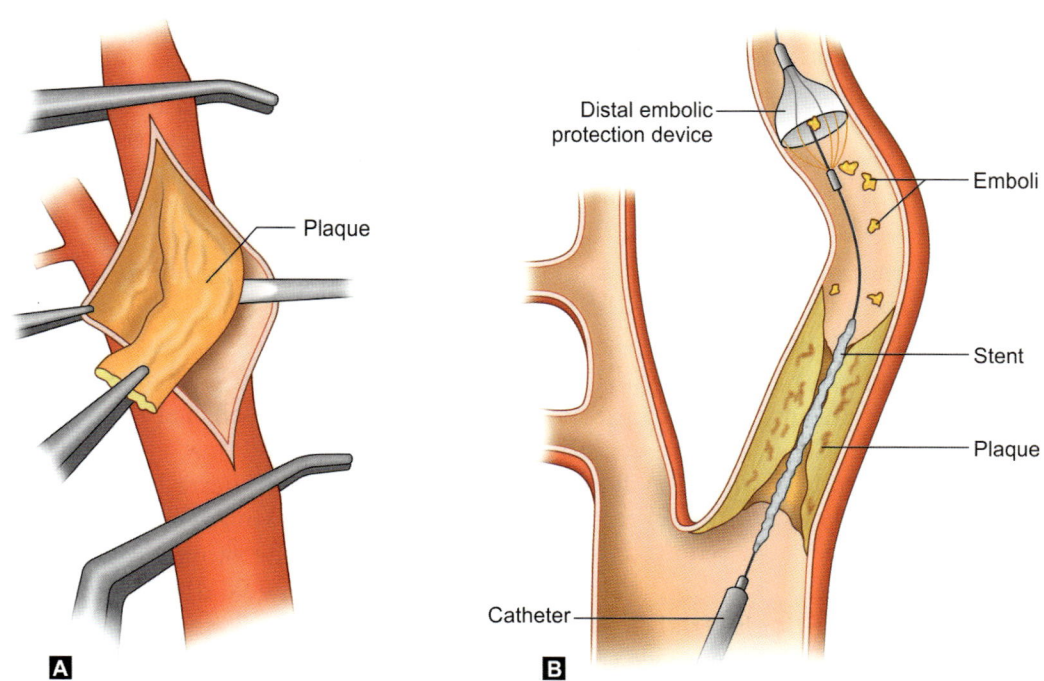

**Figs 10.3A and B:** Carotid endarterectomy versus stenting—intervention in the diseased carotid artery

NASCET investigators (1998) also demonstrated a benefit of CEA for patients with 50 to 69% carotid stenosis but not for those with less than 50% stenosis.

## European Carotid Surgery Trial [6]

A trial very similar to NASCET was undertaken at 97 centers in 12 European countries and the results reported in 1998. There were 1807 patients in the surgery group and 1211 patients in the medical management comparator group. Patients were stratified into 3 categories of mild (10 to 29%), moderate (30 to 69%), and severe (70 to 99%) carotid stenosis. The investigators found a highly significant benefit of CEA for patients with 70 to 99% stenosis but no benefit in those with milder stenosis.

## ASYMPTOMATIC PATIENTS

Patients with asymptomatic lesions are currently responsible for majority of the carotid interventions in the United States. The indications for CEA in asymptomatic patients are more controversial than those for symptomatic patients. ACAS[21] and ACST[22] evaluated the efficacy of CEA in asymptomatic patients.

## Asymptomatic Carotid Surgery Trial (ACAS)

ACST was the largest study to evaluate the efficacy of CEA for asymptomatic carotid stenosis. The 5-year risk for any stroke was 6.4% in the surgery cohort and 11.8% in the observation group. The Asymptomatic Carotid Atherosclerosis Study showed that asymptomatic patients with more than 60% stenosis have a better outcome with CEA than with medical management. ACAS demonstrated the superiority of CEA over antiplatelet therapy alone for asymptomatic patients.

## CAS TRIAL in Symptomatic Stenosis

Two large prospective randomized European trials, EVA-3S [23] and SPACE1,[24] examined the role of CAS vs CEA in neurologically symptomatic patients.

In EVA-3S the investigators compared CAS with CEA in 527 recently symptomatic patients who had carotid stenosis of at least 60%. This trial showed a statistically inferior outcome for CAS compared with CEA (stroke death, 9.5% vs 3.8%) but the study was criticized because of the relatively low level of experience required in the CAS arm.

International Carotid Stenting Study Trial (ICST),[25] enrolled 1713 patients, demonstrated an increased stroke risk for CAS (7.7%) compared with CEA (4.1%) in neurologically symptomatic patients.

## CREST [19]

The CREST trial randomly assigned 2502 patients with carotid atherosclerotic disease to endarterectomy or stenting. The proportion of enrolled patients with asymptomatic and symptomatic carotid disease was 47% and 53%, respectively. The overall effectiveness and safety of the two procedures (CAS and CEA) were similar, and the benefits were equal for men and women and for patients with asymptomatic and symptomatic carotid disease . The risk of composite primary outcome of stroke, MI, or death did not differ significantly among symptomatic and asymptomatic patients between CAS and CEA patients.

## OTHER CONSIDERATIONS

*Bilateral carotid artery disease:* When the extent of contralateral carotid disease is significant enough for bilateral CEA, mostly staged approach is prefered. When one side is symptomatic and the other asymptomatic, the symptomatic lesion is usually treated first and the asymptomatic side is treated after recovery from the first operation. If both sides are asymptomatic with similar stenosis, the lesion supplying the dominant hemisphere is first considered for intervention.

*Vascular procedures:* There are no trials of prophylactic CEA prior to major vascular procedures like aortic aneurysm repair or peripheral vascular procedures. Many vascular surgeons prefer performing prophylactic CEA in anticipation of vascular surgery involving significant hemodynamic fluctuations which will affect cerebral perfusion.

*Intracranial aneurysm:* Ipsilateral intracranial aneurysms which are distal to internal carotid artery stenosis are susceptible to sudden hemodynamic changes associated with CEA leading to aneurysm rupture. On the other hand, surgical clipping of an aneurysm distal to a severe internal carotid stenosis may increase the risk of ischemic stroke.

## Relative Contraindications for CEA

The following conditions may increase the risk of local or systemic complications:

1. History of prior neck irradiation resulting in "woody fibrosis" of the skin and subcutaneous tissues.
2. Concurrent tracheostomy
3. Prior radical neck dissection with or without radiation: Radical neck surgery poses surgical challenges because of the difficulty of exposing the artery and the relatively high risk of perioperative infection. The risk of cranial nerve injury is higher in

these situations, but the overall risks of mortality and stroke are comparable. Patients who have undergone cervical radiation therapy have an increased incidence of disease at the carotid bifurcation.

Modern radiation therapy has been designed specifically to avoid severe fibrotic tissue reactions. Several studies indicate that CEA can be performed successfully after neck radiation, although the procedure is technically challenging. In this situation, CAS may be safer to perform, but the rate of restenosis after CAS is high, ranging from 18 to 80% over 3 years.

4. Contralateral vocal cord paralysis from prior endarterectomy, because bilateral nerve palsies could compromise the airway.
5. Atypical lesion location, either high or low that is surgically inaccessible
6. Severe recurrent carotid stenosis
7. Unacceptably high medical risk

## PREOPERATIVE EVALUATION

One or more of the following factors are thought to have an association with poor outcome (stroke, myocardial infarction or death) at 30 days after CEA in a few studies:

- Age 80 years or older
- Severe heart disease
- Severe pulmonary dysfunction
- Renal insufficiency or failure
- Stroke as the indication for endarterectomy

National Surgical Quality Improvement Program of the American College of Surgeons analyzed a sample of 3949 patients to define the high risk characteristic for patients undergoing CEA. Patients with one or more "high risk" factors (age >80 years, major cardiac disease or chronic obstructive pulmonary disease) were considered to be high risk. It was observed that the 30 day stroke rate was similar for patients with and without "high risk" criteria (1.4% versus 1.7%) but the 30-day mortality was significantly higher for patients with "high risk" criteria (1.3% versus 0.4%).[26]

Risk is particularly high in those patients with acute or unstable neurological symptoms (e.g. very recent stroke or crescendo TIAs), and neurological risk is lower in asymptomatic patients or those with ocular symptoms only. Chronic renal failure, severe coronary artery or peripheral vascular disease or patients with a combination of medical risk factors also have poor perioperative outcome. Long term outcome is worse in patients who smoke, and those with diabetes or hyperlipidemia, but for these and other risk factors, for example, age or gender, the evidence is inconclusive.

*Mayo risk factor classification for CEA is as follows:*[27]

| Preoperative risk stratification for patients undergoing CEA | | |
|---|---|---|
| Risk group | Characteristics | Total Morbidity and Mortality (%) |
| 1 | Neurologically stable, no major medical or angiographic risk | 1 |
| 2 | Neurologically stable, significant angiographic risk, no major medical risk | 2 |
| 3 | Neurologically stable, major medical risk, major angiographic risk | 7 |
| 4 | Neurologically unstable, major medical or angiographic risk | 10 |

| Type of risk | Risk factors |
|---|---|
| Medical risk | Angina |
| | Myocardial infarction (<6 months) |
| | Congestive heart failure |
| | Severe hypertension (>180/110 mm Hg) |
| | Chronic obstructive pulmonary disease |
| | Age >70 years |
| | Severe obesity |
| Neurologic risk | Progressing deficit |
| | New deficit (<24 hours) |
| | Frequent daily TIA (s) |
| | Multiple cerebral infarcts |
| Angiographic risk | Contralateral ICA occlusion |
| | ICA siphon stenosis |
| | Proximal or distal plaque extension |
| | High carotid bifurcation |
| | Presence of soft thrombus |

The 2012 National Guidelines for Stroke recommend that carotid intervention for recently symptomatic severe carotid stenosis should be regarded as an emergency procedure in patients who are neurologically stable, and should ideally be performed within 48 hour of a transient ischemic attack or minor stroke and definitely within 1 week.

## CAROTID ARTERY OCCLUSIVE DISESASE IN ASSOCIATION WITH CORONARY ARTERY DISEASE

In evaluating patients with carotid arterial occlusive disease the systemic and progressive nature of athero-sclerosis must always be kept in consideration. CAD is common in patients undergoing CEA and is the one of the important cause of both early and late mortality.

According to the ACC cardiac risk stratification for noncardiac surgical procedures CEA is an intermediate risk surgery with a reported cardiac risk generally >1%

but <5%.[28] There is a high incidence of CAD in patients undergoing CEA but preoperative investigations are rarely needed for the evaluation of myocardial function except if there are major clinical predictors of increased perioperative cardiovascular risk like unstable angina, recent MI with evidence of ongoing ischemia, decompensated congestive heart failure, significant valvular disease, etc. This approach is based on the fact that randomized trials have established that CEA can prevent stroke in appropriately selected patients and it is unlikely that the results of specialized testing would lead to cancellation of the procedure. It is also believed that careful intraoperative and postoperative monitoring is standard for all patients undergoing CEA and so specialized preoperative testing has little potential to change perioperative management. Many clinicians consider the strategy to proceed with CEA without additional studies in asymptomatic stable CAD patients.

However patients having both severe CAD and severe carotid artery occlusive disease represent a management challenge because it is often controversial which disease should be treated first. The nature and severity of cerebrovascular and coronary disease must be evaluated and a decision must be made to perform either a combined or a staged procedure. A staged approach with CEA as the first procedure can lead to significant morbidity from cardiac causes whereas performing coronary revascularization first may result in a high incidence of stroke. For patients with both unstable CAD and symptomatic carotid artery disease, a combined procedure has been advocated.

Postoperative stroke complicates 1 to 2% of all isolated coronary artery bypass graft (CABG) surgery and can lead to a 3- to 6-fold increased risk of mortality and carotid artery stenosis has been recognized as a significant risk factor for perioperative stroke in this population. Increasing carotid disease burden seems to be associated with a higher risk of stroke after CABG. ACC/AHA guidelines recommend selective preCABG screening for carotid artery disease by carotid duplex ultrasound in patients who are ≥65 years old, have left main coronary disease, peripheral vascular disease, history of tobacco use, history of prior stroke/TIA, or a carotid bruit.[29] An increase in the incidence of CVA in the perioperative period for patients undergoing cardiac surgery has been demonstrated for patients with a carotid bruit, carotid stenosis of more than 50%, or a history of TIA or CVA.

In conclusion, numerous reports support a combined approach with both low morbidity and low mortality but no randomized trials have been performed to assess the benefit of combined versus staged procedures. Management of an individual patient should thereby be guided by careful assessment of the severity of the coronary and carotid disease with emphasis on both surgeon and institution specific experience. Carotid artery angioplasty plus stenting has recently been introduced as an alternative revascularization modality before staged CABG. The role of carotid artery angioplasty and stenting in this setting is unproven. When coronary intervention can be performed percutaneously, this should precede carotid intervention. A review of the literature to date suggests that CEA, followed by CABG, is associated with the lowest stroke rate, whereas combined CEA and CABG carries a higher mortality rate, and delayed CEA is associated with the lowest mortality but the highest stroke rate. In a meta-analysis, Naylor et al found that the total stroke/MI/death rate associated with any combination CEA and CABG ranges from 9 to 12%.[30]

### Medical management for the perioperative period of patients with carotid occlusive disease

Recommendations for periprocedural management of patients undergoing CEA are as follows:

*Class I*

1. Aspirin (81 to 325 mg daily) is recommended before CEA and may be continued indefinitely postoperatively (Level of Evidence: A)
2. Beyond the first month after CEA, aspirin (75 to 325 mg daily), clopidogrel (75 mg daily), or the combination of low-dose aspirin plus extended-release dipyridamole (25 and 200 mg twice daily, respectively) should be administered for long-term prophylaxis against ischemic cardiovascular events (Level of Evidence: B)
3. Administration of antihypertensive medication is recommended as needed to control blood pressure before and after CEA (Level of Evidence: C)
4. The findings of clinical neurological examination should be documented within 24 hours before and after CEA (Level of Evidence: C)

*Class IIa*

1. Patch angioplasty can be beneficial for closure of the arteriotomy after CEA (Level of Evidence: B)
2. Administration of lipid-lowering medication for prevention of ischemic events is reasonable for patients who have undergone CEA irrespective of serum lipid levels, although the optimum agent and dose and the efficacy for prevention of restenosis have not been established (Level of Evidence: B)

Patients taking combined aspirin and clopidogrel therapy in the perioperative period have a 0.4 to 1.0% higher risk of major bleeding compared with aspirin alone. Aspirin therapy alone does not have to be discontinued before CEA. The risks of periprocedural MI from aspirin withdrawal outweighs the risk of fatal or severe bleeding from aspirin use. The ACC Perioperative Guidelines endorses the continued use of aspirin before and after CEA. Patients should continue aspirin therapy after CEA indefinitely, according to recommendations for high-risk patients with atherosclerosis.

There has been a consensus that preprocedural clopidogrel should be stopped approximately 5 days before elective CABG. Recent data from a large, retrospective, multicentered clinical experience suggest that clopidogrel may be safely continued through the perioperative period without increased bleeding risk. It is therefore reasonable to individualize the management of perioperative clopidogrel therapy. There is no clear information regarding the risks or benefits of continued clopidogrel monotherapy in the periprocedural period for CEA.

One meta-analysis showed preoperative statin therapy resulted in a significant reduction in perioperative mortality in patients undergoing vascular surgery. One small randomized trial found that perioperative death, MI and stroke in patients undergoing vascular surgery was reduced in the group treated with atorvastatin. The evidence for continued use of statin therapy currently remains largely observational. Furthermore, the optimal time for starting therapy, the duration of therapy, dose or target LDL levels to be achieved still remain to be determined.

Antihypertensive, beta blocker and lipid-lowering therapy should be initiated in patients undergoing CAS according to the same recommendations for CEA. Patients should be started on dual antiplatelet therapy with aspirin (325 mg) and clopidogrel (75 mg). No randomized trial has yet compared CAS performed with dual-antiplatelet therapy vs aspirin alone. However, the published periprocedural stroke, MI and death rates in all recent clinical trials have been achieved with this combination therapy.

*Assessing the risk associated with intervention*

The risk associated with CEA and CAS can be increased with certain clinical features like:

*1. Anatomic characteristics*

a. **Lesion location:** Surgical exposure is difficult for lesions at or above the level of the C2 cervical vertebra, below the clavicle, and lesions extending outside the cervical segment of carotid artery. The high carotid artery surgical exposure may be associated with increased difficulty in directly visualizing the end point of the endarterectomy and can be associated with increased incidence of vagus nerve injury .

b. **Lesion characteristics:** Certain lesion-specific characteristics are thought to increase the risk of cerebral vascular events after CAS. Different lesion characteristic like "soft" lipid-rich plaque, extensive (15 mm or more) disease, a preocclusive lesion, heavy calcification, unstable plaque, etc. can increase the risk of embolization during placement of the wire or stent across the carotid lesion.

*2. Patient characteristics:* The risk of periprocedural events after CEA or CAS might be increased in patients presenting with severe comorbid conditions, like dialysis-dependent renal failure, New York Heart Association class III or IV heart disease, left ventricular ejection fraction less than 30%, class III or IV angina pectoris, left main or multivessel coronary disease, severe aortic valvular disease, oxygen- or steroid-dependent pulmonary disease, or contralateral carotid occlusion.

## ANESTHESIA GOALS FOR CAROTID ENDARTERECTOMY

Anesthetic management goals for CEA include the following:
1. Protection of the heart and brain from ischemic injury,
2. Hemodynamic stability with control of the heart rate and blood pressure,
3. Adequate analgesia from surgical pain
4. Adequate stress response management
5. To have an awake patient at the end of surgery for the purpose of neurologic examination

## WHAT ARE THE ANESTHETIC TECHNIQUES FOR CAROTID SURGERY?

An ideal anesthesia technique should provide optimal brain perfusion and oxygenation, optimal hemodynamic and myocardial oxygen balance, adequate stress response management, early identification of neurological injury, with good surgical and patient comfort.

The type of anesthesia depends on the predisposition of the surgeon and anesthesiologist and the cooperation of the patient.

Patients undergoing CEA are anesthetized with one of the following techniques:
1. General anesthesia (GA) with inhaled or total intravenous anesthesia or a special technique of GA

(cooperative patient general anesthesia), which is total intravenous anesthesia that is reduced to only high-dose remifentanil during carotid clamping.

2. Regional anesthesia.

*GALA Trial:* It was a parallel group, multicentre, rando-mised controlled trial of 3526 patients with symptomatic or asymptomatic carotid stenosis from 95 centers in 24 countries.[31] Participants were assigned to surgery under general (n = 1753) or local (n = 1773) anesthesia groups. The primary outcome was to analyse the proportion of patients with stroke (including retinal infarction), myocardial infarction, or death 30 days after surgery in the two groups. The trial concluded that there was no definite difference in outcomes between general and local anesthesia for carotid surgery. The two groups did not significantly differ for quality of life, length of hospital stay, or the primary outcome in the prespecified subgroups of age, contralateral carotid occlusion, and baseline surgical risk. The anesthetist and surgeon, in consultation with the patient, should decide which anesthetic techniques to be used on an individual basis.

## REGIONAL ANESTHESIA

CEA under regional anesthesia requires blocking the second, third and fourth cervical dermatome. Regional anesthesia is suitable for different surgical approaches like transverse or longitudinal incision. However, if the transverse incision crosses midline then supplemental local anesthetic infiltration will be required. Some over-lap of unanesthetized dermatomes onto the surgical field, from the contralateral side may cause patient discomfort and may require supplemental local anes-thetic. Sedation is usually supplemented with the regional block during awake CEA, as inadequate analgesia and anxiety may increase the stress response which can result in various adverse effects.

### Anatomy for Regional Anesthesia

The cervical plexus is formed by the ventral rami of the upper four cervical nerves (C1–C4). The nerves pass laterally along the corresponding transverse process. The superficial sensory branches supply the skin and subcutaneous tissues of the neck and posterior aspect of the head and the deep motor branches supply the neck muscles. Ansa cervicalis (C1–C3), is formed from the motor component of the plexus and supplies the nerves to the anterior neck muscles. The anatomical distribution of the cervical dermatomes is shown in Fig. 10.4.

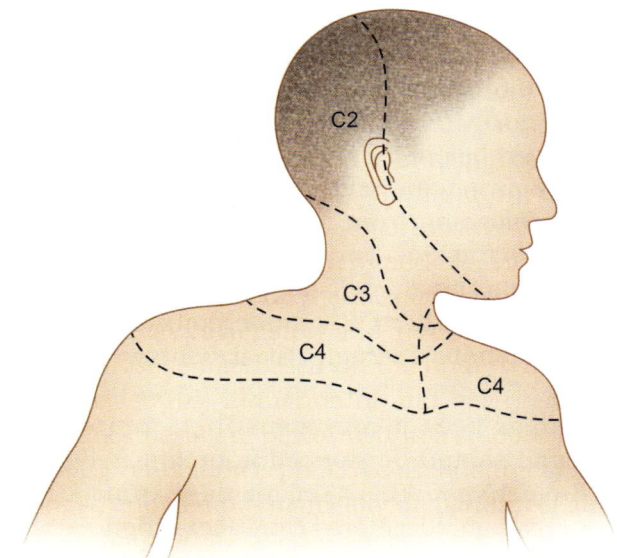

**Fig. 10.4:** Anatomy of the cervical dermatomes

The branches of the cervical plexus are as follows:

| Cutaneous branches | Lesser occipital nerve (C2,3)<br>Greater auricular nerve (C2,3)<br>Transverse cervical nerve (C3,4)<br>Supraclavicular nerve (C3,4) |
|---|---|
| Muscular branches | Ansa cervicalis (C1–3)<br>Branches to posterolateral neck muscles |

Four different techniques are commonly used:
1. Local infiltration.
2. Cervical epidural.
3. Superficial cervical plexus nerve block.
4. Superficial and deep cervical plexus nerve block.

### Advantages of Regional Anesthesia

1. Ease of neurological monitoring and identification of patients requiring shunt. Regional anesthesia is associated with a better assessment of neurologic function during surgery. The most reliable way to assess neurological function is to perform surgery under local anesthesia in an awake patient. Any change in consciousness, speech, higher mental function or muscle function after clamping of the carotid artery will provide an early sign of impending cerebral injury. Decrease in cerebral blood flow and ischemia results in deterioration of conscious level or focal deficit. Higher cortical function can be examined by minimental state questions and motor function by asking the patient to hold or squeeze objects like toy in the contra-lateral hand. If there is any sign of hypoperfusion resulting in clinical symptom a shunt can be used.

2. Regional anesthesia leads to the avoidance of expensive neurologic monitors during surgery.

3. Preservation of normal cerebrovascular reflexes with local anesthesia. Cerebral oxygenation is maintained following application of the carotid clamps during loco-regional anesthesia. This phenomenon appears to depend on a reflex rise in blood pressure that is not seen in general anesthetic compared to local anesthesia patients. The preservation of normal cerebrovascular reflexes results in less cerebral injury.

4. Greater stability of blood pressure and decreased vasopressor requirements.

5. Preserved cerebral autoregulation of perfusion: During regional anesthesia, autoregulation of brain circulation is maintained providing physiological distribution of blood flow during hypoperfusion periods that preserve oxygen balance.

6. It can avoid some adverse consequences of GA on health-related quality of life

7. Lower cardiovascular morbidity: Magnadottir et al concluded after a series of 600 cases of CEA that regional anesthesia is safer than general anesthesia in terms of cardiopulmonary complications.[32]

8. Shorter ICU and hospital stay: Papavasiliou et al found that the mean hospital stay was shorter after regional anesthesia (1.25 days ) in comparison to after general anesthesia (3.48 days).[33]

9. Lower expense: Ricotta et al demonstrated a significant cost difference while providing local anesthesia in comparison to general anesthesia. [34]

10. Local anesthesia seems to be more effective than general anesthesia for patients with contralateral carotid occlusion.

## Disadvantages of Regional Anesthesia

1. A proportion of patients are unsuitable for local anesthesia because communication with the patient to allow accurate awake testing is not possible like in patients who have residual motor weakness, dysarthria or dysphasia following a previous stroke, patients who are deaf or who do not speak the same language as the anesthetist which does not allow effective communication.

2. High degree of patient cooperation and contact is essential throughout the procedure. The following patients are not suitable candidates for a regional block: patients who are unable to remain still or follow directions; patients with joint problems, tremors, or neurologic disorders; anxious, agitated, or claustrophobic patients; and patients with a short, fat neck.

3. There is difficulty in emergency intraoperative airway control. If there is an urgent need to secure the airway for various reasons including airway obstruction, restlessness, loss of consciousness, or a grand mal seizure, tracheal intubation can be technically difficult and associated with hemodynamic instability (anesthetic-induced hypotension) and additional risks for patients.

4. Regional anesthesia may not be effective in preventing intraoperative myocardial ischemia Pain and anxiety during the procedure might increase the risk of myocardial ischemia.

5. When compared with general anesthesia, regional anesthesia may not be effective in decreasing the stress response of surgery. It may be associated with increased levels of blood catecholamines. A high incidence of tachycardia has been reported in patients undergoing regional anesthesia for CEA.

6. Certain complications are associated with regional anesthesia techniques like nerve injuries or accidental intravascular drug injection.

## Local Infiltration

The use of local anesthetic alone by the method of infiltration has been described by various authors .The anesthetist or the surgeon can anesthetize the different tissue layer by using large volumes of dilute local anestheic along the line of incision, at each dissection plane and finally into the carotid sheath.

### Advantage
- It is a simple technique.
- It is easy to perform.
- Rescue technique in case of less than adequate nerve block.

### Disadvantage
- It is a slow technique.
- May be uncomfortable to the patient and so it is not well tolerated by the patient.
- Time consuming and so the surgeon may not have the patience to use the technique effectively.

## Cervical Epidural

Originally performed by Dogliotti in 1933 for thoracic surgery, this block can provide suitable conditions for carotid surgery. An epidural catheter is inserted at C6–7 and a dilute anesthetic solution such as bupivacaine 0.25% injected.

*Technique of cervical epidural:* Patients are to be placed in the sitting position with the head flexed and resting on the thorax, in order to open the lowest cervical interspaces. The spinous process of C7, which is horizontal in this position is identified. An 18-gauge Tuohy needle is inserted by a midline approach into the C6–C7 or C7–TI interspace after cutaneous local anesthesia. The epidural space can be identified by aspiration of a saline solution drop hanging at the needle base. It should be ensured that the needle has not entered into the subarachnoid space nor penetrated an epidural vein. The epidural catheter should be inserted gently. In ASA physical status IV patients, cervical epidural insertion can be performed in the lateral decubitus position, using the loss of resistance technique. The local anesthetic solution be injected after a test dose like 2 ml of 2 percent lidocaine. An epidural catheter may be 'topped up' for prolonged procedures.

*Concerns with cervical epidural:* Bilateral cervical and upper thoracic nerve roots are affected with cervical epidural which can result in significant side-effects, including hypotension, bradycardia, and respiratory impairment.

Dural tap, epidural hematoma and direct spinal cord damage are few dangerous complications which are associated with the technique. Neurological deficit can also occur in a significant proportion of patients, but the incidence of permanent neurological deficit is correspondingly low. However, it is emphasized that the experience of the technique is essential to prevent the highly dangerous complications which may occur occasionally.

*Superficial cervical plexus nerve block:* Superficial block is performed superficial to the investing layer of deep cervical fascia. A superficial block alone is seldom sufficient for CEA. The deep branches supplying the neck muscles cannot be blocked making surgery on the deep structures difficult.

It can be performed by either of the following two techniques:

1. *Landmark technique:* The patient is in a supine position with the head facing away from the side to be blocked. The primary landmarks which need to be identified for performing this block include the following:

   A. Mastoid process
   B. Clavicular head of the sternocleidomastoid
   C. The midpoint of the posterior border of the sternocleidomastoid

   The landmark are shown in Fig. 10.5.

   The needle is inserted along the posterior border of the sternocleidomastoid and three injections of 5 ml of local anesthetic are injected behind the posterior border of the sternocleidomastoid muscle subcutaneously, perpendicularly, cephalad, and caudad in a 'fan' shaped manner. The direction of the needle is shown in Fig. 10.6.

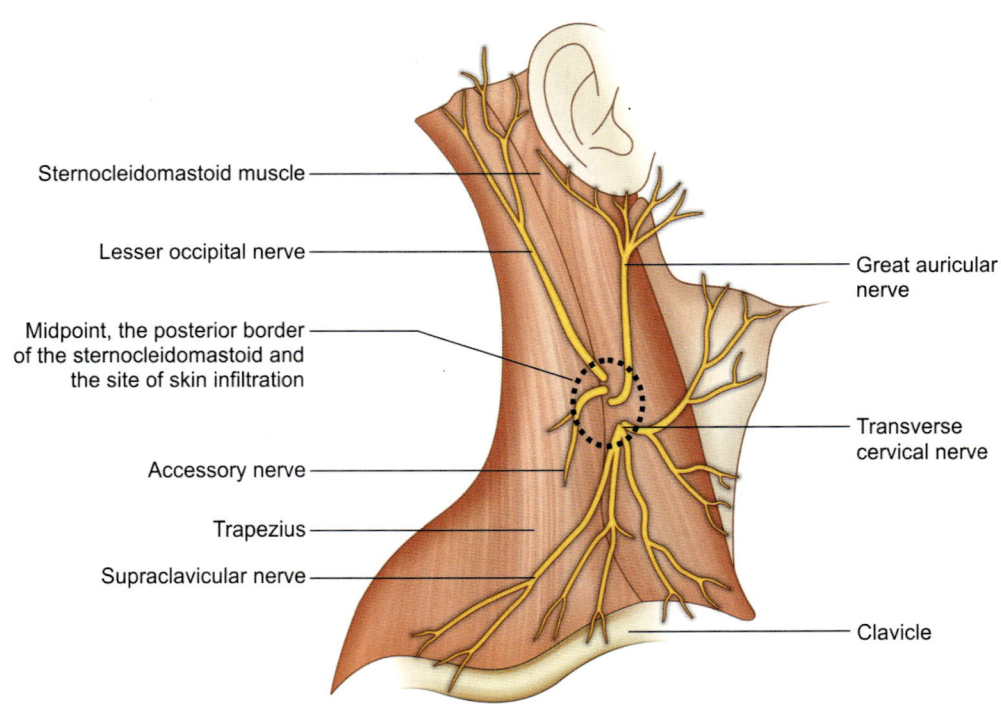

**Fig. 10.5:** Anatomical landmark for superficial cervical plexus block

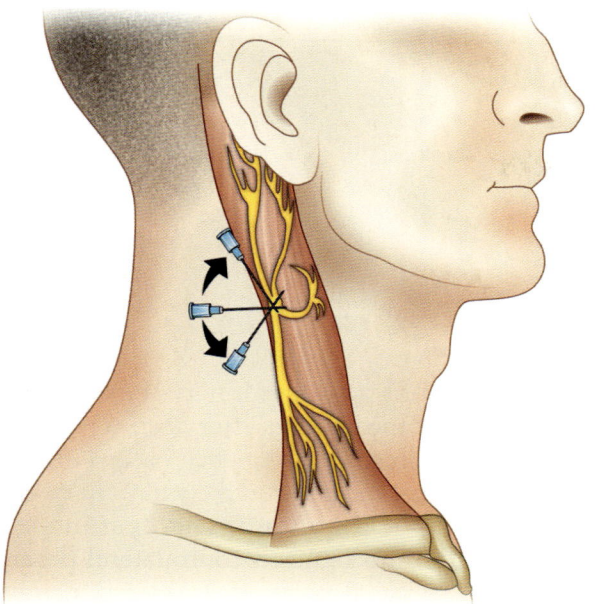

**Fig. 10.6:** Three different directions of needle for injection along the posterior border of sternocleidomastoid muscle to provide a complete superficial cervical plexus block

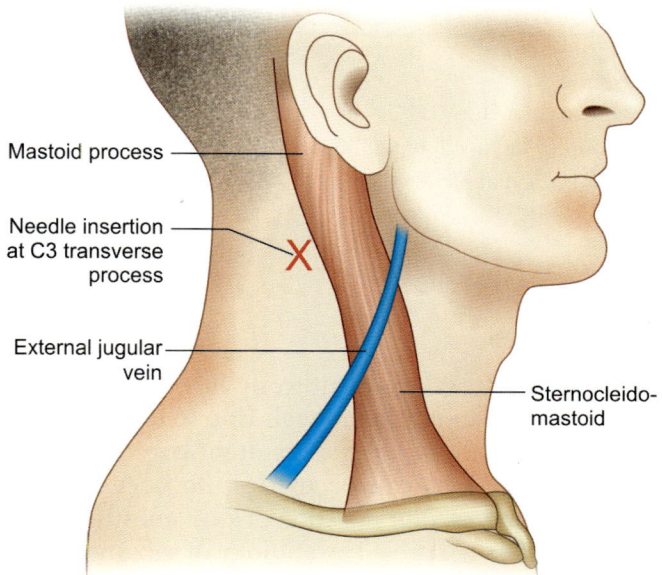

**Fig. 10.7:** Surface marking for deep cervical plexus block

2. *Ultrasound-guided superficial cervical plexus block:* Ultrasound guidance for regional anesthesia is in widespread practice as a means to improve quality and safety. Ultrasound can demonstrate the cutaneous branches of the superficial cervical plexus and their relation to the surrounding anatomy. The advantages over the landmark technique include the ability to visualize the spread of LA in the correct plane and to avoid inadvertent damage to neighbouring structures. However, ultrasound guidance has not been shown to improve the success of superficial cervical plexus blocks.

## DEEP CERVICAL PLEXUS BLOCK

This block is performed as a single or multiple injection technique. It can be performed by either of the following two techniques:

1. *Landmark technique:* The three landmarks for a deep cervical plexus block are as follows:
   - Mastoid process
   - Chassaignac's tubercle (transverse process of C6)
   - Posterior border of the sternocleidomastoid muscle

   The patient is in the same position as for the superficial cervical plexus block. The surface marking for the block is shown in Fig. 10.7.

   The cervical transverse processes is palpated behind the sternocleidomastoid muscle. After skin disinfection and intradermal infiltration with lidocaine, 25 G block needle is usually introduced in a slightly caudal and posterior direction until the cervical transverse process is encountered. A slightly caudal orientation of the needle is important to prevent inadvertent insertion of the needle toward the cervical spinal cord and the needle should never be oriented cephalad.

   Nerve stimulators can serve as a useful method in identifying the deep cervical plexus. Responses which may be elicited from nerve stimulator for deep cervical plexus identification include neck muscle contractions; scapular movements like elevation and internal rotation; paresthesia over the upper arm, shoulder, neck, etc.

2. *Ultrasound-guided deep cervical plexus block:* The transverse process are easily visualized subcutaneously with ultrasound The neck is scanned from the mastoid process to Chassaignac's tubercle to allow identification of the relevant anatomy.

### Pharmacology of Cervical Plexus Block

Most local anesthetic agents have been used for cervical plexus block. Ropivacaine and levobupivacaine are less potent than bupivacaine, but have a safer profile with regard to LA toxicity. Ropivacaine has the advantage of offering longer postoperative pain relief compared with mepivacaine and causing less vasodilatation than levobupivacaine.

## COMPLICATIONS OF REGIONAL ANESTHESIA

| Superficial plexus block | Deep plexus block | Cervical epidural anesthesia |
|---|---|---|
| ■ Intravascular injection | ■ Intravascular injection | ■ Hypotension/bradycardia |
| ■ Recurrent laryngeal nerve block | ■ Subarachnoid injection with brainstem anesthesia | ■ Respiratory failure |
| ■ Partial brachial plexus block | ■ Phrenic nerve block | ■ Dural puncture |
| | ■ Recurrent laryngeal nerve block | ■ Bloody tap |
| | ■ Vagus nerve block | |
| | ■ Horner syndrome | |

1. *Toxic reactions:* Can result from either intravascular injections or high blood levels due to large volumes of local anesthetic with a resultant overdose. Intra-aterial injections can occur despite negative aspiration. Intravascular injection of local anesthetic drug can result in seizures. The etiology of seizures during CEA is multifactorial which includes causes like LA overdose, direct intravascular injection of local anesthetic, cerebral ischemia, etc.

2. *Cervical plexus block complication:* It is observed that more complications result in patients undergoing deep cervical plexus block and combined deep and superficial cervical plexus block in comparison to superficial block alone. The higher success rate of USG guided block is yet to demonstrated in large clinical trials for cervical plexus block . Complications include subarachnoid and epidural injections at the cervical level and it usually occurs when the needle is not kept in a slightly caudad direction during injection. There is also a possibility of intraspinal puncture and subsequent injury to the spinal cord. It is also possible for the local anesthetic to spread into the neuraxis by means of direct penetration of the intervertebral foramen of the cervical spine producing total brainstem anesthesia.

3. *Cardiovascular complications:* In GALA trial no difference was seen in myocardial infarction between the GA and LA groups. Cardiac complications are relatively common in arteriopaths presenting for any type of surgery, so the development of cardiac complications after administration of cervical plexus block may not necessarily imply a causal relationship. Accidental surgical manipulation of the vagus nerve, which lies within the carotid sheath, can lead to profound hemodynamic disturbance, including nausea and vomiting, bradycardia, hypotension, and even cardiovascular collapse. In patients undergoing CEA under cervical plexus blockade, ST-segment depression occurring during clamping or shortly after declamping is highly predictive of adverse cardiac complications.

4. *Airway complications:* Phrenic nerve block may occur in up to half of the patients after deep cervical block. It is of little clinical consequence except in patients with severe chronic obstructive pulmonary disease or contralateral diaphragmatic dysfunction. In patients with unrecognized contralateral phrenic or recurrent laryngeal nerve damage from previous cardiac or neck surgery, cervical plexus block may result in respiratory distress or obstruction. Airway compromise after CEA may be life-threatening. Airway edema is demonstrable in all patients undergoing CEA. It may be due to local trauma and interference with venous and lymphatic drainage.

4. *Nerve injuries:* Nerve injuries can occur as a result of the regional block or the surgery itself and may be asymptomatic. The nerves at risk of injury are the marginal mandibular branch of the facial, laryngeal, accessory, hypoglossal, the sympathetic chain (Horner's syndrome) and the radial nerve. The cutaneous sensory nerves supplying the second, third and fourth dermatomes can also be damaged. Most cranial nerve injuries probably result from stretching, retraction, clamping, or imprudent use of diathermy and resolve within four months. Dexamethasone has been shown to be effective at decreasing the incidence of temporary post-CEA cranial nerve dysfunction. Facial nerve block has also been described after superficial cervical plexus block and must be distinguished from a cerebrovascular event.[7]

## GENERAL ANESTHESIA

Oxygenation, the airway, systemic arterial pressure and blood carbon dioxide tensions may be controlled effectively under general anesthesia, allowing the anesthetist to influence over factors which improve surgical outcome; namely cerebral blood flow and cerebral metabolism.[35,36] Some degree of cerebral protection is another benefit of the carefully managed general anesthetic. General anesthesia is usually maintained with a combination of volatile anesthetic (typically isoflurane, desflurane, or sevoflurane) and opioid. Neuromuscular blockade is maintained throughout the procedure. Propofol infusion is a reasonable alternative. The use of remifentanil, an ultrashort-acting opioid, has also become popular as an adjunct to general anesthesia for CEA. Its short duration of action facilitates titration of anesthesia and promotes early emergence, particularly when used in combination with short-acting volatile anesthetic drugs such as desflurane and sevoflurane.

## Advantages

1. It provides a safe airway throughout the procedure with controlled ventilation and arterial carbon dioxide concentrations.

2. Pharmacological cerebral protection by general anaesthetic agents: Both inhalation and intravenous agents have theoretical neuroprotective effects which may help in decreasing the cerebral injury.

3. Patients can find CEA under regional anesthesia stressful. They must lie still with their head turned to one side for 90 min or more and the positioning of the drapes may be profoundly unpleasant for a claustrophobic patient.

4. General anesthesia provides the surgeon with better operating field, motionless operating area and better visualization.

5. Stress reduction with general anesthesia may benefit patients with unstable cardiovascular conditions.

## Disadvantages

1. Complications of GA ranging from major airway problems to "minor" complications including headache, sore throat, nausea and vomiting.

2. In patients undergoing GA, the development of a new stroke is recognized only after recovery from anesthesia. The residual effects of GA in the early postoperative period can mask the symptoms or signs of neurologic complications from surgery.

3. Neuromonitoring methods used with general anesthesia have relatively low sensitivity and specificity for detecting inadequate cerebral perfusion and intraoperative stroke, with the chance of false-positive and false-negative results in comparison to an awake patient under regional anesthesia.

## Monitoring during CEA

1. *ECG:* Continuous ECG monitoring is mandatory. Five-lead ECG monitoring should be used and two ECG leads (usually II and V5) should be displayed. Automated ST-segment analysis should be used if available. Continuous ECG monitoring is necessary to detect arrhythmias myocardial ischemia. Depression of the ST segment >1 mm may indicate myocardial ischemia, prompting interventions to improve myocardial oxygen supply and reduce myocardial oxygen demand (e.g. raising diastolic blood pressure or decreasing heart rate).

2. *Invasive blood pressure:* An indwelling arterial catheter is usually inserted in the contralateral radial artery. It is used for direct monitoring of systemic arterial pressure in order to rapidly detect and treat hypotension or hypertension and collection of blood for arterial blood-gas analysis and other laboratory tests. The Australian Incident Monitoring Study established the superiority of direct arterial blood pressure monitoring over indirect monitoring techniques for the early detection of intraoperative hypotension.

3. *Pulse oximeter:* The pulse oximeter provides not only a continuous estimate of blood oxygen saturation, but also the detection of a peripheral pulse.

4. *Temperature monitoring:* It is a useful aid to maintenance of cardiovascular stability and also to estimation of appropriate timing of awakening and antagonism of neuromuscular block.

5. *Central line or pulmonary artery catheter:* As large blood losses or fluid loads are not usually associated with the procedure, central venous or pulmonary artery catheterization is unnecessary unless the cardiovascular system is unstable (recent myocardial infarction) or there is a history of congestive heart failure or poor left ventricular function.

## Airway Management

The operation may be performed with a laryngeal mask airway. In view of difficult access to the airway during surgery and with the head turned to one side, most anesthesiologists prefer the definitive airway control offered by endotracheal intubation.

## Patient Positioning

If general anesthesia is being considered, positioning of the patient's head is an important consideration. Many patients have cervical spondylosis, vertebro-basilar insufficiency, or both, and inappropriate operative positioning may exacerbate or cause neurological damage.

## PHARMACOLOGICAL CEREBRAL PROTECTION BY ANESTHETIC AGENTS

*Barbiturates:* The primary mechanism by which barbiturates provide cerebral protection include the ability of barbiturates to reduce oxygen metabolism ($CMRO_2$) and thereby the oxygen demand, by decreasing the electrical activity. Other mechanisms include redistribution of regional cerebral blood flow, reduction in intracranial pressure, prevention of oedema and inhibition of $Ca^{++}$ influx. However large doses can cause both cardiovascular and respiratory complications.

*Etomidate and propofol:* They may also provide cerebral protection by similar mechanisms (reduction in $CMRO_2$, redistribution of cerebral blood flow, inhibition of free fatty acid liberation). The side effect of etomidate include adrenocortical suppression and myoclonus.

*Inhalational agents:* Many consider sevoflurane, the volatile agent of choice for neuroanesthesia. Desflurane has been shown in an animal model to cause marked vasodilation increasing cerebral blood volume, and hence intracranial pressure. Although both sevoflurane and isoflurane can provide rapid recovery, sevoflurane produces less vasodilation than isoflurane at the same depth of anesthesia.

### Preconditioning

It is known that both volatile and intravenous anesthetics have a role in anesthetic preconditioning and postconditioning, but it seems that sevoflurane and propofol have different energy-related mechanisms for preconditioning. Sevoflurane directly affects ATP synthesis through regulation of cytochrome oxidase (complex IV) and ATP synthase, so that the protective effects of sevoflurane in ischemic conditions are related to its energy-preserving effect while propofol has a role in mitochondrial localization of cytochrome c and in maintaining mitochondrial membrane potential. Volatile anesthetics provide major improvement in ischemic outcome, and the dose needed to achieve this neuroprotection is within a clinically relevant range, while higher doses actually may worsen outcome. Volatile anesthetics protect against both global (e.g. complete cessation of blood flow to the brain) and focal (e.g. obstruction of flow distal to the circle of Willis) ischemia. However, in focal ischemia the improvement in outcome is persistent, whereas in global ischemia the improvement in outcome is transient.

### Role of Nitrous Oxide

The use of nitrous oxide should be avoided if possible. Nitrous oxide increases the cerebral metabolic rate and produces a concomitant increase in middle cerebral artery blood flow velocity. It causes increase in cerebral blood flow in the presence of both the volatile anesthetic agents and propofol. The administration of nitrous oxide is controversial as a result of reports of potential adverse effects on cerebral metabolism and increased risk of postoperative vomiting.

*$pCO_2$ manipulation:* In the 1960s it was believed that general anesthesia with hypercapnia was the preferred technique for CEA. Hypercapnia causes vasodilatation leading to increase global cerebral blood flow and so hypoventilation was one of the perceived methods to increase the cerebral blood flow. It was thought to provide cerebral protection. This technique is not followed now for two reasons. First, intracerebral steal may occur with the diversion of blood supply from compromised tissue to relatively normal tissue, leading to hypoxic brain damage. Second, because of the deleterious effects on the heart of increased carbon dioxide tension. Myocardial ischemia and arrhythmias may develop. However, no studies have proved any clinical benefit of manipulating carbon dioxide so most anesthetist maintain normocarbia during the procedure.

*Hyperglycemia:* Hyperglycemia worsens ischaemic brain damage and should be avoided. Emphasis should be on maintenance of normoglycemia during surgery. A few authors suggest that it may be beneficial to maintain a blood glucose level below 200 mg/dL in patients undergoing CEA. The Johns Hopkins Hospital found that operative-day glucose greater than 200 mg/dL at the time of CEA was associated with an increased risk for perioperative stroke or transient ischemic attack, MI, and death.[37] However, if insulin is used to treat preoperative or intraoperative hyperglycemia then there should be careful monitoring of the blood glucose level to avoid the dangers of hypoglycemia.

*Blood pressure manipulation:* The high incidence of associated risk factors like ischemic heart disease, heart failure, diabetes mellitus, etc. in patients undergoing CEA predisposes the patients to increased cardiovascular risk and so it is reasonable to control arterial pressure as precisely as possible. Cerebral blood flow in patients with carotid stenosis depends on collateral circulation and autoregulation of cerebral blood flow may be impaired, especially in hypertensive patients. Vigorous antihypertensive treatment in these circumstances can predispose to cerebral ischemia.

*Pathophysiology of hemodynamic instability:* The arterial baroreflex is the reflex alteration in sympathetic and parasympathetic activity due to acute changes in arterial pressure which is mediated by the carotid baroreceptors. Baroreflex function is mostly altered in patients undergoing CEA causing increased association of hemodynamic instability during CEA. Surgical manipulation of the carotid sinus, alterations in the renin–angiotensin system, central catecholaminergic activity, have been advocated as a few theories for impaired baroreceptor reactivity. Impaired baroreflex and cerebrovascular reactivity are considered to be predictors of long-term adverse outcomes. Surgical removal of a carotid atherosclerotic plaque and stripping of sensory nerve endings from the arterial lumen causes immediate partial disruption of baroreceptor reactivity leading to hypertension and increased arterial pressure instability. This may last for several hours or days after surgery.

*Effects of carotid cross-clamping and shunting:* Cross-clamping of the carotid artery leads to decrease in cerebral blood flow, which is accompanied by a compensatory increase in arterial pressure mediated by baroreceptor reflexes and an increase in sympathetic nervous activity. Use of shunt or unclamping at the end of surgery leads to restoration of such changes. These changes may be less observed in patients undergoing CEA under deep general anesthesia (GA) as both baroreceptor function and cerebral autoregulation may be attenuated. The duration of cross-clamping may also have an effect on hemodynamic stability.

*Perioperative management of blood pressure:* If a patient is diagnosed to have preoperative hypertension before surgery then it is reasonable to take time to achieve good control of the arterial pressure in patients who have a preoperative systolic blood pressure consistently above 180 mm Hg, who do not have severe bilateral disease, and are not having frequent neurological events. But in certain situations like patients having severe bilateral disease and having frequent TIA, it seems appropriate to proceed to surgery even if the hypertension is not controlled. Preoperatively, it is important to control and maintain arterial pressure but avoid excessive decrease in cerebral perfusion distal to a carotid stenosis. Vigorous antihypertensive treatment before surgery or hypotension during anesthesia in these circumstances can cause ischemic stroke due to cerebral hypoperfusion. Preoperative hypertension is found to be associated with postoperatve hypertension. Consequently, it may also lead to postoperative wound hematoma formation with possibility of airway obstruction.

Intraoperative goals are to maintain cerebral perfusion pressure and collateral flow during a period when cerebral pressure autoregulation is impaired. Cerebral blood flow may be impaired by carotid clamping or by surgery itself. It is probably beneficial to avoid hypotension if possible, particularly during the period of carotid cross-clamping, whereas after restoration of flow, it is preferable to avoid hypertension. Complication like 'watershed' stroke during the period of carotid cross-clamping have lead to pharmacological manipulation to increase the blood pressure which in many cases has shown to reverse neurological deterioration during cross-clamping in patients. However, patients with cerebrovascular disease often have ischemic heart disease such that perioperative cardiac adverse events may be precipitated with increase in arterial pressure. Blood pressure and heart rate are controlled within individualized ranges during the surgery with short-acting agents whenever possible (esmolol, phenylephrine, nitroglycerin, and sodium nitroprusside). Blood pressure preservation or augmentation can be accomplished by maintaining light levels of general anesthesia or by administering sympathomimetic drugs such as phenylephrine and ephedrine.

Postoperatively, cerebral circulation distal to the surgical site is increased compared to preoperative values. The new endarterectomy site is also a potential site for the formation of hematoma.

## ANTICOAGULATION

Heparin is administered in the intraoperative period before cross-clamping of the carotid artery to reduce the risk of thromboembolic complications. It may be given as a fixed dose of heparin (often 5000 units) or as weight-based dose.[38] Fixed heparin dosing achieves safe and efficacious anticoagulation in the majority of patients having CEA, with 5000 units expected to result in 15-minute ACT of 175 to 425 seconds but there may be a wide variation in the intraoperative activated clotting times. Weight-based heparin dosing (85 IU/kg) may reduce the incidence of subtle complications like hematoma formation, decline on neuropsychometric tests. However, there is no statistically proven clinical advantage of either dosing regimen. The antiplatelet action of aspirin may be reduced during the intraoperative period after the administration of heparin and it has been suggested that this may account for some perioperative thromboembolic events. The decision of whether or not to reverse heparin following CEA is controversial. The potential reduction of the risk of thrombosis at the endarterectomy site with non-reversal has to be measured against a potential increase in the risk of wound hematoma. Some authors suggest that the use of protamine may be associated with an increased incidence of stroke. When protamine is used it should always be administered slowly, while monitoring for an adverse reaction (hypotension due to histamine induced vasodilation or a more severe anaphylactic reaction) which may compromise cerebral circulation.

## NEUROLOGICAL MONITORING

Stroke is the most common major complication of CEA. Its incidence was 5.5% in the North American Symptomatic CEA Trial (NASCET) and 6.5% for patients with moderate stenosis in the European Carotid Surgery Trial.

Stroke during CEA can occur due to various mechanisms. The two most important causes of perioperative stroke include embolism and hemodynamic compromise. Embolic stoke remains the most important cause of perioperative stroke. It can occur during different phases of surgery like the dissection phase of the surgery, at shunt insertion, at clamp release or during the 12-hour period immediately after surgery. While performing the endarterectomy there is temporary occlusion and opening of the affected artery and during this interval there is a risk that collateral cerebral blood flow to the ipsilateral hemisphere via the circle of Willis may not be sufficient to maintain neuronal integrity, resulting in hemodynamic stroke. If there is an associated contralateral carotid occlusion, there is a risk of global cerebral ischemia as collateral flow becomes entirely dependent on the vertebrobasilar system and leptomeningeal arteries which may not be able to supply both the cerebral hemispheres.

The role of cerebrovascular monitoring during CEA should be seen in the context of improving the outcome of the operation.[39] Assessment of cerebral ischemia may be unreliable in predicting perioperative stroke. The routine use of cerebrovascular monitoring during CEA is not universally accepted. Controversy remains concerning methods of intraoperative monitoring, criteria for shunt placement and optimal anesthetic technique. Different practical issues like availability of different cerebrovascular monitors, the availability of trained personnel in the operating room, cost, etc. affects the type of neurological monitoring performed in different institutes. The utility of cerebral monitoring is mainly to identify patients in need of carotid artery shunting and patients who may benefit from blood pressure augmentation or change in surgical technique.

The different techniques of neurological monitoring include:

1. *Awake patient:* The awake patients is regarded as the gold standard for intraoperative monitoring. An awake patient can be easily monitored to detect any ischemic episode as well as postoperative neurological examination is facilitated. Anxiety in awake patient can increase the sympathetic response which subsequently increases the risk for myocardial ischemia in patients already prone to cardiac events.

2. *Stump pressure:* Stump pressure (SP) is the pressure measured distal to the surgically occluded carotid artery and is thought to equal the collateral perfusion pressure via the circle of Willis. Stump pressure is usually measured after occlusion of the common and external carotid arteries using a 20 gauge catheter introduced in the common carotid artery proximal to the carotid plaque and connected to a transducer It is often used to determine the need of shunt placement. A number of thresholds for the stump pressure, ranging between 25 and 70 mm of Hg, have been proposed below which shunting would be appropriate. Stump pressure measurement using a 50 mm Hg cut-off has been reported to be a reliable predictor of ischemia necessitating a shunt placement. The advantages of carotid stump pressure monitoring are inexpensive, relatively easy to obtain and continuously available during carotid clamping. However, in practice a few centers employ stump pressure monitoring because the accuracy in determining adequacy of collateral flow and the need for selective shunting have been questioned. Ischemia may occur in the operative site in spite of adequate stump pressure if there is middle cerebral artery stenosis on that side. Studies in patients who underwent surgery under general anesthesia suggest stump pressure to be specific but not sensitive at identifying patients who develop EEG changes consistent with cerebral ischemia upon carotid cross-clamping.

3. *EEG:* EEG changes with ischemia. Two issues influence the efficacy and reliability of processed EEG as a monitor for cerebral ischemia during CEA. Firstly, the minimum number of channels (or areas of the brain) to be monitored. The 16-channel unprocessed EEG is clearly a reliable and sensitive monitor for intraoperative cerebral ischemia during CEA, but 16-channel EEG monitored by a dedicated technician is not possible in the majority of operating rooms. Therefore, processed EEG using fewer than 16 channels is utilized much more commonly. Clinical experience suggests that the minimum number of

channels for adequate sensitivity and specificity are four channels (two per side). The second issue is the experience level of the observer monitoring the processed EEG.

EEG monitoring is initiated prior to induction of anesthesia because anesthetic agents may impact the EEG recording. The American Society of Neurophysiological Monitoring recommends a baseline EEG prior to induction of anesthesia. After induction, a second baseline EEG is obtained under general anesthesia before any carotid manipulation has occurred. Subsequently, EEG waveforms are obtained from scalp electrodes during the procedure.

**Changes in EEG waves with ischemia include the following:**

- Decreased high frequencies
- Increased low frequencies
- Decreased amplitude
- Isoelectric EEG

When EEG is used for monitoring during CEA, a stable physiologic state is necessary. Inhalational agents like isoflurane, desflurane and sevoflurane produce similar EEG changes at equipotent levels and, when used at 0.5 MAC, allow for more reliable EEG cerebral ischemia monitoring. The clinical utility of intraoperative EEG monitoring during CEA is limited by different factors. First, the EEG may not be able to detect subcortical or small cortical infarcts. Second, false-negative results are not uncommon. Patients with pre-existing stroke or reversible neurologic deficits may have a particularly high incidence of such results. Third, the EEG is not ischemia specific and may be affected by changes in temperature, blood pressure and anesthetic depth. Fourth, false-positive results (no perioperative neurologic deficit with significant ischemic EEG changes intraoperatively) occur because not all cerebral ischemia uniformly proceeds to infarction.

4. *Somatosensory evoked potentials*: Somatosensory evoked potential monitoring is based on the response of the sensory cortex to electrical impulses from peripheral sensory nerve stimulation. The sensory cortex, being primarily supplied by the middle cerebral artery, is at risk during carotid artery clamping. SSEP monitoring, unlike EEG, is able to detect subcortical sensory pathway ischemia.[40] Characteristic SSEP tracings (decrease in amplitude and/or increase in latency) occur with decreased regional cerebral blood flow. No specific amplitude reduction or increase in latency has been established as a physiologic marker of impaired regional cerebral blood flow under operative conditions in humans. Anesthetics, hypothermia and blood pressure may affect SSEP significantly. SSEP is usually recorded from median nerve (wrist) or posterior tibial nerve (ankle) Somatosensory evoked potentials (SSEPs) offer theoretical advantages over the EEG for cerebral ischemia monitoring. This type of monitoring examines not only the cortex but the deeper structures of the brain. Stimulation from a peripheral nerve passes through first- and second-order neurons and brainstem synapses before evoking a response in the somatosensory cortex. It may be superior in patients whose baseline EEG is not easily interpretable because of a previous stroke. It should however be borne in mind that the volatile anesthetic agents can reduce the amplitude of SSEP signals

5. *Transcranial Doppler (TCD)*: TCD utilizes pulsed wave Doppler to measure blood velocities in the middle cerebral artery. The sensitivity and specificity of this technique is unreliable for detection of cerebral ischemia, since changes in blood flow velocity may reflect changes in arterial diameter rather than blood flow changes. Available data strongly suggest that a decrease of 85% of the ipsilateral middle cerebral artery flow velocity at cross-clamping and 25 emboli per 10-minute interval or 50 emboli per hour during the immediate postoperative period are associated with brain infarction. These criteria cannot be considered definitive at the present time and the there is a need for appropriately designed studies to establish definitive transcranial Doppler criteria.

Ackerstaff et al[41] reported that intraoperative monitoring with transcranial Doppler can identify patients at an increased risk for perioperative stroke. The authors found that certain transcranial Doppler variables were independently associated with perioperative stroke. These are embolism during the dissection and wound-closure phases of surgery, a drop of 90% in the middle cerebral flow velocity at cross-clamping and an 100% increase in the pulsatility index at clamp release.

In contrast to other moitoring techniques TCD is able to detect emboli. The majority of perioperative neurological events are embolic or thrombotic rather than hemodynamic in nature. TCD monitoring is undoubtedly operator-dependent.

6. *Regional CBF:* Intracarotid Xenon133 in saline is used for detection of regional blood flow. Regional cerebral blood flow measurements during CEA are obtained by intravenous or ipsilateral carotid artery injection of radioactive xenon and analysis of decay curves obtained from detectors placed over the area of the ipsilateral cortex supplied by the middle cerebral artery. Measurements are typically obtained before, during and immediately after carotid clamping. The disadvantages of this monitoring technique include the expense and the expertise required to interpret these blood flow measurements.

7. *Cerebral oxygenation:* Direct monitoring of cerebral oxygenation can be obtained with jugular bulb venous monitoring and near infrared spectroscopy.

Jugular bulb venous monitoring allows determination of the arterial—jugular venous oxygen content difference and jugular venous oxygen saturation. It therefore provides information on global cerebral oxygen metabolism. Jugular venous samples are obtained from a catheter inserted into the jugular bulb ipsilateral to the surgical site. Continuous fiberoptic jugular venous oximetry catheters are available as well. Significant technical and methodologic shortcomings have limited the clinical application of this monitoring during CEA.

*Near infrared spectroscopy:* Near infrared spectroscopy (NIRS) gives a value for regional cerebral oxygenation ($rSO_2$) which is a composite measure of arterial venous and capillary oxygenation, although the predominant influence is the venous blood. Carotid cross-clamping produces a decrease in $rSO_2$. Unfortunately, this change is not consistently related to changes in other measures of cerebral blood flow. The advantage of NIRS is that it is easy to use and that it offers a real-time and noninvasive means for the assessment of cerebral oxygenation. The low spatial resolution of the measurement system placement over the parietal middle cerebral artery territory, as advocated by Williams and coworkers might lead to a better agreement between SEP monitoring and NIRS.[42] However, this approach is hampered by the necessity of shaving an area of the patient's head equal to the size of the sensor pad, which will probably not be acceptable to many of the patients undergoing the procedure for investigational purposes.

*Shunting during CEA:* There are three schools of practice
• Shunt routinely.
• Shunt never, or very rarely.

• Shunt selectively, based on monitoring to detect cerebral ischemia.

There are different types of carotid shunt but all are essentially a length of plastic tubing to carry the blood from the common carotid to the internal carotid artery, which will maintain blood flow during the course of surgery as shown in Fig. 10.8. It may seem to be a useful technique to maintain cerebral blood flow in those patients who have a contralateral carotid stenosis or a compromised circle of Willis. The complications associated with shunt insertion include air or plaque embolization, intimal tears, carotid dissection, hematoma, nerve injury, infection and late carotid restenosis. For all these risks, flow through the shunt may be inadequate to meet cerebral oxygen requirements.

### Emergence

Emergence should be designed to avoid excessive coughing or straining and surges in systemic blood pressure, which might open the freshly closed arteriotomy. Many surgeons prefer patients to be awake and the patient to be extubated at the conclusion of the procedure to facilitate neurologic examination in the early postoperative period. Neurologic deficits on emergence require immediate attention about the need for angiography, reoperation or both. The period of emergence and extubation may be associated with marked hypertension and tachycardia, which may require aggressive pharmacologic intervention.

### Complications

Major perioperative complications of CEA include stroke, myocardial infarction, and death. Other postoperative complications are cranial nerve injuries, wound hematoma, hypertension, hypotension, hyperperfusion syndrome, intracerebral hemorrhage, seizures and recurrent stenosis.

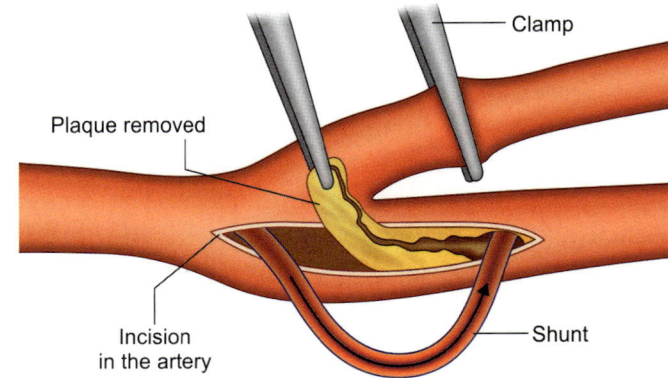

**Fig. 10.8:** Use of shunt during the procedure of carotid endarterectomy

Postoperative problems after CEA include the following:

1. Cardiovascular
   - Hypotension
   - Hypertension (particularly after carotid sinus nerve section or local anesthetic block)
   - Arrhythmia
   - Myocardial ischemia
2. Airway obstruction caused by edema and hematoma
3. Neurological deficit—requires immediate surgical opinion
4. Cranial nerve injury
5. Hyperperfusion syndrome—headache, seizures, hemorrhage

### Stroke, Myocardial Infarction and Death

The overall mortality for CEA was reported to be 1.3 to 1.8% in 2 large systematic reviews. The risk of stroke or death is related mainly to the patient's preoperative clinical status.

Symptomatic patients have a higher risk than asymptomatic patients, as do those with hemispheric versus retinal symptoms, urgent versus elective operation, reoperation versus primary surgery. Patients having high-risk anatomic criteria, such as restenosis after CEA and contralateral carotid arterial occlusion also have higher perioperative stroke/death rates.

### Stroke

Stroke is the most common major complication of CEA. Endarterectomy has an inherent risk of perioperative stroke, precisely the event which it is meant to prevent. Differences in accuracy of diagnosis, definition of stroke, study design and other factors have lead to a wide range in reported risk, from 1 to 20%.[43] Its incidence was 5.5% in the NASCET and 6.5% for patients with moderate stenosis in the European Carotid Surgery Trial. The CREST trial reported a 2.3% incidence of periprocedural or ipsilateral stroke within 30 days of operation. Although both embolism and hemodynamic compromise can lead to perioperative brain ischemia, embolism is increasingly considered the more common mechanism. Unexpected incidents, such as intraoperative internal carotid artery thrombosis, can occur and lead to distal ischemia. In a small percentage of patients a hyperperfusion syndrome develops postoperatively, leading to brain edema and hemorrhage.

Mechanisms of stroke after CEA:
- Ischemic hemorrhagic
- Restenosis or reocclusion
- Embolization
- Luxury perfusion syndrome
- Shunt injury
- Hypoperfusion
- Thrombus formation

Some investigators have initiated either intravenous dextran-40 or platelet glycoprotein IIB/IIIA receptor antagonist therapy during the immediate postoperative period and have shown a subsequent decrease of the emboli count and a reduction of perioperative morbidity.

Several large, multinational randomized controlled trials (RCTs) have shown that for carefully selected patients operated on by experienced surgeons, CEA plus medical therapy reduced the risk of stroke and death compared to existing medical therapy alone.

## RISK FACTORS

Many authors have reported that the incidence of perioperative stroke rate is lowest in patients who are symptom free before endarterectomy, higher for patients diagnosed with TIA and highest for patients diagnosed with stroke. Tu and colleagues performed a population-based review to identify risk factors for perioperative stroke and death after CEA.[44] Thereby, Ontario CEA Registry analysis has suggested the following risk factor scoring system for assessing the risk factors for death or stroke after CEA:

| Number of points | Risk factor |
|---|---|
| 1 | History of stroke or TIA within 6 months of surgery |
| 1 | Contralateral occlusion of the carotid artery |
| 1 | History of atrial fibrillation |
| 1 | History of CHF |
| 1 | History of diabetes |

Total: 0 to 5. Add up the number of points to calculate the risk score

Patients with risk scores of 2, have a particularly high risk of perioperative complications. The investigators suggested a simple scoring method to estimate the potential 30-day risk of stroke or death after CEA, calculated by adding the number of pre-existing risk factors, with a rate for 3.3% for no risk factors and a higher rate of 15.8% for four risk factors.

Halm and colleagues in the New York Carotid Artery Surgery Study in 2009 suggested that several socio-demographic, neurological and comorbidity risk factors can predict perioperative death or stroke after CEA.[45] The risk of death or stroke increases with increasing neurological severity, distant cerebrovascular disease, TIA or stroke as the indication for CEA. Several other indicators of severity of carotid and neurological disease (contralateral stenosis $\geq$50%, admitted from the emergency department and severe disability) also increased the risk of adverse outcomes.

Recently published primary data from the Carotid Revascularization Endarterectomy Versus Stenting Trial (CREST) showed no difference in the composite end point of stroke, myocardial infarction (MI) or death during the periprocedural period and ipsilateral stroke over 4 years of follow-up. However, the risk of periprocedural stroke was found to be higher with CAS versus CEA (4.1 vs 2.3%), and the risk of periprocedural MI was higher with CEA than with CAS (2.3% vs 1.1%).

## Myocardial Ischemia

Atherosclerosis of the carotid bifurcation is commonly associated with coronary atherosclerosis, so myocardial ischemia is a major cause of perioperative complications, including nonfatal MI and late mortality in patients undergoing CEA.

Different trials consider different evidence of myocardial ischemia like chest pain or equivalent symptoms consistent with myocardial ischemia or ECG evidence of ischemia, including new ST-segment depression or elevation >1 mm in ≥2 contiguous leads or new pathological Q waves in ≥2 contiguous leads, troponin T ≥0.10 or elevation of CK-MB or troponin I >2 times the detection limit or with an upward trend at any quantitative level. In NASCET and ECST, the incidence of perioperative MI was 0.3 and 0.2%, respectively. Myocardial infarction was not a component of the primary end point for the endarterectomy versus angioplasty in patients with symptomatic severe carotid stenosis (EVA-3S) trial or in the stent-supported percutaneous angioplasty of the carotid artery versus endarterectomy (SPACE) trial. In EVA-3S, SPACE, and the International Carotid Stenting Study (ICSS), cardiac biomarkers were not specified per protocol. Accordingly, the reported rates for MI were much lower than in CREST. Specifically, the rate of MI was 0.4% for CAS and 0.8% for CEA in EVA-3S and 0.4% for CAS and 0.6% for CEA in ICSS. In ICSS, fatal MI events occurred in 3 of 853 patients (0.4%) with CAS, and 5 nonfatal MIs occurred in 821 patients with CEA (0.6%). Only in the high-surgical-risk, randomized stenting and angioplasty with protection in patients at high risk for endarterectomy (SAPPHIRE) trial, which incorporated systematic collection of CK and CK-MB, there was a higher rate of MI detected: 5.9% for CEA and 2.4% for CAS. In particular, patients with known cardiovascular disease or renal insufficiency were more prone to periprocedural MI. Candidate approaches might include high-dose statins, which have shown benefit in reducing periprocedural MI after percutaneous coronary intervention, or more robust dual antiplatelet therapy, as is used for

CAS. Many authors have shown that the natural history of carotid and coronary artery occlusive diseases are clearly intertwined. Patients requiring surgical revascularization for extracranial cerebrovascular disease should be carefully evaluated for coronary artery disease.

## Wound Hematoma

Wound hematomas are relatively common following CEA.In the NASCET study 5.5% of patients had documented wound hematomas. The majority are relatively small and cause little discomfort. Larger hematomas or those that expand precipitously require emergency treatment. If there is no loss of airway, the patient should undergo emergency evacuation of the hematoma in the operating room. If the airway has been obstructed by a hematoma, some prefer to open the wound at the bedside. A significant wound hematoma may compromise the patient's airway, resulting in a need for emergency reintubation and reoperation. This event is associated with higher in-hospital mortality, stroke, and myocardial infarction.Wound hematoma is more likely to occur when anticoagulation is not promptly reversed or in patients with poorly controlled postoperative hypertension.

## CRANIAL NERVE INJURY

The vagus nerve lies posterior and lateral to the internal and common carotid but may be positioned around the carotid artery. Trauma to the nerve may occur if the dissection is not kept close to the wall of the artery. The recurrent laryngeal nerve can be injured if it follows an anomalous course, traversing behind the common carotid. Vagus and recurrent laryngeal nerve injury will result in vocal cord palsy. Trauma to the superior laryngeal nerve will result in difficulty in swallowing, and change in the quality of the voice due to cricothyroid muscle dysfunction. The hypoglossal nerve descends along the course of the internal carotid passing medially over the more superficial external carotid, traction on the nerve can cause tongue deviation to the side ipsilateral to the endarterectomy. The ansa hypoglossus injury is inconsequential. The carotid sinus nerve, stimulation leads to hypotension and bradycardia. The marginal mandibular nerve itself may be injured if the incision is carried too cephalad.

## POSTOPERATIVE HYPERTENSION

About 21% of normotensive patients may have increased blood pressure after CEA. The particular peak of risk is highest in the first 48 hours after surgery. The pathophysiology of this usually episodic hypertension might be related to surgically induced abnormalities of carotid baroreceptor sensitivity. Particular attention is important during dissection of the common carotid artery to avoid damaging the vagus nerve and the carotid sinus and to prevent carotid baroreceptor dysfunction. Although instability in blood pressure is a temporary phenomenon and persistence of hypertension is quite rare, an increase in blood pressure and its variability 12 weeks after surgery has recently been demonstrated and characterized as baroreflex failure syndrome. Occurrence of this syndrome after CEA is associated with bilateral surgical procedures.

In patients undergoing CEA, untreated preoperative hypertension is associated with postoperative hypertension.

## CEREBRAL HYPERFUSION SYNDROME (CHS)

Reactive hyperemia was first described in 1925 during reperfusion after vascular occlusion of limbs, over-abundant cerebral blood flow relative to metabolic needs was termed "luxury perfusion syndrome" in 1966. CHS can occur after CEA or carotid angioplasty with stenting. The reported incidence of CHS reported is about 0–3% in most studies. The clinical symptoms associated with CHS includes throbbing ipsilateral frontotemporal or periorbital headache, and sometimes diffuse headache, eye and face pain, vomiting, confusion, macular edema, visual disturbances, focal motor seizures with frequent secondary generalisation, focal neurological deficits, and intracerebral or subarachnoid hemorrhage. Although most patients have mild symptoms and signs, it can progress to severe and life-threatening symptoms. Patients with CHS may be misdiagnosed with other complications like thromboembolism as CHS is a diagnosis based on several nonspecific signs and symptoms. If not treated properly it can result in severe brain edema, intracerebral or subarachnoid hemorrhage, and death. CHS is most common in patients with increases of more than 100% in perfusion compared with baseline after CEA and is rare in patients with increases in perfusion less than 100% compared with baseline. The risk factors are diminished cerebrovascular reserve, postoperative hypertension and hyperperfusion lasting more than several hours after carotid intervention. Patients at greatest risk include those who already have a reoperative reduction in hemispheric CBF owing to bilateral high-grade carotid stenoses, unilateral high-grade carotid stenosis with poor collateral cross-flow, or unilateral carotid occlusion with contralateral high-grade stenosis. The syndrome is thought to result from restoration of perfusion to an area of the brain that has lost its ability to autoregulate as the result of a chronic decrease in CBF. The restoration of CBF leads to a state of hyperperfusion that persists until autoregulation is reestablished, usually over a period of days. Impaired autoregulation due to endothelial dysfunction mediated by generation of free oxygen radicals is one of the proposed mechanism in the pathogenesis of CHS. Treatment strategies are aimed towards regulation of blood pressure and limitation of rises in cerebral perfusion.

## ANESTHESIA FOR CAS

Percutaneous carotid revascularization with balloon angioplasty was pioneered in the early 1980s. The advent of stent technology in the mid 1990s allowed protection against dissections.

Its safety and efficacy relative to CEA, particularly with respect to perioperative and long-term neurologic outcome, is currently the subject of several multicenter studies. CAS techniques have been progressively modified as new technologies become available to include self-expanding stents and cerebral-protection devices. With ongoing advances in endovascular technology and increasing experience with CAS of interventionalists, CAS is challenging CEA as a treatment option for patients with carotid artery disease. Advocates of CAS suggest that the technique offers advantages in patients who have high-risk medical conditions and those who have surgically inaccessible carotid disease (e.g. previous neck irradiation, intracranial stenosis).

## INDICATIONS FOR CAS

According to American Heart Association guidelines for secondary prevention of stroke, CAS is reasonable when performed by operators with established periprocedural morbidity and mortality rates of 4–6%, similar to that observed in trials of CEA and CAS. In the United States, CAS with embolic protection device is considered to be reasonable and appropriate for symptomatic patients with carotid stenosis ≥70% at high risk for surgery. The conditions considered under high risk conditions are as follows:

- Congestive heart failure NYHA class III/IV
- Left ventricular ejection fraction <30%
- Unstable angina
- Contralateral carotid occlusion
- Recent myocardial infarction
- Previous endarterectomy with recurrent stenosis
- Earlier radiation treatment to the neck

## Contraindications

Contraindications to CAS include the following:

- History of allergic reaction to intravenous (IV) contrast material
- Unfavorable anatomy
- Unstable carotid plaque
- Unstable aortic arch plaque

The primary limitation for performing CAS is unfavorable anatomy. Unfavorable aortic arch types, vascular anomalies such as bovine anatomy, proximal and distal tortuosity and other specific arterial lesions can reduce success with this approach. Poor candidates for CAS also include patients with incomplete collateral circulation or so-called isolated hemispheres who are intolerant of the reversal of flow.

## Outcomes after CAS

In the carotid and vertebral artery transluminal angioplasty study (CAVATAS),[46] a multicenter clinical trial in which 504 patients with carotid stenosis were randomly assigned to undergo either CEA (253 patients) or CAS (251 patients), there was no substantial difference in the rate of ipsilateral stroke over a 3-year follow-up period. The study was criticized by the interventionalist community for the low stenting rate (26%) and by surgeons for the high event rates in the surgical arm. The Stenting and angioplasty with protection in patients at high risk for endarterectomy (SAPPHIRE) trial is the first randomized trial comparing CEA and CAS with (embolic protection device) EPD.[47] The study focused on patients at high risk for surgery with ≥50% symptomatic or ≥80% asymptomatic carotid stenosis. Among the 334 patients randomized, major adverse events occurred in 12.2% in the stent group and in 20.1% in the CEA group ($p = 0.053$) at 1 year. A recently published subanalysis of the CREST trial showed that restenosis and occlusion rates were similar up to 2 years after CEA and CAS.[48]

## Technique for CAS

*Carotid stent devices:* Carotid stents can be grossly divided into two groups: Open stent architecture (e.g. Acculink) and closed stent architecture (e.g. Exact). Most registry studies have failed to demonstrate any clinically important advantages of one stent type over another.[49] Drug-eluting stents, which are widely used for coronary artery disease are rarely used in the carotid circulation because of the low rate of restenosis with bare metal stents due to the larger diameter of the carotid arteries.

*Stents (balloon-expandable and self-expanding)*

There are 2 basic types of stents—balloon-expandable and self-expanding.

Balloon-expandable stents are mounted on a balloon catheter and passively enlarged to the desired diameter at the implantation site by dilating the balloon. They are better suited for proximal carotid artery and innominate artery lesions and offer greater precision during CAS. Their collapsed diameter is slightly larger than that of self-expanding stents; therefore, it is often difficult to cross a lesion with them unless the stenosis is predilated.

Self-expanding carotid stents are used as a minimally invasive alternative to CEA. They open actively after being released from the delivery system. Their self-expanding character depends either on the braiding structure or on the type of alloy (usually nitinol or stainless steel)

*Embolic protection devices:* The purpose of cerebral protection devices (CPDs) is to capture atherosclerotic emboli during catheter manipulation, angioplasty, and stenting. The risk of atheroembolization is greatest during balloon angioplasty of the stenosis and when the lesion is crossed by a wire. Embolic protection device technology (EPD) continues to evolve. There are two basic types of devices: filter and retrograde flow devices. Filter designs allow continuous antegrade flow through the internal carotid artery during stent placement. Filter type EPDs are more commonly used, but their effectiveness remains debated. Flow reversal designs promote flow of blood, including particulate matter, retrograde away from the internal carotid artery.

*Filter devices:* Devices that occlude filter distal blood flow are designed to catch debris dislodged during stent placement. Although filter devices are the most commonly used type of EPD, they have several disadvantages. They must pass across the stenosis and tight lesions may require unprotected predilatation before the distal device can be placed, a process that may dislodge emboli. The presence of the EPD in the distal carotid artery may induce vasospasm that can severely compromise outflow and cause stroke if prolonged. Spasm can be treated with an intra-arterial vasodilator such nitroglycerine, but such treatment can lead to hypotension. Filter-type EPDs may cause complications related to vessel wall injury or to difficulty in removal of the device once the carotid stent has been placed. The benefit of EPDs has not been definitively established in randomized trials and the available evidence is conflicting. The most likely explanation for the inability of EPDs to prevent all perioperative strokes is that they do not prevent all emboli from reaching the distal cerebral vessels.

*CAS procedure:* CAS can be performed in an angiography suite or appropriately equipped operating room. The patient should receive antiplatelet therapy prior to the procedure.

*Approach:* Access for CAS (CAS) can be obtained through a variety of approaches, as follows:

- *Femoral:* This is the most preferred approach. It avoids technique-related angulation and offers improved guide wire and catheter maneuverability.

- *Brachial/radial:* Brachial approach is associated with a risk of damaging the median nerve; moreover, owing to the extreme angulation, manipulation of the catheter is difficult with this approach.

- *Carotid:* Both percutaneous and direct open exposures have been reported and both are associated with the risk of causing inadvertent dissection and inadvertent crossing of the stenotic lesion; these approaches have largely been abandoned.

With femoral access, an arch aortogram should be performed unless the arch anatomy is already known from preoperative imaging, such as computed tomographic angiography or magnetic resonance angiography.

*Stent insertion:* The femoral pulsation is palpated, and a micropuncture needle is inserted 1 finger breadth below the inguinal ligament. Upon entry into the artery, a hydrophilic wire is inserted through the needle by means of the Seldinger technique. The needle is removed and is replaced by a sheath. A guide wire is advanced into the aorta under direct fluoroscopy. An H1 catheter is placed over the guide wire and positioned in the aortic arch. Heparin 80 IU/kg is administered. An aortogram is obtained in the left anterior oblique position at 45° of angulation. The aortic arch, innominate artery, left common carotid artery, and left subclavian artery are identified. Selective catheterization of the left or right common artery is performed. The guide wire is placed in the external carotid artery, and the H1 catheter is then placed in the external carotid artery. The guide wire is replaced with a stiffer wire. A shuttle sheath is advanced to the common carotid artery. A carotid arteriogram is obtained (in anteroposterior, lateral, and intracerebral views). The lesion is crossed with wire. CPD is positioned with a monorail system. Predilatation is performed with a 2- to 3-mm balloon. The stent is placed across the lesion and deployed (Fig. 10.9). A repeat arteriogram is performed. Any residual stenosis

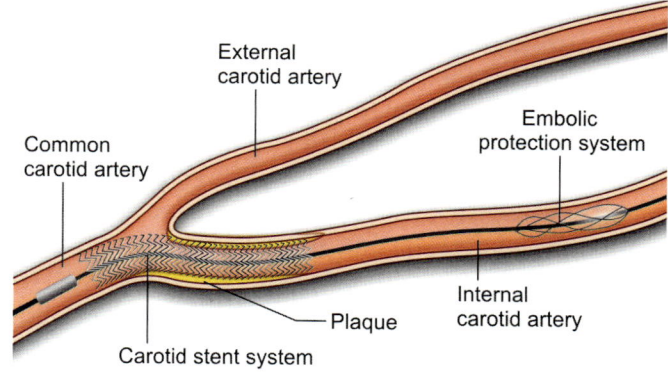

**Fig. 10.9:** Carotid artery stenting

exceeding 30% is treated with balloon angioplasty. Sheaths and wires are removed, and an access site closure device is deployed.

*Anticoagulation:* Before manipulation of the guidewires and catheters within the carotid artery, the patient should be anticoagulated with heparin to maintain the activated whole blood clotting time (ACT) at 250 to 300 seconds. *Bivalirudin* can be used as an alternative to heparin and may be associated with a lower incidence of bleeding compared with heparin.

*Embolic protection device placement:* Embolic protection devices (EPDs) are deployed following placement of the guide wire and sheath and are removed once the carotid artery stent has been positioned, deployed and expanded. Two general types (i.e. distal or proximal) of EPDs are available.

*Stent placement and dilation:* With the EPD in position, the carotid artery stenosis is predilated (if needed), and the carotid stent positioned and then deployed. A poststenting angioplasty is performed within the stent to ensure its full deployment and apposition against the arterial wall. During carotid stenting, balloon inflation to expand the carotid stent may lead to excessive stimulation of the carotid baroreceptor resulting in perioperative hemodynamic instability. Bradycardia due to baroreceptor activation can occur and lead to hypotension. The reaction is usually transient but may require the administration of *atropine.* Repeat carotid arteriography should demonstrate brisk flow through the previously stenotic carotid artery. The procedure of carotid artery stenting is as follows:

## Perioperative Care and Anesthesia Technique

*Antibiotic prophylaxis:* Antibiotic prophylaxis prior to CAS is usually a standard practice by most clinicians.

*Antiplatelet therapy:* For CAS, many centers employ a dual antiplatelet regimen similar to that used for percutaneous coronary intervention; however, there is limited evidence regarding the effectiveness of dual antiplatelet. In the Carotid Revascularization Endarterectomy versus Stenting Trial (CREST), patients were treated with aspirin (325 mg twice daily) and clopidrogel (75 mg twice daily) starting at least 48 hours before the CAS. Those scheduled for CAS within 48 hours received aspirin 650 mg and clopidogrel 450 mg at least four hours before the CAS procedure. Following CAS, treatment included aspirin 325 mg once or twice daily and clopidogrel 75 mg daily for at least 30 days, with a recommendation to continue aspirin indefinitely (at least one year). Some authors suggest continuing dual antiplatelet therapy with *aspirin* and *clopidogrel* for six weeks following the CAS procedure. Aspirin should be continued indefinitely. Radiated patients are at high risk for recurrent carotid stenosis following CAS, as high as 30% in some series.

*Perioperative statins:* Statin therapy is recommended for patients with coronary risk equivalents. Statin use is associated with significantly fewer embolic particles. Statin use stabilizes atherosclerotic plaque, resulting in a more fibrous plaque that is less vulnerable to embolise.

*Choice of anesthesia:* Most carotid stenting procedures are performed with local anesthesia and minimal or no sedation, but some operators employ general anesthesia

Anesthesia for percutaneous carotid interventions differs from that used for carotid surgery. Protection of the brain from ischemic insult is paramount, and attention to physiological factors influencing cerebral blood flow is mandatory. The anesthesiologist plays a crucial role in maintaining hemodynamic stability, adjusting anticoagulation, and monitoring neurological status. The anesthetist has to work closely with the interventionist/surgeon in planning a percutaneous carotid procedure. Anesthesiologist must evolve a plan that maximizes the therapeutic benefit while minimizing morbidity and meet the basic goals of anesthesia—ablation of pain, protection against ischemic injury to the heart and brain and obtain a motionless field. The anesthetic management differs depending on the access route, and the anesthesiologist must be prepared for a change to the alternative technique should the initial approach fail. The anesthesiologist should always be prepared to induce general anesthesia and perform endotracheal intubation if the surgeon must abandon a percutaneous access altogether and proceed to an open procedure. When the patient is awake, the anesthesiologist should keep close contact with the patient and

constantly assess mental status, as well as motor and sensory performance. The most crucial time for an ischemic event is during balloon inflation and stent deployment, when the patient must hold breath and keep the neck stable. The anesthesiologist must evaluate vital signs and check activity on the contralateral side during the procedure. Direct carotid access is usually accomplished with the patient under general anesthesia and intubated. This guarantees the motionless field requisite to this approach and allows the patient's head to be hyperextended and rotated laterally with the shoulder on the affected side elevated. Short acting drugs are selected because the patient must be awake immediately following the procedure. The vigilance in hemodynamic and neurological monitoring exercised during anesthesia must continue in the intensive care unit. The events most likely to occur are circulatory instability, respiratory insufficiency, hematoma formation and onset of new neurological deficits.

CAS is associated with a number of periprocedural events, including hypotension and vasovagal and vasodepressor reactions. Thereby, continuous electrocardiogram and blood pressure monitoring has become routine. Different pharmacological agents have been used for such situations during CAS. Atropine, 0.5 to 1 mg given intravenously, may be administered prophylactically before the angioplasty or stent portion of the procedure to avoid or attenuate bradycardia. Rarely, persistent bradycardia may require insertion of a temporary transvenous pacemaker. Sustained hypotension requires adequate hydration and careful adjustment of antihypertensive medication immediately before the procedure. Persistent hypotension, requires intravenous phenylephrine (1 to 10 mcg/kg/min) or dopamine (5 to 15 mcg/kg/min) for treatmemt. Hypertension occasionally develops immediately before, during, or after the procedure, and maintenance of systolic blood pressure below 180 mm Hg is advised to minimize the risk of intracranial hemorrhage or the hyperperfusion syndrome.

## Risks Associated with CAS

The risks and potential complications of CAS are as follows:

- Neurological deficits,
- Injury of the vessels accessed to approach the lesion, the artery in the region of stenosis, and the distal vessels,
- Device malfunction,
- General medical and access-site complications,
- Restenosis, and
- Mortality.

## CONCLUSION

CEA is a validated intervention for stroke prevention associated with high-grade carotid stenosis.

Attention to comorbidities, patient selection, and monitoring techniques may lead to better outcomes. CAS may overcome anatomical surgical challenges and minimize risk of myocardial infarction. The choice of regional or general anesthesia is important in the clinical management of the patients. Regional anesthesia for carotid surgery has evolved over the last 15 years with new regional techniques, new methods of locating the cervical plexus, new drugs, and better management of the patient but regional anesthesia has not been shown to be associated with better outcome than GA. Our challenges for the future will include management of the 'urgent carotid', optimizing arterial pressure control, and developing clinical protocols to avoid perioperative complications to decrease the overall perioperative morbidity and mortality. The anesthetist has an important role in controlling perioperative risk associated with both CEA and CAS.

## REFERENCES

1. Heart Disease and Stroke Statistics—2009 Update. Dallas, Texas: American Heart Association.

2. Petty G, Brown RD Jr, Whisnant JP, Sicks JD, O'Fallon WM, Wiebers DO. Ischemic stroke subtypes: A population-based study of incidence and risk factors. Stroke 1999; 30(12): 2513–16.

3. Goldstein LB, Adams R, Alberts MJ, et al. Primary prevention of ischemic stroke: a guideline from the American Heart Association/American Stroke Association Stroke Council: Cosponsored by the Atherosclerotic Peripheral Vascular Disease Interdisciplinary Working Group; Cardiovascular Nursing Council; Clinical Cardiology Council; Nutrition, Physical Activity, and Metabolism Council; and the Quality of Care and Outcomes Research Interdisciplinary Working Group: The American Academy of Neurology affirms the value of this guideline. Stroke 2006;37:1583–633.

4. Morasch MD, Parker MA, Feinglass J, et al. Carotid endarterectomy: Characterization of recent increases in procedure rates. J Vasc Surg 2000;31:901–9.

5. North American Symptomatic Carotid Endarterectomy Trial (NASCET) Collaborators: Beneficial effect of carotid endarterectomy in symptomatic patients with high-grade carotid stenosis. N Engl J Med 1991; 325:445–53.

6. European Carotid Surgery Trial: Randomised trial of endarterectomy for recently symptomatic carotid stenosis: final results of the MRC European Carotid Surgery Trial (ECST) Lancet 1998;351:1379–87.

7. Sacco RL, Adams R, Albers G, et al. Guidelines for prevention of stroke in patients with ischemic stroke or transient ischemic attack: a statement for healthcare professionals from the American Heart Association/American Stroke Association Council on Stroke: co-sponsored by the Council on Cardiovascular Radiology and Intervention. Stroke 2006; 37:577–617.

8. Wolf PA, Clagett GP, Easton JD, et al. Preventing ischemic stroke in patients with prior stroke and transient ischemic attack: A statement for healthcare professionals from the stroke council of the American Heart Association. Stroke 1999;30:1991–4.

9. The Sixth Report of the Joint National Committee on prevention, detection, evaluation, and treatment of high blood pressure. Arch Intern Med 1997;157:2413–46.

10. Vasan RS, Beiser A, Seshadri S, Larson MG, Kannel WB, D'Agostino RB, Levy D. Residual lifetime risk for developing hypertension in middle-aged women and men: The Framingham Heart Study. JAMA 2002;287:1003–10.

11. Adult Treatment Panel II: Summary of the second report of the National Cholesterol Education Program (NCEP) Expert Panel on Detection, Evaluation, and Treatment of High Blood Cholesterol in Adults. JAMA 1993;269:3015–23.

12. Albers GW, Hart RG, Lutsep HL, et al. AHA Scientific Statement. Supplement to the guidelines for the management of transient ischemic attacks: A statement from the Ad Hoc Committee on Guidelines for the Management of Transient Ischemic Attacks, Stroke Council, American Heart Association. Stroke 1999;30:2502–11.

13. Antiplatelet Trialists' Collaboration: Collaborative overview of randomised trials of antiplatelet therapy. I: Prevention of death, myocardial infarction, and stroke by prolonged antiplatelet therapy in various categories of patients. BMJ 1994;308:81–106.

14. Taylor DW Barnett HJ, Haynes RB, et al. Low-dose and high-dose acetylsalicylic acid for patients undergoing carotid endarterectomy: A randomised controlled trial. Lancet 1999;353:2179–84.

15. CAPRIE Steering Committee. A randomised, blinded, trial of clopidogrel versus aspirin in patients at risk of ischaemic events (CAPRIE). Lancet 1996; 348:1329–39.

16. Diener HC, Bogousslavsky J, Brass LM, Cimminiello C, Csiba L, et al. Aspirin and clopidogrel compared with clopidogrel alone after recent ischaemic stroke or transient ischaemic attack in high-risk patients (MATCH): Randomised, double-blind, placebo-controlled trial. Lancet 2004; 364:331–337.

17. Bhatt DL, Topol EJ. On behalf of the CHARISMA Executive Committee. Clopidogrel added to aspirin alone in secondary prevention and high-risk primary prevention. Rationale and design of the Clopidogrel for High Atherothrombotic Risk and Ischemic Stabilization, Management, and Avoidance (CHARISMA) trial. Am Heart J 2004;148:263–8.

18. Diener H, Cunha L, Forbes C, Sivenius J, Smets P, Lowenthal A. European Stroke Prevention Study 2: dipyridamole and acetylsalicylic acid in the secondary prevention of stroke. J Neurosci 1996;143:1–13.

19. Brott TG, Hobson RW 2nd, Howard G, Roubin GS, Clark WM, Brooks W, et al. CREST investigators. Stenting versus endarterectomy for treatment of carotid-artery stenosis. N Engl J Med 2010;363:11–23.

20. Brott TG, Halperin JL, Abbara S, Bacharach JM, Barr JD, Bush RL, et al. 2011 ASA/ACCF/AHA/AANN/AANS/ACR/ASNR/CNS/SAIP/SCAI/SIR/SNIS/SVM/SVS guideline on the management of patients with extracranial carotid and vertebral artery disease. A report of the American College of Cardiology Foundation/American Heart Association Task Force on Practice Guidelines, and the American Stroke Association, American Association of Neuroscience Nurses, American Association of Neurological Surgeons, American College of Radiology, American Society of Neuroradiology, Congress of Neurological Surgeons, Society of Atherosclerosis Imaging and Prevention, Society for Cardiovascular Angiography and Interventions, Society of Interventional Radiology, Society of NeuroInterventional Surgery, Society for Vascular Medicine, and Society for Vascular Surgery. Circulation 2011;124:e54–130.

21. Executive Committee for the Asymptomatic Carotid Atherosclerosis Study. Endarterectomy for asymptomatic carotid artery stenosis. JAMA 1995;273:1421–28.

22. Halliday A, Mansfield A, Marro J, et al. MRC Asymptomatic Carotid Surgery Trial (ACST) Collaborative Group. Prevention of disabling and fatal strokes by successful carotid endarterectomy in patients without recent neurological symptoms: randomized controlled trial. Lancet 2004; 363:1491–1502.

23. Mas JL, Trinquart L, Leys D, et al. Endarterectomy Versus Angioplasty in Patients with Symptomatic Severe Carotid Stenosis (EVA-3S) trial: results up to 4 years from a randomised, multicentre trial. Lancet Neurol 2008;7:885–92.

24. Eckstein HH, Ringleb P, Allenberg JR, et al. Results of the Stent-Protected Angioplasty versus Carotid Endarterectomy (SPACE) study to treat symptomatic stenoses at 2 years: A multinational, prospective,randomised trial. Lancet Neurol 2008;7:893–902.

25. Ederle J, Dobson J, Featherstone RL, et al. Carotid artery stenting compared with endarterectomy in patients with symptomatic carotid stenosis (International Carotid Stenting Study): an interim analysis of a randomised controlled trial. Lancet 2010;375:985–97.

26. Leichtle SW, Mouawad NJ, Welch K, et al. Outcomes of carotid endarterectomy under general and regional anesthesia from the American College of Surgeons' National Surgical Quality Improvement Program. J Vasc Surg 2012; 56:81.

27. Mayo score Sundt TM Jr, Sandok BA, Whisnant JP. Carotid endarterectomy. Complications and preoperative assessment of risk. Mayo Clinic Proc 1975;50:301–6.

28. Fleisher LA, Beckman JA, Brown KA, et al. ACC/AHA 2007 guidelines on perioperative cardiovascular evaluation and care for noncardiac surgery: a report of the American College of Cardiology/American Heart Association task force on practice guidelines (writing committee to revise the 2002 guidelines on perioperative cardiovascular evaluation for noncardiac surgery). Circulation 2007;116:e418–e500.

29. Hillis LD, Smith PK, Anderson JL, et al. Special articles: 2011 ACCF/AHA guideline for coronary artery bypass graft surgery: Executive summary: A report of the American College of Cardiology Foundation/American Heart Association task force on practice guidelines. Anesth Analg 2012; 114(1):11–45.

30. Naylor AR, Bown MJ. Stroke after cardiac surgery and its association with asymptomatic carotid disease: An updated systematic review and meta-analysis. Eur J Vasc Endovasc Surg 2011;41(5):607–24.

31. GALA Trial Collaborative Group, Lewis SC, Warlow CP, et al. General anaesthesia versus local anaesthesia for carotid surgery (GALA): a multicentre, randomised controlled trial. Lancet 2008;372:2132.

32. Magnadottir HB, Lightdale N, Harbaugh RE: Clinical outcomes for patients at high risk who underwent carotid endarterectomy with regional anesthesia. Neurosurgery 1999;45:786–92.

33. Papavasiliou AK, Magnadottir HB, Gonda T, et al. Clinical outcomes after carotid endarterectomy: Comparison of the use of regional and general anesthetics. J Neurosurg 2000; 92:291–6.

34. Ricotta JJ, HargadonT, O'Brein-Irr M. Cost management strategies for carotid endarterectomy. Am J Surg 1998;176: 188–92.

35. Leichtle SW, Mouawad NJ, Welch K, et al. Outcomes of carotid endarterectomy under general and regional anesthesia from the American College of Surgeons' National Surgical Quality Improvement Program. J Vasc Surg 2012; 56:81e3–88e3.

36. Schechter MA, Shortell CK, Scarborough JE. Regional versus general anesthesia for carotid endarterectomy: The American College of Surgeons National Surgical Quality Improvement Program perspective. Surgery 2012;152:309–14.

37. McGirt MJ, Woodworth GF, Brooke BS, et al: Hyperglycemia independently increases the risk of perioperative stroke, myocardial infarction, and death after carotid endarterectomy. Neurosurgery 2006;58:1066–73.

38. Poisik A, Heyer EJ, Solomon RA, Quest DO, Adams DC, Baldasserini CM, et al. Safety and efficacy of fixed-dose heparin in carotid endarterectomy. Neurosurgery 1999;45: 434–41.

39. Pennekamp CW, Moll FL, de Borst GJ. The potential benefits and the role of cerebral monitoring in carotid endarterectomy. Curr Opin Anaesthesiol 2011;24:693–7.

40. Beese U, Langer H, Lang W, Dinkel M. Comparison of near-infrared spectroscopy and somatosensory evoked potentials for the detection of cerebral ischemia during carotid endarterectomy. Stroke 1998;29:2032–7.

41. Ackerstaff RG, Moons KG, van de Vlasakker CJ, et al. Association of intraoperative transcranial Doppler monitoring variables with stroke from carotid endarterectomy. Stroke 2000;31:1817–23.

42. Williams IM, Picton A, Farrell A, Mead GE, Mortimer AJ, McCollum CN. Light-reflective cerebral oximetry and jugular bulb venous oxygen saturation during carotid endarterectomy. Br J Surg 1994;81:1291–5.

43. Goldstein LB, Moore WS, Robertson JT, Chaturvedi S. Complication rates for carotid endarterectomy: A call for action. Stroke 1997;28:889–90.

44. Tu JV, Wang H, Bowyer B, et al. Risk factors for death or stroke after carotid endarterectomy: Observations from the Ontario Carotid Endarterectomy Registry. Stroke 2003;34:2568–7.

45. Halm EA, Tuhrim S, Wang JJ, et al. Risk factors for perioperative death and stroke after carotid endarterectomy: results of the new york carotid artery surgery study. Stroke 2009 Jan;40(1):221–9.

46. Endovascular versus surgical treatment in patients with carotid stenosis in the Carotid and Vertebral Artery Transluminal Angioplasty Study (CAVATAS): A randomised trial. Lancet 2001;357:1729–37.

47. Yadav JS, Wholey MH, Kuntz RE, et al. Protected carotid-artery stenting versus endarterectomy in high-risk patients. N Engl J Med 2004;351:1493–501.

48. Lal BK, Beach KW, Roubin GS, Lutsep HL, Moore WS, Malas MB, et al. Restenosis after carotid artery stenting and endarterectomy: a secondary analysis of CREST, a randomised controlled trial. Lancet Neurol. Sep 2012;11(9):755–63.

49. Bates ER, Babb JD, Casey DE Jr, Cates CU, Duckwiler GR, Feldman TE, et al. ACCF/SCAI/SVMB/SIR/ASITN 2007 clinical expert consensus document on carotid stenting: A report of the American College of Cardiology Foundation Task Force on Clinical Expert Consensus Documents (ACCF/SCAI/SVMB/SIR/ASITN Clinical Expert Consensus Document Committee on Carotid Stenting). J Am Coll Cardiol 2007 Jan 2;49(1):126–70.

# CHAPTER 11

# Monitoring in Vascular Surgery

Arindam Choudhury

## INTRODUCTION

Monitoring of physiological parameters is an integral part of safe conduct of anesthesia. Various monitoring systems are employed during comprehensive anesthesia management for vascular surgeries. Some are routine (ASA standards of monitoring) and some are specific to the vascular procedure/surgery contemplated. The cardiovascular monitoring devices include but are not limited to electrocardiography (ECG), invasive pressure monitoring [arterial blood pressure (ABP), central venous pressure (CVP), pulmonary artery pressure (PAP), etc.], various cardiac output measuring and monitoring devices. Apart from this, there are other important monitored parameters, with which we keep a vigil on different physiology/system such as temperature regulations, body fluids homeostasis through urine output monitoring, cerebral and neurological functions monitoring and coagulation systems monitoring.

### Basic Concepts of Physiological Measurements

Accurate measurements of physiological parameters during anesthesia for vascular surgery are very critical and it enables the clinician to deliver safe and optimum care to the patient. Monitoring devices along with basic clinical inputs from the patient are essential tools in the specialized clinical environment. It is essential to keep a record of the 'measurands' provided by these monitors. In the process of measurement, a measurand should be compared to a predefined standard. Challenges offered by the measurement systems involve the maintenance of precision and accuracy. The readings obtained from these measurement devices are also prone to human interpretation and cognition errors. The basic principles involved in data acquisition, processing, display and storage are discussed briefly in the following sections.

## Components of an Ideal Measurement System

Each measurement system should contain following vital components for data acquisition, components that allow the measured variables to be compared to the standards and displayed.

a. Sensor or transducer
b. Signal processing
c. Output or display
d. Control or feedback

a. *Sensor:* This is a device that undergoes physical or chemical changes in response to variations in the measured parameters. It also allows conversion of signal into more meaningful and interpretable readings. It is also known as transducer when it converts one form of energy into another and their examples are shown in Table 11.1.

   Most transducers generate electrical signals and these signals are processed further before display. Simpler 'non-electrical' monitoring devices rely on a calibrated linear scale and they require very little processing before display (e.g. sphygmomanometer).

**Table 11.1:** Examples of transducer types and their conversion methods used in medical practice

| Physiological parameters | Transducer | Conversion |
|---|---|---|
| **Pressure** | Electro-mechanical | Resistance/capacitance changes |
| **Temperature** | Thermistor | Resistance changes |
| **Oxygen saturation** | Optical | Potentiometric changes |
| **ECG, EEG and EMG** | Ag/Ag chloride electrode | Potentiometric changes |

b. *Signal processing:* Electrical signals generated by the transducers are generally weak and too small for display. Therefore, they require amplification to bring about an increase in their scale. The ratio of signal strength at output after amplification compared to the original input signal strength is called the **gain**. Another important aspect of an amplifier is their ability to reduce interference from other electrical devices, which tend to distort the measurand. This interference is known as **noise** and elimination of noise is done by a process called **common mode rejection.** Other methods of increasing **signal to noise ratio** is by utilizing electrical filters, shielding cables, etc. For individual biological signals, the amplifiers must conform to the frequency range or **bandwidth** measured signals.

Digitization of measurand is done with analogue-to-digital converter (ADC) and these digitized signals are less prone to electrical interference. They can be easily compressed, thus large amount of data can be easily stored. They can be converted back to analogue signal for display using a digital-to-analogue converter (DAC).

c. *Display:* Simple non-electric monitors rely on linear or non-linear scale for display. With the advancement of electronics, digital display and linear encoders are superseding the mechanical and old-fashioned display. All digitized physiologic measurands are displayed in the video display unit (VDU) with capability of showing alphanumeric characters. A monitor screen or VDU is generally made up of cathode ray ocsillographs or liquid crystal display (LCD) unit that can effectively communicate with a central processing unit.

d. *Feedback control:* Like biofeedback mechanisms, a feedback control is very important in every monitoring device. It allows the measured signals to be interpreted and necessary changes made by a knowledgeable observer or an enabled device controlled by an appropriate algorithm. However, it is important in the first place that the monitoring device be accurate and auto-calibrated.

*Calibration:* In a truly accurate monitoring system, linearity would exist between the measured value and the actual value. The linearity of a system is a measure of how well the measured variables represent the true value. Non-linearity prevails when the relationship between measured value and the true value differ from each other. In reality, most monitoring device are not perfectly linear. Most frequently, baseline drift or offset drift occurs in transducers that describes a change within

it leading to over or underestimation of the measured value. This is a fixed deviation from the true value throughout the measurement range and is commonly due to changes in the ambient temperature as the semiconductors employed in such systems can be extremely sensitive to temperature changes. Some measurement systems are able to compensate for non-linearity errors electronically all by itself. This auto-calibration happens intermittently at a set interval. Calibration checks for linearity by comparing measured value with known values at preset points. For example, an arterial pressure transducer is calibrated at 0, 100 and 200 mmHg. These transducers are calibrated at the factory and in clinical settings a one point calibration at 0 mmHg (**Zeroing**) is usually sufficient.

### The Units of Measurements

The system internationale (SI) units are a logical strategy of measurement based on metric or decimal system that ascribes value to certain numerical figures. The value of a quantity is usually expressed in terms of a number and a reference unit. The SI system identifies seven fundamental or base units, two supplementary units and 22 derived units (Table 11.2).

The gram was the fundamental unit of mass in the centimeter-gram-second (CGS) system (1874) but this was replaced by the kilogram in meter- kilogram-second (MKS) system (1889), and subsequently was incorporated into the SI system. The dimensionless supplementary units are the radian (rad) and steradian (sr) for plane and solid angles respectively. Derived units are functions of one or more of the base units, e.g. the unit of force (m.kg. $s^{-1}$) is also called the newton (N). Decimal multiples and submultiples of the base units are expressed by adding appropriate prefixes (Table 11.3).

### ELECTROCARDIOGRAPHY

For obtaining a good ECG display, one has to fulfill certain minimum requirements as mentioned below:

a. Good quality ECG electrodes preferably (silver chloride gelled electrodes)

b. A good contact with the skin over the bony prominences.

c. Skin should have minimum impedance to electric current transmission. This can be achieved by lightly scrapping the stratum corneum with a dry gauge piece.

d. A five lead system of electrodes are utilized for maximum information with minimum inconvenience and encroachment in the surgical field.

**Table 11.2:** The seven fundamental SI units

| Base | Dimensional symbol | SI unit name | SI Symbol | Definition |
|---|---|---|---|---|
| **Length** | L | Meter | m | 1 m is the length of the path travelled by light in a vacuum during 1/ 299792458s |
| **Mass** | M | Kilogram | kg | I kg is the mass of a platinum-iridium prototype preserved at the BIPM, Paris. |
| **Time** | T | Second | s | 1 s is the duration 9192631770 periods of radiation corresponding to the transition between two levels of the ground state of cesium −133 atom. |
| **Electric current** | I | Ampere | A | 1 A is the constant current which would produce a force of $2 \times 10^{-7}$ newton/m between two straight parallel conductors of infinite length of negligible CSA in vacuum. |
| **Thermodynamic temperature** | Θ | Kelvin | K | 1 K is the 1/273.16 of absolute temperature of the triple point of water |
| **Amount of substance** | N | Mole | mol | 1 mol is the amount of substance that contains as many elementary substances as there are in 0.012 kg of Carbon-12 |
| **Luminous intensity** | J | Candela | cd | 1 cd is the luminosity in a given direction from a source that emits monochromatic radiation at $540 \times 10^{12}$ Hz and has radiant intensity in that direction of 1/683 watt per steradian. |

CSA—cross-sectional area, BIPM—international bureau of weight and measures.

**Table 11.3:** Some SI prefixes in common use in anesthesia

| Factor | Name | Symbol | Factor | Name | Symbol |
|---|---|---|---|---|---|
| $10^1$ | deca | da | $10^{-1}$ | deci | d |
| $10^2$ | hecto | h | $10^{-2}$ | centi | c |
| $10^3$ | kilo | K | $10^{-3}$ | mili | m |
| $10^6$ | mega | M | $10^{-6}$ | micro | m |
| $10^9$ | giga | G | $10^{-9}$ | nano | n |
| $10^{12}$ | tera | T | $10^{-12}$ | pico | p |

e. As the operation room is replete with many different types of electrical equipment electrical interference is common occurrence; most notable among them is the ECG interference due to electrosurgical unit (commonly referred to as electro-cautery equipment), which operates at 60 Hz. So, proper 'earthing' of all the equipments and an ECG system having the capability of eliminating all these electrical interference will provide the best display of the electrical activities of the heart.

The five electrodes (one in each extremities and one precordial unipolar lead) utilized in 5 lead system allow simultaneous recordings of the six standard frontal limb leads as well as at least one precordial unipolar lead. The later is dependent on the location of the chest electrode relative to the position of the heart after positioning the patient for the surgery. Current practice standards recommend continuous monitoring of frontal limb lead II and unipolar chest lead IV, as they best detect any arrhythmia episode and for ischemic events (sensitivity >90%) by continuous real-time ST- segment monitoring.[1] But patient position, location of the surgical incision (oblique thoracotomy, etc.) can make placing of the 'true' lead IV monitoring impractical in this subset of patients. Moreover, modification in the monitoring equipment is yet to occur to incorporate $V_4$ monitoring exclusively or along with $V_5$ unless these practical hindrances are overcome.[2]

## INVASIVE PRESSURE MONITORING

### Arterial Pressure Monitoring

During vascular anesthesia case management, intra-vascular pressure measurements are commonly obtained. Arterial pressure is obtained by inserting a catheter inside the arterial lumen (usually a peripheral artery). Pressure waves displayed on the monitor represents the transmitted force that was generated within left ventricle. Estimation of the force requires a device that converts the mechanical energy into electrical signals and such a device is called a (electromechanical) transducer.

Most non-invasive methods of blood pressure measurement require detection of blood flow past an occlusion cuff and they do not display a waveform and provide data at an interval. Intra-arterial catheter based pressure monitoring remains a gold standard because of the following advantages:

i. Vascular surgery is always associated with wide swings in BP and rapid fluid shifts as a result of surgical manipulations and underlying cardio vascular diseases. Therefore, Intra-arterial blood pressure monitoring provides beat-to-beat measurements of BP and waveform analysis a must for these operations.

ii. More over arterial trace provides a wealth of information apart from instantaneous BP readings when it is most needed. The upstroke slope analysis in terms of pressure changes over time (dp/dt) correlates with myocardial contractility while in high SVR situations there will be an increase in the upstroke slope and a decrease in the down stroke slope of the arterial waveform. During IPPV the respiratory phasic variations of amplitude of the arterial traces gives an indications of hypovolemia along with a visual indication of narrowed pulse pressure in the tracings of the arterial waveform (stroke volume variation).

iii. Another advantage is the multiple blood samples that can be obtained when an arterial catheter is in situ.

iv. Selective site (e.g. right radial artery) cannulations provide a good measure for upper body perfusion pressure during femoro-femoral bypass. This is utilized during thoraco-abdominal aneurysm surgeries as the upper body is selectively perfused through a separate axillary artery cannula.

v. Depending on the site of arterial cannulation for monitoring purpose any accidental clamping or ligation can also be detected and consequent

mishaps can be avoided specially during surgeries involving the isthmus of the aorta like PDA ligations, coarctation of aorta, double arch, vascular ring, etc. In this situation we routinely cannulate femoral artery along with the right radial artery. Some time during dissection and vessels identification, these arterial lines proves immensely helpful for confirmation before ligating PDA or any aberrant vessel not supplying the lower body and vital organs.

### Site of Cannulation

a. *Radial artery and ulnar artery:* During vascular surgery, radial artery is one of the most commonly chosen sites for monitoring due to factors like superficial locations, easily accessible and presence of collateral circulation. The ulnar artery provides the major supply of oxygenated blood in about 90% of individuals. The radial and ulnar arteries are feeders of the palmer arch and it provide collateral flow in the unfortunate event of radial artery occlusion/thrombosis. Although the value of preoperative Allen's test has been challenged we routinely perform this test for both palmer arch preoperatively. This test is performed by occluding both radial and ulnar artery with manual compression, while the patient is asked to open or close his/her fist until it becomes pale. Releasing the compression restores the ulnar artery flow and the time of reperfusion and restoration of normal color is observed. With normal collateral circulation the color returns within 5 sec (Fig. 11.1). If it is delayed for 15 seconds or more, cannulation of radial artery is relatively contra-

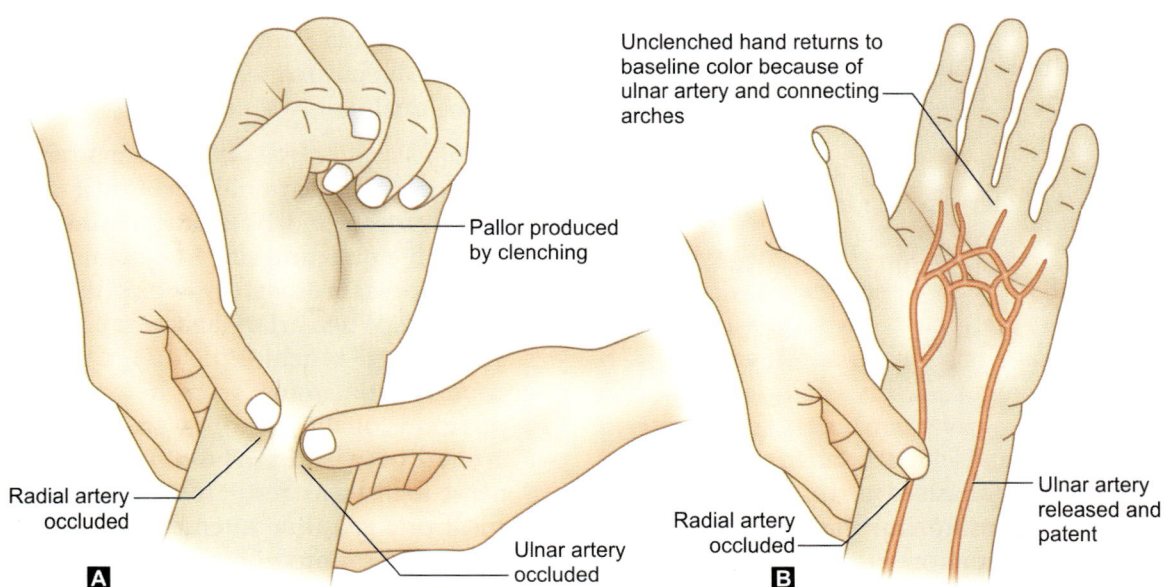

**Figs 11.1A and B:** A demonstration of Allen's test performed at the bedside

indicated. The modified Allen's test can be performed with Doppler probe or pulse oximeter to document collateral flow, which is a more objective method.

**Site selection:** The following issues are to be taken into consideration, before attempting any arterial cannulation.

  i. Proximal arterial cut down (e.g. radial artery cannulation distal to ipsilateral brachial artery cut down site) may result in dampened wave form or vascular thrombosis.

 ii. The vessel requiring clamping during surgery (ipsilateral branch vessels are obviously not a good choice for cannulation for monitoring purpose).

iii. Any history of ischemia or prior surgery of the limb.

 iv. Presence of A-V fistula/Shunt created for hemodialysis, the limb is generally avoided.

  v. In absence of above factors we choose the radial artery of the non-dominant hand of the patient for cannulation for monitoring and sampling purposes. The predictive value of Allen's test is questionable and there are many reports of hand ischemia requiring digital amputation following radial artery cannulations despite normal pre-operative Allen's test.[3]

b. *Brachial and axillaries arteries:* This artery courses medial to the bicipital tendon in the antecubital fossa along with the median nerve. There is little collateral circulation to the arm if brachial artery gets occluded. Therefore, it should be avoided as far as possible. Cut down results in more number of complications as compared to brachial arterial cannulation.[4]

   The axillary artery course along with the brachial plexus inside the brachial sheath and it is usually cannulated at the junction of deltoid and pectoralis muscle where it is prominently felt. Because the tip of 15 cm long catheter may lie in the aortic arch, it has limited role in surgeries involving the ascending and the arch of the aorta. Axillary artery cannulations may be necessary in peripheral vascular disease and the left side is preferable over the right side to minimize the chance of cerebral embolism during flushing the catheter.

c. *Femoral artery (FA) and dorsalis paedis artery (DPA):* Patient with vascular disease the femoral artery cannulations for monitoring may not be a good choice. Aortic obstruction may decrease arterial pressure in the FA or the FA may be the area of operation it self. Patients undergoing thoraco-

abdominal aortic reconstructive surgery, one of the femoral artery may be utilized for perfusion of organs and tissue distal to the aortic cross clamp during partial left or right heart bypass. This is done in order to preserve the blood flow of spinal cord. During partial bypass it is important to measure distal aortic pressure in addition to arterial pressure monitoring in one of the upper extremities.

## Complications

  i. *Haemorrhage:* The arterial pressure monitoring catheter carries the potential risk of death from exsanguination if the catheter is open to atmosphere due to accidental disconnections. The use of luer lock connector and constant vigilance decrease the risk of this complication. Presence of stopcock in the monitoring system (transducers) also increases the chance of bleeding due to inadvertent opening of control lever that would open the transducers to the atmosphere.

 ii. *Thrombosis:* Distal ischemia following radial artery cannulations is relatively rare but when it occurs the patient may land up with amputation of thumb and index finger. Any evidence of ischemia should call for aggressive investigation and early therapy involving the services of vascular, hand and plastic surgeon. Also, streptokinase, heparin, anti-platelet agents and stellate ganglion block are the other modalities of treatment of digital ischemia.

iii. *Embolisation:* Air and other particulate matter can be forcefully flushed into an artery through the catheter in situ. Cerebral embolism is more likely from the right axillary artery catheter although it is also possible through brachial and radial artery. Factors directly related are the volume and rapidity of the flush.

 iv. *Hematoma and nerve injury:* Hematoma formation is common after arterial puncture if it is not immediately occluded by counter pressure directly above the puncture site. In patients with coagulopathy pressure has to be applied for a longer duration. When artery and nerve lie together in a sheath (e.g. brachial plexus), chances of nerve compression injury from hematoma following puncture of the artery is greatly increased. As arterial cannulation is a blind procedure, direct nerve injury may result from needle trauma, more so during multiple attempts at arterial cannulations. For example, median nerve is commonly injured as it lies in close proximity to the brachial artery.

v. *Risk of infection:* There is always an element of risk of infection whenever an invasive catheter is inserted and left in contact with the blood stream. The possible sources may be—(a) poor manufacturing standards, (b) poor aseptic technique of insertion, (c) contaminated flushing solution, etc. Other avoidable causes of infection include reusable dome transducer, dextrose containing flushing solution and the length of indwelling catheter placement. Catheter is an inert foreign body, so any amount of antimicrobial drug administration cannot make it sterile in vivo. Therefore, the best possible step is the removal of the catheter whenever infection is detected at the cannulation site or patient continues to have signs of infection with unknown source.

## Central Venous Pressure Monitoring

A catheter is inserted inside one of the large central veins to estimate the filling pressures of the right atrium. For vascular surgical patients, right internal jugular vein (IJV) is commonly cannulated for monitoring purposes unless there is any contraindication.

## Technique of CVP Insertion

Central venous cannulation can be achieved by the catheter-through-needle, catheter over guide-wire or catheter over the needle technique. We most commonly perform the Seldinger's catheter over the guide-wire technique. Alternatively, vascular ultrasonography may be used to guide venous puncture and passing of the guide-wire inside the venous lumen under vision. The introducer needle can be marked or unmarked for the ease of the operator for an error free procedure.

a. **Indications:** A 'hydrocath' or central venous catheter is inserted primarily to know the status of intravascular volume. The accuracy and reliability as an indication of left heart filling pressure depends on factors like:
   i. Pulmonary vascular resistance.
   ii. Functional status of the ventricles
   iii. Integrity of the valves (especially Tricuspid valve)
   iv. Ventilatory factors like application of positive end expiratory pressure (PEEP).

b. **Site of cannulation**
   i. In cardiovascular surgery, the right IJV is generally preferred by all the anesthesiologists because of its easy access and its straight course. Absence of valve till the superior vena cava (SVC) and relatively clean and unsoiled area are the other factors for its preference over the other site.

The success rate is also higher compared to other sites. IJV cannulation is relatively contraindicated in patients who had previous neck surgery and absolutely contraindicated in cases of local infection near the puncture site.

ii. External jugular vein is a less preferred site for reaching the SVC as the success rate is lower because of its tortuous drainage, although a 'J tipped' guide-wire and slight traction of the ipsilateral arm at the shoulder joint allows negotiation of the catheter past the obstructions and increases the success rate. This vein is easy to perforate and if perforation occurs in the intrathoracic segment, any hematoma or extravasations can be missed. There were cases of hydrothorax following lately detected extravasations. Therefore, while using multilumen catheters, confirmation by aspiration of freely flowing venous blood from all the lumens is very important, should be practiced routinely and incorporated in any checklist (vide infra).

iii. *Femoral vein:* This vein is rarely cannulated in adult patients. Yet, this site may be the only available option in a subset of patients. The cannulations technique is relatively simple and Seldinger technique may be necessary at times. The incidence of catheter related sepsis and thrombophlebitis is slightly higher as compared to other central venous access sites. In superior vena cava syndrome, femoral vein needs to be cannulated who require CVP monitoring and a long catheter is inserted to reach the intrathoracic segment of IVC.

iv. *Subclavian vein:* This vein can be approached either through a supra- or infra-clavicular puncture. The success rate is higher than external jugular but lower than that of (R) IJV approach. This approach is usually avoided by Cardiac Anesthesiologist because of relatively higher incidences of complications[5] and if sternal retractor is applied after sternotomy, the catheter have higher chances of getting entrapped and obstructed between the inferior margin of clavicle and the anterior surface of the first rib. But, in patients requiring carotid artery surgery and CVP monitoring during the procedure, subclavian vein cannulation can be a suitable site for CVP monitoring.

v. *Anti-cubital vein:* The cephalic or the brachial vein is frequently utilized for CVP monitoring. Although it is advantageous to utilize this vein for cannulation as there is less likelihood of any complication, the disadvantages are that it is difficult to ensure the placement of catheter tip into the central vein and failure to advance the catheter past the shoulder or 'malplacement' in the ipsilateral IJV are other common problems with this approach.

## Common Pitfalls

1. Arterial puncture involving central venous cannulation is not uncommon and it happens more frequently in the inexperienced hands. The reason for this is all deep veins lie in close proximity with major arteries. Other reason can be highly variable course of the veins. Therefore, whenever puncture is unsuccessful with standard landmark technique, USG guided cannulation should be practiced to ensure successful venous puncture without injuring other adjacent vital structures. When using landmark technique without USG guidance, it is advisable to use smaller gauge (e.g. 22G) needle as a 'pilot' puncture device to minimize hematoma formation.

   A large hematoma may form if the inadvertent arterial puncture is too large, and direct pressure is not applied for 30 minutes or the patient is on anti-coagulation therapy or the patient has coagulopathy. Venous obstruction occurring in the area of large formations of AV fistula is also reported in the literatures.

2. Hemothorax, pnumothorax and hydrothorax: Hemothorax is a potential complication of subclavian vein cannulation if the subclavian artery is accidentally injured. Hemothorax may also develop if the catheter in situ erodes through a venous wall into the plural cavity.

   If the pleural cavity is entered and the lung parenchymal is punctured during central venous cannulation, a pneumothorax will be produced. A pneumothorax is frequent complication of subclavian approach of central venous cannulation as opposed to internal jugular venous cannulation.

   If the cathether tip erodes the vessel wall and lodges itself inside the pleural cavity, all the fluid that is administered (without the knowledge of the administrator that the fluid is not reaching the vascular compartment) through the catheter will accumulate in the pleural cavity resulting in hydrothorax.

3. Embolism: Air can be entrained in a spontaneously breathing patient when he generates enough negative intra-thoracic pressure during inspiration. One has to be careful for air embolism when cannulating a central vein in a spontaneously breathing patient and

this is a potentially fatal complication. Occasionally, 'spallation' can occur during inserting of catheter through needle technique and the fragments may embolise into the right side of the heart or the pulmonary arterial tree.

4. Pericardial effusion and temponade: If the right atrium or the right ventricle is perforated during central venous cannulation, it can result in pericardial effusion or rarely a temponade. The risk of this type of complications increases when a rigid guide wire is used.

5. Nerve injury: Stellate ganglion, phrenic nerves and brachial plexus, all lie in the vicinity of the IJV. Any needle injury can produce permanent nerve damage during central venous cannulation.

6. Other complications: Sometimes tissue punch biopsy of the vessel wall being cannulated may occur and the piece of tissue may prevent free movement of the guide wire inside the Seldinger needle and may even jam the former inside the needle leading to unsuccessful cannulations. The author recommends aspiration of sufficient quantity of freely flowing venous blood so that any punched tissue fragment may be cleared from the needle before insertion of the guide wire.[6]

## Pulmonary Artery Catheterization

In patients with normal pulmonary arterial tone and no structural defects or valvular abnormality, pulmonary artery diastolic press (PAD) and pulmonary capillary wedge pressures (PCWP) correlates well with left atrial pressure (LAP) which in turn is a surrogate for left ventricular end diastolic pressure (LVEDP). LVEDP is an estimate of left ventricular end diastolic volume (LVEDV), which reflects the true LV preload. The relationship between "LVEDP and LVEDV is best understood by the LV compliance curve or the LV pressure volume loop.

Patients undergoing vascular surgery have high incidence of coronary artery disease (CAD) and unlike healthy subjects, CVP in them is not a reliable surrogate for the left sided filling pressures. Unfortunately, CAD patients can have mitral valvular disease, in such situations PCWP/PAD does not correlate well with LVEDP.

## Indications of PAC in Vascular Surgery Patients

i. Major vascular procedure involving large fluid shifts and/or blood loss in patients with ventricular dysfunction.

ii. Patients with recent myocardial infarction or unstable angina

iii. Patients with hypovolemia, cardiogenic or septic shock with multi-organ failure.

iv. Severe trauma patients

v. Patients requiring ionotropes and IABP counter pulsation

vi. Patients undergoing surgery of the aorta requiring application of aortic cross clamp

vii. Patient planned for endovascular repair of the aorta with a possibility of conversion to open procedure

viii. Patient undergoing liver transplantation

## Contraindications

### Absolute contraindications

i. Tricuspid atresia or pulmonic valve stenosis

ii. Right atrial or ventricular mass (e.g. tumours, thrombus, etc.)

iii. Tetralogy of Fallot

### Relative contraindications

i. Severe arrhythmia (ventricular tachyarrythmias, significant ventricular ectopics, long QT syndrome, etc).

ii. Clinically significant coagulopathy

iii. Newly inserted pacemaker wire

## Site of Cannulation

As PA catheter is usually slided through a long sheath of appropriate caliber, the sheath is usually inserted into IJV, which is usually inserted into the IJV that offer a valve-less straight course for the sheath. The right IJV remains the most convenient route although other route such as femoral and axillary veins are also described and practiced. PAC insertion is always guided by real-time pressure monitoring (Fig. 11.2) as its tip traverses different vessel and chambers of the heart (a near alternative for procedure under vision). The balloon tipped catheter is easily floated in the blood stream from RA to the pulmonary artery and into one of its branches for wedging.

## Complications

All complication discussed for the central venous cannulation are also relevant for PA catheterization. Apart from them, other important complications exclusive to PAC are highlighted below:

i. Arrhythmias: The most common/frequent arrhythmia is PVCs, however life threatening ones like VT/VF are also reported. A positional maneuver with 5° reverse Trendelenburg and slight

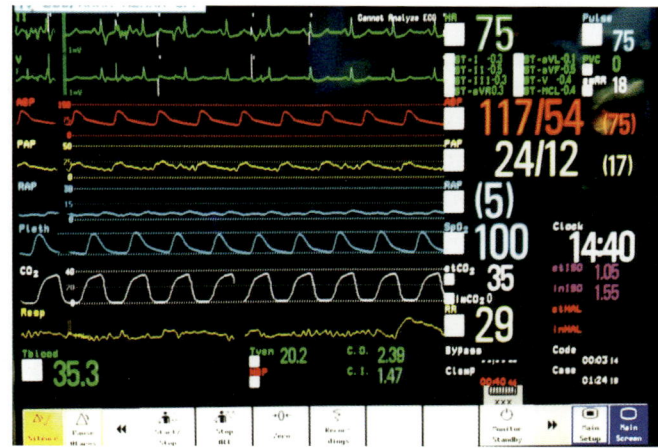

Fig. 11.2: A multi-parameter monitor is very essential for successful insertion of PA catheter

right lateral tilt eases the safe migration of the balloon tip across the infundibulum into the PA.

ii. Conduction defects: Complete heart block may develop in a patient with pre-existent LBBB. The incidence of RBBB is 3%. Pacing option should be kept open in such patients.

iii. Endobronchial hemorrhage and pulmonary infarction: The risk factors include advanced age, distal tip placement, pulmonary hypertension, mitral stenosis, coagulopathy and balloon hyper inflation. Most of the time, right pulmonary artery was injured. Pulmonary infarction is not common nowadays, as unlike previously, we never keep the balloon inflated and in the wedge position. It is only inflated when the wedge pressure is required to be estimated.

iv. Catheter knotting: This usually occurs as a result of coiling of the catheter within the right ventricle. This can be un-knotted with a guide wire under fluoroscopic guidance or knot is tightened and withdrawn along with the sheath. Alternately, if the patient's right atrium can be open to release the knotted segment and the catheter is then withdrawn under vision.

## CARDIAC OUTPUT MONITORING

This is one of the most important components of hemo-dynamic monitoring for the vascular surgical patients. Devices that are used for measuring cardiac output (CO) ranges from highly invasive to semiinvasive to totally noninvasive technologies. It provides information with connotation for the management of preload, afterload, heart rate and contractility. In nutshell, CO reflects status of the total circulatory system.

Nowadays, the preference is shifting towards less invasive technologies like TEE, Vigileo (pulse contour analysis of arterial waveform), etc. for assessment of CO. The different technologies and their principles are described below:

i. Thermodilution method: This is one indicator dilution technique based on the principle that same quantity of indicator administered/injected at a point in circulating blood should be detected downstream when measured at a different point. *Stewart and Hamilton* described this principle mathematically as:

$I = CO \times \int c\, dt$ or, $CO = (I \times 60)/\int c\, dt$, where $I$ = amount of indicator injected, $\int c\, dt$ is the indicator concentration over time, CO is the cardiac output in liters per minute and 60 converts seconds into minutes.

The PAC has a thermistor near its tip, which measures the change in temperature of a given bolus of indicator (viz 10 cc of cold saline). For the measurement of CO by the thermodilution (TDCO), the modified Stewart-Hamilton equation needs to be applied.

$CO = [V\,(T_b - T_i) \times C_1 \times C_2] \times 60 \int_0^\infty \Delta T_B(t)\, dt$, where, CO is the cardiac output, V is the volume of injectate, $T_b$ is the initial blood temperature, $T_i$ is the initial injectate temperature, $C_1$ is the density factor, $C_2$ is the computation constant and $\int_0^\infty \Delta T_B(t)\, dt$ is the integral of blood temperature change over time.

Factors that determine the accuracy are:

1. Deviation from the protocol defined for the measurements markedly influence the accuracy. For example, when more indicator is administered then the computer was programmed for, the system will under estimate the CO measurement. Similarly, loss of indicator and rapid re-circulation results in erroneously high values.

2. The speed of injection: The speed of indicator administration also influences the accuracy.

## Limitations

i. The 'tail-end' of the temperature curve may be influenced by spontaneous variation in temperature in PA.

ii. Intermittent determination requires repeated injection of indicator which may lead to fluid overload.

iii. Measurement is labour intensive.

## CONTINUOUS THERMODILUTION CARDIAC OUTPUT (CCO)

In this method cold saline (fluid) is not required to be administered; rather the temperature is raised by a heating element in the proximal segment of the catheter and detected by heat sensor at the tip. This method employs pseudo-random stochastic analysis of the temperature decay in the blood stream.[7]

Although intermittent TDCO is fraught with many limitations and is labour intensive, it still holds its place as 'gold standard' of CO measurement in the clinical settings. All the limitations mentioned in TDCO is taken care of in the CCO but it is more expensive (almost double in price). It is still a question whether this price is worth spending, as routine monitoring of CO in cardiac surgery patients could not establish a clear benefit and improved outcome.

## OTHER SEMI INVASIVE METHODS

1. **Pulse contour cardiac output measurement**: Arterial waveforms are analysed and allow the calculation of CO. The pulse waveforms are derived from the invasive arterial catheters. The waveforms are analysed (e.g. area under the curve, etc.) to derive the measure of cardiac output. The principle of stroke volume calculation from pulse pressure is described by Erlanger and Hooker and it assumes that the rate of blood flow from the arterial tree to the venous system is proportional to the rate of pressure decline. Newer image processing and digital signal processing methods are incorporated for better correlation of CO with the gold standard. Although this method is less cumbersome, there are certain drawbacks of this technology worth a mention. First, this system requires calibration against a standard technique. Damping of arterial system is another issue that may lead to falsely low CO values. In addition to this, certain other conditions like arrhythmia, body position and arterial pathologies may provide us false CO values.

2. **Thoracic impedance cardiometry:** In electrical cardiometry, a continuous low ampere, high frequency electrical current is delivered across two electrodes, which is simultaneously sensed through another pair of electrodes. This is based on the principle of thoracic bio-impedance measurement first utilized by national aeronautics and space administration (NASA) for the estimation of cardiac output without requiring a transducer system in 'zero' gravity situation/environment (e.g. outer space, ISS international space station, etc.). Changes in thoracic impedance are induced by pulsatile blood

flow through the intrathoracic segment of the aorta, ventilation status (positive pressure ventilation, negative pressure ventilation, etc.). The primary measured parameters in this technology are heart rate, stroke volume (SV) and rest of the hemodynamic parameters are derived based on formulae and algorithms feeding extraneous measured variables. For calculation of SV, only the pulsatile component of electrical impedance changes across the aorta (dz/dt) is analyzed. Validation of CO measurement against the 'gold standard' is in progress and only large multi-centric studies with sufficient power will prove its worthiness for clinical monitoring as far as CO measurement is concerned. Factors affecting the CO measurement are pulmonary edema, massive pleural effusion, rhythm disturbances such as atrial fibrillation and intracardiac shunts. The electrical cardiometry device can continuously monitor CO and also help us promptly recognize any hemodynamic changes in patients undergoing vascular surgery.

3. **Carbon dioxide rebreathing technique:** Carbon dioxide ($CO_2$) rebreathing can be used for estimating CO using Fick's principle. By estimating oxygen consumption for $CO_2$ production, capnographic $CO_2$ measurement can be used to determine CO.

   a. *Pre-requisites:* Patient should be sedated, intubated and mechanically ventilated. The capnographic equipment need to be connected to estimate the CO.

   There are controversies regarding the correlation between this method and the standard CO measurement technique. Both studies refuting the correlation as well as citing good correlation exists in the literature.

4. **Ultrasound based cardiac output measurement:** With the advent of three-dimensional (3-D volume scan) echocardiography, estimation of left ventricular volume has become more realistic and accurate. With the help of automated border detection algorithm, endocardial surfaces are traced inside a volume scan data pile to give us the LV cavity volume.

   a. *USCOM:* This is a cardiac output monitor particularly designed to derive stroke volume by utilizing Doppler shift principle. Analysis of Doppler frequency shift in the reflected echo signals from the moving RBCs. Blood flow velocity, direction and the rate of change of velocity can be determined and from all these information, SV and hence the CO can be calculated as:

$$SV = VTI \times CSA$$

   where VTI is Doppler velocity time integral (area under the curve of spectral Doppler), and CSA is cross-sectional area of the site of flow measurement.

Stroke volume can be multiplied by the heart rate to provide us the CO. Depending on the velocity being measured; a pulsed wave or continuous wave Doppler can be applied. Theoretically, CO can be determined at all anatomic sites in the heart, (e.g. aortric, mitral and pulmonary positions).

The usual site of transducer placement in USCOM is the suprasternal notch. Calculation of CSA at LVOT is done assuming it as a tubular structure. In reality, it may not be so and hence some degree of error does exist. Doppler beam must be aligned parallel to the blood flow as far as possible. An angle correction of 20° is permissible as the error factor is limited to 5% only.

## Transesophageal Echocardiography (TEE)

A state of the art technology, increasingly gaining acceptance and recognition as an intraoperative (real time) monitoring device of cardiovascular status both in terms of function and anatomy. TEE can very well visualize and delineate the pathologies of the ascending aorta, descending thoracic aorta from dissection to calcification. Moreover, it can assess the effect of aortic cross clamping on the left ventricle as well as act as monitor for myocardial ischemia. If any new regional wall motion abnormality is detected after aortic cross clamping, the proximal pressure should be decreased with the help of a vasodilator till the RWMA resolves. TEE for vascular surgeries is dealt in greater details elsewhere in this book. (Chapter 12)

## *Perfusion and Respiratory Monitoring*

*a. Peripheral oximetry:* Monitoring of oxygen saturation in the peripheral circulation utilizing infrared sensor has tremendous value in vascular surgical patients. Pulse oximetry incorporates plethysmography, which characterizes pulsatile flow in the peripheral circulation. It is also a visual indicator of pulse and left ventricular ejection. Pulse contour analysis and CO measurements are tried with success using peripheral plethysmography. It is good indicator of perfusion to a particular limb. The caveats are peripheral pulse is influenced by the vasoconstriction due to hypovolemia, hypothermia and local obstruction to blood flow. The principle of transmittance pulse oximetry allow for distinction between pulsatile and non-pulsatile vessels carrying oxygenated blood. Prior to 1995, most $SpO_2$ measurement techniques used to utilize two wavelengths of light 660 nm (red) and 940 (infra red) nm. These pieces of equipment had hard times estimating $SpO_2$ in low flow/hypoperfusion states. Latest advancements in $SpO_2$ technology incorporate novel signal processing algorithms developed by Masimo Inc. and they call it 'signal extraction technology'. With this new probe, venous/capillary blood signals are efficiently filtered and provide most reliable $SpO_2$ values in low signal to noise ratio situation.

*b. Aterial blood gas analysis:* Arterial blood gas (ABG) analysis is a type of lung function test, which assesses the performance of lung in terms of oxygenation and carbon dioxide ($CO_2$) removal from the blood. In addition it tells us about the acid–base status of an individual's blood in health and disease. Thus, any patient who is mechanically ventilated during general anesthesia for major vascular surgeries will immensely benefit from ABG analysis as 'one lung ventilation' is very common during such procedures. The principle behind this test utilizes Nernst equation for pH estimation, polarographic method (Clark's electrode) for estimation of partial pressure of oxygen and Stowe's electrode for partial pressure of carbon dioxide in blood. There are two types of ABG analyser (a) point of care (POC) or bedside devices using specific cartridges and (b) centrally located high performance analyzers. The later type can handle large number of samples and requires calibration at regular interval. There are certain pitfalls of ABG analysis: (i) Sampling errors can after result and subsequent patient management, therefore, proper training and education is necessary before reading ABG result. For interpretation, ABG trends rather that a single value would be more appropriate. (ii) Error in result might surface due to alteration in temperatures, e.g. pH is highly temperature sensitive so is solubility of $CO_2$. The readers are referred to other sources of arterial blood gas analysis for alpha stat and pH stat management as it is beyond the scope of the present chapter.

## Neuromonitoring

*Regional oximetry:* Other major oximeter that utilizes reflected light from living tissue in an attempt to estimate oxyhemoglobin ($HbO_2$) saturation in other organ. For example, cerebral oximeter may be able to measure mean brain $HbO_2$ saturation, a balanced oxygenation among tissue capillary, venous and arterial blood. These tissue oxygen saturation monitors are of great value when arch vessels are manipulated under guidance of cerebral oxygen monitoring (right or left sided). Near infra red spectroscopy (NIRS) is routinely applied to bilateral fore head during surgery involving the arch vessels. Two flat disposable sensors emitting 700–900 nm infrared and red light on forehead and two separate channels are displayed on the monitor. The accepted minimum value for viable cerebral average tissue oxygenation is 45%. Anything between 20 and 40% $ScO_2$ indicates disturbed perfusion and $ScO_2$ between 0–20% infer brain damage. The normal $ScO_2$ range between 60 and 80% and between 80 and 100% is considered as luxury perfusion. $ScO_2$ 45–60% is considered buffer value, which is below normal yet the neurophysiological function remains intact. Thus the brain continues to function despite less than normal tissue oxygenation (under anesthesia). It is important to understand the limitation of this technology before making clinical decisions. For the brain, the relationship between the area of tissue damage and neurological outcome is not commensurate. *For example, a very small infarct* (say, 3 mm³ lacunar infarct) in thalamus can produce a severe neurological deficit (e.g. hemiparesis), whereas very large tissue loss (frontal lobe resection) may produce minimal or no neurological deficit. Nevertheless, recent evidence indicates that NIRS

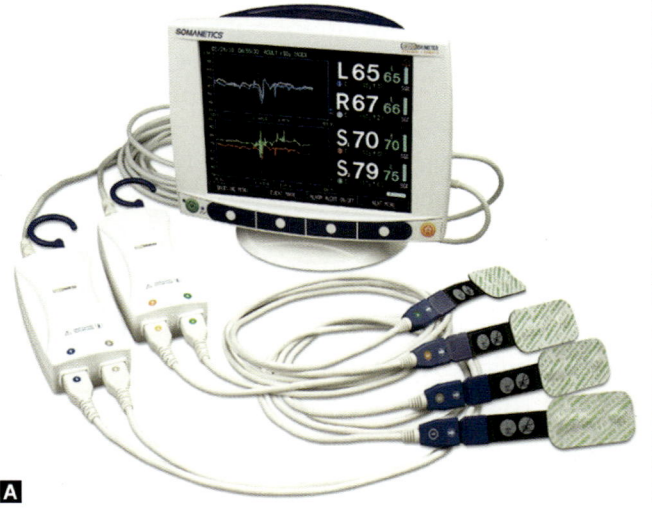

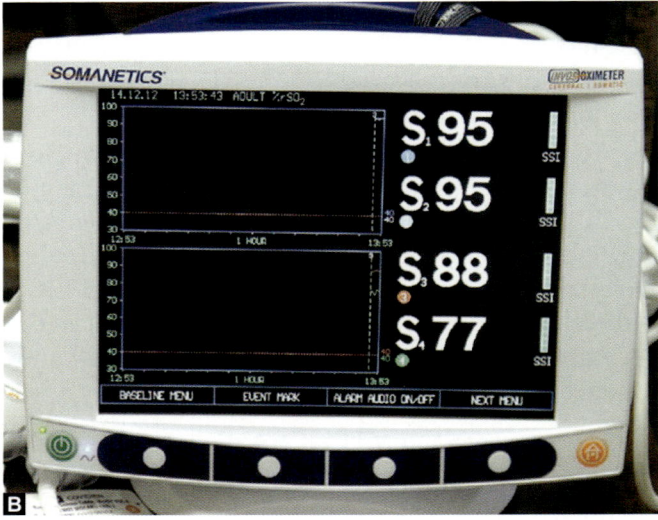

**Figs 11.3A and B:** Near infrared spectroscopy monitor and its sensors (different available sizes shown in A)

monitoring can detect inadequate perfusion in real-time, identifies as significant decrease in cerebral $SO_2$ value (Fig. 11.3). Failure to restore $rSO_2$ value or a sustained decrease of $ScO_2$ less than 60% is associated with poor neurological outcomes.

### Somatosensory Evoked Potential

Somatosensory evoked potential (SSEP) may be used as a part of neurophysiologic intraoperative monitoring (NIOM) for the assessment of functional integrity of the somatosensory pathways. Surgery of the descending thoracic aorta poses highest risk of injury of the spinal cord with incidence of paraplegia reaching almost 40%.[8] Monitoring of SSEP tells us about the function of the dorsal column and it can act as surrogate marker for global spinal cord function.

*Technique:* The selection of nerve to be stimulated for SSEP depends on the surgical procedure planned. For surgery involving the levels below $C_8$–$T_1$ segments, posterior tibial nerve (PTN) or common peroneal nerve (CPN) is stimulated. Stimulation of PTN at the ankle is preferred because it is easily accessible.

*Placement of electrodes:* The cathode should be placed over the medial malleolus 1–2 cm posteriorly. The anode is placed 1–2 cm distal to the cathode behind the ankle. Stimulation of CPN is technically difficult but it becomes useful when PTN cannot be stimulated due to peripheral neuropathy of BK amputation. The technique is similar to nerve stimulation and is described for PTN as below:

- Stimulation of PTN will produce planter flexion of the great toe and/or cupping of the respective sole. A stimulus of 20 mAmp is sufficient to elicit a response in a pharmacologically paralysed patient.

- A stimulation rate of 2–10 Hz is recommended for intraoperative monitoring. A stimulation rate in multiple of main AC current frequency (i.e. 60 Hz in Indian subcontinent) should be avoided, otherwise noise artifacts may appear in the SSEP recording (Fig. 11.4).

- SSEPs are obtained independently in both limbs. Current equipment standard permits right and left stimulation and their recordings to be displayed simultaneously. If the signal from one limb is weak, the response recording of bilateral SSEP is of great help, but at times unilateral injuries of the cord may go undetected.

- Cortical SSEPs are near field, short latency evoked potentials (EPs) recorded from the scalp over the underlying sensory cortex using bipolar scalp-to-scalp derivations. Subcortical SSEPs are near field EPs recorded using scalp to non-cephalic electrode derivation. Typical analysis time is 75–150 ms and the analysis time should be at least twice the latency of the last waveform of interest.

- A sufficient number of repetitions must be averaged to produce an interpretable and reproducible SSEP. Roughly, 250–1000 trials are needed, if this exceeds there will be delay in providing feedback to the surgeon. Modification of montage may yield higher signal to noise ratio of the cortical waveforms.

- Sterile subdural needle electrodes (screw type) or standard disk EEG electrodes are normally used (Fig. 11.3). The former is easy to use as head need not be shaved off hair, but they are more likely to get dislodged (Fig. 11.4).

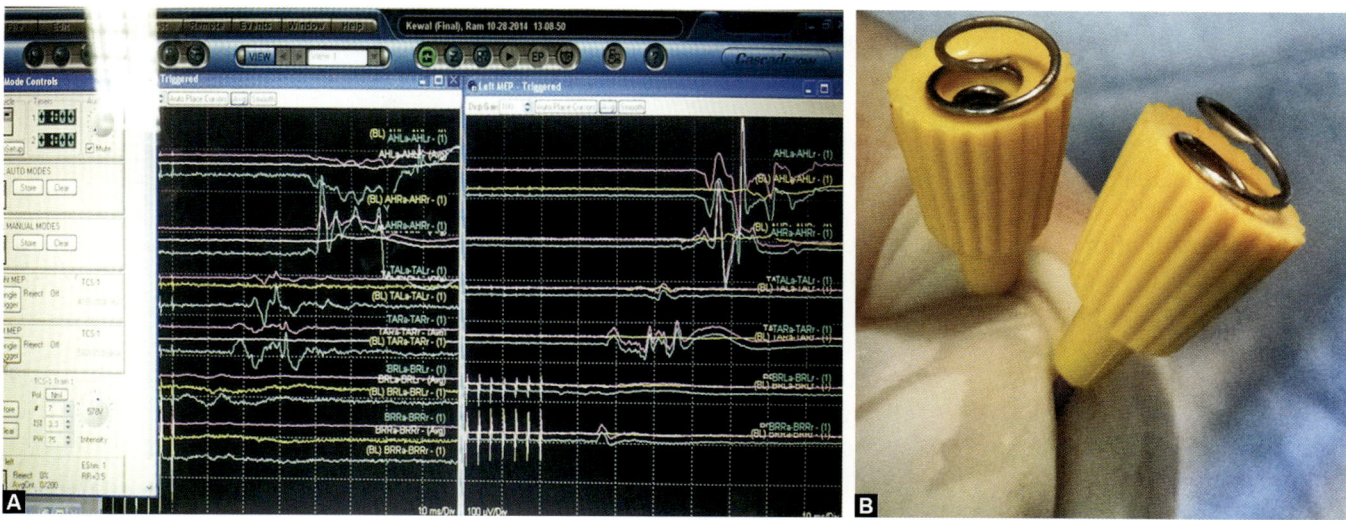

**Figs 11.4A and B:** A neurophysiologic monitor display panel and screw type electrodes for better signal transmission

• When NIOM with tibial SSEP is done, it may be useful to obtain CPi, CPc, Cz, FPz, $P_2$ montage referred to either chin or EPc electrodes. This allows for selection of best montage.

Typically, a 50% drop in amplitude and a 10% prolongation in latency are considered a significant change in SSEP. However, smaller and clearly distinct changes may also be significant. Any alterations in SSEPs are immediately brought to the notice of the surgical team and the anesthesiologist as a warning that the neural function is in jeopardy.

### Motor Evoked Potential

Motor evoked potential (MEP) is one of the most important tools in the NIOM armamentarium especially for thoracic aneurysm surgeries. Surgeons are always concerned about discharging an ambulatory patient after a successful surgery. MEP directly monitors the functional integrity of the motor neural network starting from motor cortex to peripheral nerves carrying motor fibers till the muscle end plate of their target muscles. As mentioned above, surgery of the descending thoracic aorta carries greater risk of ischemic insult to the spinal cord and disruption of functional integrity at any level will cause paralysis. This is because the lateral column and anterior horns of the spinal cord encases cranial nerves, corticospinal tracts and second order motor neutrons respectively. Monitoring MEP warns us about highest impairment of neural function of the motor nerves that may occur during such surgeries.

*Technique*: The most important technical consideration about MEP is the interference of anesthetic agent with the synaptic transmission. Most commonly stimulation is performed transcranially, although direct cortical stimulation is also possible (as in neurosurgery with exposed motor cortex). The outputs resulting from the transcranial electrical stimulations are usually recorded from two points along the motor pathways; (a) directly from the spinal cord, (b) as compound muscle response from the target muscles. Muscle relaxants are used only during induction of anesthesia for facilitating endotracheal intubation. During the maintenance phase, only propofol and opioid infusions can be used to maintain deep sedation and analgesia (Table 11.3). A transcranical cortical stimulation induces a D wave followed by series of I waves. I waves are usually lost during anesthesia, but trains of D wave generated by pulse-train stimulation can produce depolarisation of alpha motor neuron.

*Electrode placement*: Transcranial cortical stimulation is best carried out using cork-screw type electrodes

which are self retaining subdermal needles (Fig. 11.4). They are inserted over the central scalp region over the 'motor strips' according to the international 10–20 system of electrode placement (Fig. 11.5). Usually the anode is always placed over the motor cortex as the anodal stimulation activates the corticospinal axons at lower stimulation threshold as compared to cathodal stimulation. Usually one electrode is placed in the C1 and the other at the C2 position for bilateral stimulation.

• Stimulation may be constant current or constant voltage type but in the former, output limit of the stimulator may not be high enough to produce reliable response for some systems.

• Constant voltage stimulation in the setting of low impedance can overcome these limitations. Typical stimulation intensities are 200 mA and 400 V with duration of stimulation being 0.5–1 msec.

• Stimuli are delivered in trains of four to nine with an interstimululs interval of 2–5 msec. These settings may vary depending on the target muscle group, anesthetic depth and from patient to patient.

• In the event that single train stimulus is unable to produce reliable potentials (e.g. patient with neurologic deficit), certain maneuver is used. The most common of these technique is the double train or multi-train technique, where more than one train is applied before the actual stimulus train. This is known as 'facilitation'.

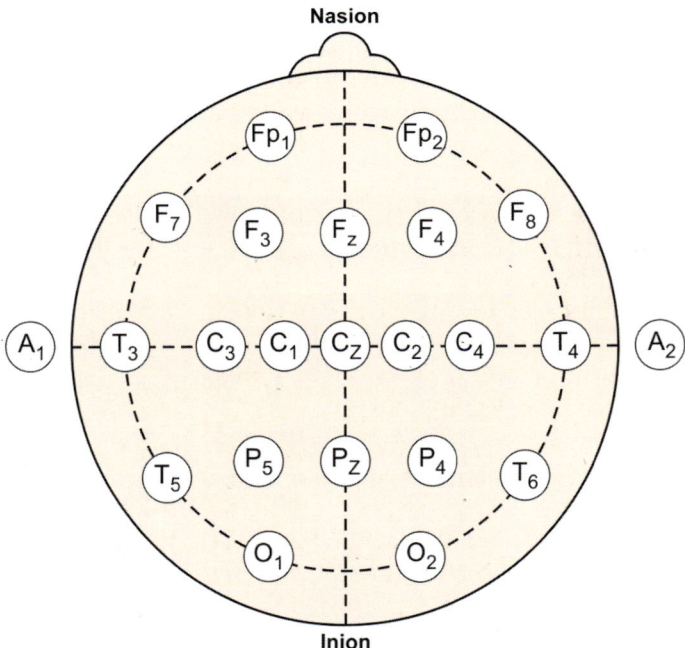

**Fig. 11.5:** International standard 10–20 system of electrode placement for NIOM. For eliciting MEP by trans cranial stimulation, needles are typically inserted in C1–C2 or C3–C4 positions

- When evaluation MEPs, it is important to distinguish evoked potentials from spontaneous muscle action potentials.
- A 50% reduction in D-wave amplitude indicates a permanent deficit, whereas <50% reduction in amplitude may suggest a transient motor deficit that will recover with time.

## Temperature Monitoring and Thermoregulation during Vascular Surgery

Core temperature monitoring is essential during most vascular surgery under general anesthesia as they involve invasion and exposure of body cavity and hence more heat loss. Temperature monitoring facilitates detection and quantification of hypothermia or hyperthermia. Intraoperative hyperthermia is more common than 'malignant hyperthermia (especially in this part of the world) and causes include excessive warming, infectious fever, bleeding inside the fourth ventricle and mismatched blood transfusion. All said and done, by far most common perioperative thermal disturbance is inadvertent hypothermia. As such, the core temperature decreases 0.5 to 1.5°C within half an hour of induction of general anesthesia due to factors such as obtundation of normal thermoregulatory response caused by the anesthetic agents as well as the ambient temperature. Operating room temperature is the most critical factor influencing heat loss because it determines the rate at which metabolic heat is lost by radiation and convection from the skin and by evaporation from the surgical incision and exposed visceras.

*Thermometers:* There are principally three types of thermometers available: (1) Temperature measurement based upon expansion of material as its temperature increases (e.g. mercury-in-glass thermometers). Mercury is liquid form of a metal (at room temperature) with high specific heat, whose expansion can be calibrated as the metal increases in volume at constant pressure depending on the changes in temperature. Mercury thermometers have two disadvantages of clinical significance; first, they require 2 to 3 minutes for thermal equilibration and second, the mercury enclosed in glass tubes may break and can be injurious. Therefore, mercury thermometers are universally replaced with electronic systems. (2) Electric technique of measuring temperature variation can be subdivided into: (a) **Resistance thermometers** (e.g. platinum wire resistor) works on the principle that resistance to electric current increases with increase in temperature which can be calibrated to temperature. (b) **Thermistor** is a semi-conductor with opposite behavior, because resistance decreases as the temperature increases. Most thermometers used in anesthesia practice from esophageal probes to one used in PA catheter tips are thermistors. (c) **Thremocouples** are conductors that generate voltage in response to changes in temperature. (3) **Thermopiles** are devices that convert infrared emissions from any object into temperature (e.g. tympanic membrane temperature monitor used in recovery room, pediatric wards, etc.). The infrared detectors produces electric signal that is proportional to the fourth power of the difference in absolute temperature (in Kelvin) of the object. This thermometer is fraught with lack of calibration, improper placement as the probe is too bulky to be used in the operation theaters and hence error prone.

*Temperature monitoring sites:* The core thermal compartment is composed of highly perfused tissues whose temperature is uniform and high compared to the rest of the body. Temperature in this compartment can be monitored in the PA, distal esophagus, nasopharynx and tympanic membrane. During cardiopulmonary bypass, core temperature monitoring site remains valid even during deliberate cooling and re-warming. Rectal temperature also correlates well with the core temperature changes but it lags behind in absolute terms. Skin surface temperature is lower than core temperature and is affected by peripheral vasoconstrictions.

Guidelines for temperature monitoring:[9]

i. Core temperature should be monitored in most surgical patients who are given GA for longer than 30 minutes.

ii. Core temperature should be measured during regional anesthesia also when changes in body temperature are intended, anticipated or suspected.

iii. Effort should be made to maintain intraoperative core temperature above 36° C (unless therapeutic hypothermia is planned for protection against ischemia and consequent injury). In thoracic aortic surgery, deep hypothermic (usually around 18°C) circulatory arrest may be required to operate upon the arch vessels. While rewarming gradually, a core temperature to the heat exchanger gradient should not exceed 10° C. Moreover, current guidelines advise to avoid cerebral hyperthermia (nasopharyngeal temperature not to exceed 37.5° C). Sometimes retrograde cerebral perfusion (RCP) is performed by infusing cold oxygenated blood into the SVC at temperatures of 8–14°C through CPB pump with a flow rate of 200–600 ml/min. The potential benefits of RCP include supply of metabolic substrate, embolic washout and maintenance of cerebral hypothermia. All the above examples testify the importance of core temperature monitoring in safe conduct of thoracic aortic surgery under GA.

## Point of Care Testing for Coagulation Monitoring

Patient with cardiovascular disease can have array of hemostatic disorders that predispose them to develop many hemorrhagic and thromboembolic diseases. Those patients, who undergo vascular procedures, invariably receive anticoagulant for technical reasons. A sizable number of such procedures conducted under cardio-pulmonary bypass and hypothermic circulatory arrest may also induce coagulation disturbances. Therefore, it becomes imperative on our part to quantify and monitor the extent of such hemostatic derangement and offer appropriate therapy based on results of such laboratory testing. Because rapidity of obtaining result matters a lot when a patient is fast exsanguinating, the entire laboratory facilities are available bedside in the modern era, and this is the philosophy behind popularity of point of care (POC) testing. The majority of POC devices today can perform multiple coagulation tests.

## Heparin Monitoring

*Activated clotting time (ACT):* The ACT is the most frequently used POC test for measuring heparin anticoagulation and it is ubiquitous in cardiac surgical theaters. The modern ACT system is a modification of Lee-White method of measuring clotting time following systemic heparinization. In this method, blood sample used to be mixed with an activator (viz, celite, kaolin, glass beads or a combination of these) in a glass test tube and the tube with a stopper used to be tilted back and forth manually until clot was formed and the time noted. Currently the two most commonly available automated systems are Hemotech (Medtronic, MN) and Haemocron (International technidyne corp., USA). The former uses a pair of plastic cuvettes (called cartridges) containing kaolin (along with calcium-chloride, sodium azide and HEPES buffer) as activator and a 'flag like' plunger pegged at the bottom of each cartridge. Blood (0.4 ml) is introduced into each cartridge and an actuator lifts the plunger up and down repeatedly. This continues till the rate of descent is slowed by the formation of clot and the decrease in velocity of the plun ger is detected by a photo-optical syst em that terminates the test and notes the time (sec) from initiation to end of test. The average of the two individual tests is also displayed on the front panel of the device. The potential limitation of the test is that the cartridge has to be pre-heated to $37 \pm 0.50°$ C. Also, it cannot estimate the heparin concentration during CPB especially during hypothermia and/or hemodilution. Other factors altering ACT values includes thrombo-cytopenia, presence of platelet inhibitors, GPIIb/IIIa and use of anti-fibrinolytic like aprotinin (only with Celite). Blood loss and transfusion requirement after CPB can be reduced with accurate control of heparin reversal guided by ACT POC test.

*Cascade system:* This POC test is a variant of ACT and it utilizes disposabie cards with celite activator to measure heparin activity. It is also known as heparin management test (HMT). The card contains para-magnetic iron oxide particle that migrates in response to an oscillating magnetic field. When clot is formed, movement of these particles is decreased. This test is capable of measuring PT and aPTT with specific activators like rabbit brain thromboplastin and magnesium aluminum silicate activators respectively. The blood moves by capi llary action and mixes with paramagnetic particles and the reagent. The decreased movement of the particles is detected optically as the samples clot and the result is displayed as time (sec) and as international normalised ratio (INR) as well for PT. HMT correlates well with anti-Xa heparin activity in CPB and is less variable than standard ACT.

## Viscoelastic Test for Clot Formation

*Thromboelastography:* The Thromboelastography (TEG) is a test for the visco-elastic properties of blood and this technology was developed as early as 1948. It examines the time taken for initiation, acceleration through clot control and lysis of fibrin clot. A small amount (0.35 ml) of blood is placed in an oscillating cuvette and a piston is lowered into the blood sample. As the blood begins to clot, the elastic forces exerted on the piston are translated to a signature tracing. These tracings are popularly known as a thromboelastogram. Currently, an activator (celite, kaolin, tissue factor, etc.) are used to accelerate the process of clot formation so that the test becomes more meaningful for POC settings. Every thromboelastogram reveals information regarding fibrin formation, fibrin-platelet interactions, platelet clot strength and fibrin lysis. There are five parameters in the tracings (viz. R, K, $\alpha$ angle, maximum amplitude or MA and MA60) that give all the above information. The normal values vary depending on the activator used. TEG can be used to predict postoperative bleeding in cardiac surgery and appropriate therapy initiated (Table 11.4). A limitation of TEG is its inability to document platelet dysfunction induced by antiplatelet agents. Also, it is extremely sensitive to vibration and external shock. The development of platelet mapping assay has overcome this disadvantage of TEG.

*Platelet mapping assay:* This technological development tries to overcome the shortcomings of the TEG and it allows measurement of platelet function in patients on antiplatelet therapy. Platelet mapping utilizes three

**Table 11.4:** Theranostic potentials of TEG (From Royston and von Kier)

| TEG variables | Implications | Therapy |
|---|---|---|
| R >14 and <21 mm | ↓ Clotting factors | One fresh frozen plasma |
| R >21 and <28 mm | ↓↓ Clotting factors | Two fresh frozen plasma |
| R >28 mm | ↓↓↓ Clotting factors | Four fresh frozen plasma |
| MA < 48 mm | ↓↓ Platelet number/function | One pooled platelet |
| MA < 40 mm | ↓↓↓ Platelet number/function | Two pooled platelet |
| Lys 30 >7.5% | Increased lysis | Aprotinin |

cuvettes. One incorporates thrombin to activate platelets and overrides the inhibition of other activation pathways such as arachidonic acid, ADP and GPIIb/IIIa. A second cuvette contains reptilase and factor XIII to create a fibrinogen clot or 'thrombin-less' clot which is weaker in strength. The third cuvette incorporates the fibrinogen clot and ADP (clopidogrel) or arachidonic acid (aspirin) is added back to stimulate the platelets. If the MA is increased in response to clopidogrel/aspirin, it indicates drug induced platelet inhibition via the respective pathway.

*Rotational thromboelastometry:* The rotational thromboelastometry (ROTEM) is another POC test to measure the viscoelastic property of blood. A small quantity of whole blood (0.3 ml) is added along with an activator to a disposable cuvette, which is placed in a temperature controlled cuvette holder. A disposable pin (sensor) fitted over a rotating shaft is lowered into the sample. A small mirror attached to the shaft reflects away an incident light. A detector records the rotation over time and this rotation is translated into a graph called thromboelastogram. The primary parameter is **CT**, which calculates time (sec) elapsed from beginning of the reaction to a 2 mm increase in amplitude. This represents initiation of clotting, thrombin formation and beginning of clot polymerization. **Clot formation time** (CFT) is represented by time required for further increase in amplitude to 20 mm. This implies fibrin polymerization and clot stabilisation with platelet and factor XIII. **Maximum clot firmness** (MCF) is proportional to the maximum amplitude (MA) attained, which correlates with fibrinogen concentration platelet count and function. **Maximum lysis** (ML) is the ratio of lowest amplitude (ohm) after MCF to that of MCF and it is a measure of fibrinolysis. The Alpha (α) angle as in TEG is the angle formed by a tangent to the ROTEM curve through the 2 mm point and the meaning is same as that of CFT, i.e. clot growth kinetics.

*Sonoclot:* The sonoclot analyser provides accurate information about the entire hemostasis process including fibrin gel formation, clot retraction (platelet function), fibrinolysis and other coagulation factors. This device consists of a probe that oscillates up and down in side the blood sample. The viscous force of the blood creates impedance to ultrasonic vibrating probe as it clots. This is converted into electronic output signal. Post-signal processing this is reported as the 'clot signal' or sonoclot signature. The sonoclot signature is the plotted values of clot function over time. The quantitative results include a lag period (called SonoACT), which corresponds to the activated clotting time (ACT), and a second peak that occurs as a result of cross-linkage of fibrin (clot rate).

*Impact cone platelet analyzer (CPA):* In this POC test, whole blood is subjected to uniform shear by a spinning cone. This allows for platelet function testing under condition akin to natural blood flow kinetics. Platelet adhesion to cone surface after automated staining is examined by image analyzing software. The ability of CPA in screening primary haemostatic abnormality and platelet response to aspirin, clopidogrel and other GPIIb/IIIa antagonist has been successfully demonstrated. Experience with CPA is currently limited as it is a relatively new technology. However, recent studies suggest that CPA has potential to detect perioperative platelet dysfunction and predict postoperative blood loss.

### POC Platelet Function Tests

*Platelet function analyser (PFA-l00):* It is a modified quantitative in vitro bleeding time estimator under artificially created high shear stress conditions. Whole blood is placed on a test cartridge and vacuum perfuses blood across a collagen-coated membrane. The shear force on whole blood activates platelet and promotes platelets adherence and aggregation. A punch whole is made on the membrane in the presence of either epinephrine or ADP as agonist. The time it takes for a clot to form in side the cartridge and prevent further blood flow is measured as closure time. It depends on platelet GPIb and GPIIb/IIIa, von Willebrand factor, platelet count and haematocrit. The response to epinephrine can detect aspirin-induced platelet dysfunction. Both channels (epinephrine and ADP) accurately detect platelet dysfunction in von Willebrand's disease.

*Varify now:* This POC test is a turbidimetric-based optical detection system that measures agonist induced agglutination of whole blood. The activated GPIIb/IIIa receptors on the platelets bind to adjacent platelets via fibrinogen beads supplied in the mixing chamber and cause agglutination of blood and the beads. Light transmittance in the chamber is measured, and which increases as agglutination increases similar to platelet aggregometry (gold standard). Aspirin and clopidogrel drug effects can be measured using appropriate 'VarifyNow' cartridges.

*Platelet works:* Platelet works (Helena laboratoeies, Baeumont, Texas) is a whole-blood assay that uses the principle of platelet count ratio to assess platelet reactivity. This instrument is a coulter counter that compares platelet counts in a standard EDTA tube versus a citrated tube after aggregation either with ADP or collagen. When blood is added to these agonist tubes, platelets get activated; they adhere to the tube and are effectively eliminated from the count. The ratio of activated to the non-activated platelet count is an indicator of the reactivity of the platelets. Platelet works is capable of measuring platelet dysfunction that accompanies cardiopulmonary bypass. Platelet function can be assessed in the static phase, dynamic phase and as a response to anagonist. Static function tests such as mean platelet volume are not very useful information as they capture function at a single point in time. Dynamic tests like viscoelastic tests and the response to a platelet agonist are more reflective of platelet function over time and are more useful for assessing drug induced platelet dysfunction.

## Conclusion

There are wide varieties of cardiovascular monitoring devices available these days. One need to choose the appropriate method that is best suited for the individual hospital settings. While choosing them one needs to keep in mind that they have to be compliant with the existing technology as well. One of the important physiological parameters which keep a vigil on physiologic homeostasis during vascular surgery, are temperature regulation and body fluids homeostasis with the help of temperature and urine output and cardiac filling pressure monitors. Point of care tests are available nowadays for blood gases, blood coagulation pathways as well as hematology parameters, which are very important for decision making while managing patients undergoing vascular surgery. Lastly, it is also very important to understand 'economics' of individual monitors and the maximal data interpretation and inference derived out of them for better management of these subset of patient population.

## REFERENCES

1. Landesberg G, Mosseri M, Wolf Y, Veselov Y, Weissman C. Perioperative myocardial ischemia and infarction: Identification by continuous 12 lead with online ST-segment monitoring. Anesthesiology 2002, 96:264–70.

2. London MJ. Multilead precordial ST-segment monitoring: "The next generation?" Anesthesiology 2002;96(2):259–61.

3. Mangano DT, Hickey RF. Ischemic injury following uncomplicated radial artery catheterization. Anesthesia analgrsia 1979;58:55–57.

4. Brown RW, Foster E, Jensen GA, et al. Safety of brachial artery catheters as monitors in the intensive care unit-prospective evaluation with the Doppler ultrasonic velocity detector. Anesthesiology 1976;44:260.

5. Kastler A, Chabbane R, Azamoush K, Cosserant B, et al. Arterial injury complicating subclavian central venous catheter insertion. J Cardiothorac Vasc Anesth 2012;26: 101–3.

6. Choudhury A, Agarwal A, Dhiraaj S. An unusual case of guidewire impaction during internal jugular venous cannulation. Anesth Analg 2005;100:1217–18.

7. Hogue CW, Rosenbloom M, McCawley C, Lappas DG. Comparison of cardiac output measurement by continuous thermodilution with electromagnetometry in adult cardiac surgical patients. J Cardiothorac Vasc Anesth 1994;8:631.

8. Husain AM, Ashton KH, et al. Thoracic aortic surgery: A practical approach to neurophysiologic intraoperative monitoring, (Ed.) Husain AM, New York, Demos 2008, pp. 227–59.

9. Sessler DI. Temperature monitoring in Miller's Anesthesia Miller RD (Ed), 8th edn. Saunders, Philadelphia, 2009, pp. 1533–56.

10. Hiratzka LF, Bakris GL, Beckman JA, et al. ACC/AHA/AATA/ACRA/ASA/SCA/SIR/STS/SVM Guidelines for the diagnosis and management of patients with thoracic aortic disease: Executive summary. A report of the ACC foundation, AHA task force on practice guidelines, American association of Thoracic surgery, American college of radiology, American stroke association, Society of Cardiovascular Anesthesiologists, Society for cardiovascular angiography and intervention and Society for vascular medicine. JAAC 2010;55:1509–1544.

11. Royston D, von Kier S. Reduced hemostatic factor transfusion using heparinase-modified thromboelastography during cardiopulmonary bypass. BV. J Anaesth 2001;86:575–8.

# CHAPTER 12

# Transesophageal Echocardiography for Aortic Surgery

Neeti Makhija

## INTRODUCTION

In the present era an increasing number of patients are being benefited by surgery on thoracic aorta due to better diagnostic modalities. Combination of echocardiography, angiography, computed tomography (CT), and magnetic resonance imaging (MRI) studies have helped in the diagnosis, timing the surgical repair, the type of surgical repair, risk evaluation, and as well as post-repair evaluation.

Previously, angiography was considered as the gold standard for diagnosing the aortic pathologies. But presently, multidetector computed tomography (MDCT) scans have become gold standard. The advantage of computed tomography (CT) is not only quick and easy access but other pathologies in the chest can also be diagnosed; and in case of polytrauma, a whole body CT can be done simultaneously. The CT has a high sensitivity of 83 to 100%, with a specificity as high as 100% for diagnosing dissection of aorta. But CT does not provide information about aortic regurgitation (AR). The MRI for aortic pathology has an advantage over CT, as there is lack of radiation and avoidance of contrast agents. But the procedure interferes with pacemakers, aneurismal clip, orthopedic hardware, is time consuming and not feasible in emergency and hemodynamically unstable patients. Echocardiography has an important role in urgent situations. Transesophageal echocardiography (TEE) has the advantage over transthoracic echocardiography (TTE), for assessment of thoracic aorta, because thoracic aorta being in close proximity to the oesophagus permits high resolution images. Not only in diagnosis but TEE has extensive role intra-operatively in decision making regarding aortic cannulation site, decision as to extent of repair required,

guide wire positioning for cannulaion and stent placement. Also, TEE is helpful intraoperatively in the post-repair assessment. At the very outset, it is essential to understand the anatomy of thoracic aorta.

## ANATOMY OF THORACIC AORTA

Aorta is the largest artery carrying oxygenated blood from the left ventricle of the heart to all parts of the body. Aorta begins at the left ventricular-aortic valve junction just to the right of the midline. Thereafter, it initially ascends superiorly and anteriorly, arches to the left in posterior direction with cephaloid convexity. Thereafter, it descends just distal to origin of left subclavian artery (LSCA) and is named as descending thoracic aorta (DTA). At the level of 4th thoracic vertebra, it courses slightly anterior and to the right towards the diaphragm. It thus traverses the thorax, then through the diaphragm into the abdomen; it thereafter continues as abdominal aorta, gives off branches and finally bifurcates into the two iliac arteries (Fig. 12.1).

The thoracic aorta can be divided into segments namely the ascending aorta comprising of aortic root and the ascending tubular part, the aortic arch and the descending thoracic aorta. Segment of aorta from the annulus of the aortic valve up to the origin of innominate artery is called the ascending aorta. The origin of the innominate artery marks the beginning of the aortic arch. The aortic arch is the segment of the aorta between the innominate artery and the left subclavian artery, beyond which is the descending thoracic aorta (Fig. 12.1).

The beginning of the aorta is from aortic root. The aortic root comprises of aortic valve annulus, aortic cusps or leaflets, sinuses of Valsalva (sinus segment) and up to the sinotubular junction. The fibrous basal ring at

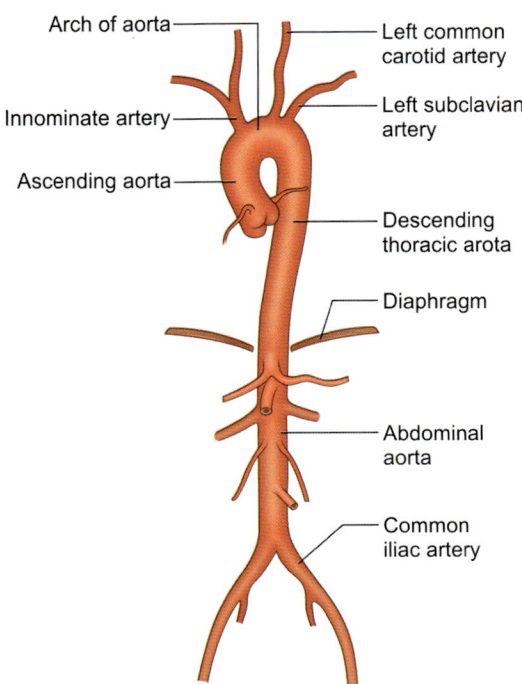

**Fig. 12.1:** Anatomy of the aorta along with its major branches

the junction of the aortic root and the left ventricle is called the aortic annulus. The annulus is not necessarily circular and may be oval or elliptical in shape. The normal aortic valve has three semilunar shaped cusps. The base of each cusp is attached to the annulus. The free margins of the cusps join its base at the point called commissure. The three aortic valve cusps lie along the three corresponding sinuses of Valsalva. These are the out pouching or dilatation on the wall of aorta. These are named as left cusp and sinus, right cusp and sinus and non-coronary cusp and sinus. The left main

coronary artery arises from the left aortic sinus and the right coronary artery from the right coronary sinus. The sinuses form the weakest segment of the aorta (Fig. 12.2). The sinotubular segment is the junction where sinus segment joins the tubular part of the ascending aorta.

The tubular part of ascending aorta begins from the sinotubular junction, travels cephalad and extends up to the origin of innominate or brachiocephalic artery.

The aortic arch or transverse aorta begins at the origin of innominate artery and normally takes a leftward and a backward curve. It travels horizontally and extends till the origin of left subclavian artery. The aortic arch thus contains the origins of innominate, left common carotid and the left subclavian artery. The most common variation among arch vessels is the presence of bovine arch in about 20% of individuals.[1] Bovine arch is defined as the common origin of innominate and the left common carotid artery.

The descending thoracic aorta (DTA) begins at the beginning of the left subclavian artery and ends at diaphragm where it becomes abdominal aorta. Just distal to origin of left subclavian artery is aortic isthmus at the site of ligamentum arteriosus. Aortic isthmus is common site of aortic coarctation, patent ductus arteriosus and traumatic aortic injury.

The DTA gives off paired intercostals arteries. The celiac trunk, superior mesenteric artery, renal artery and lumber segmental arteries arise from abdominal aorta. The abdominal aorta bifurcates into two common iliac arteries.

From the surgical and echocardiography point of view the thoracic aorta is divided into the six zones.[2] First three zones within the ascending aorta, zones 4

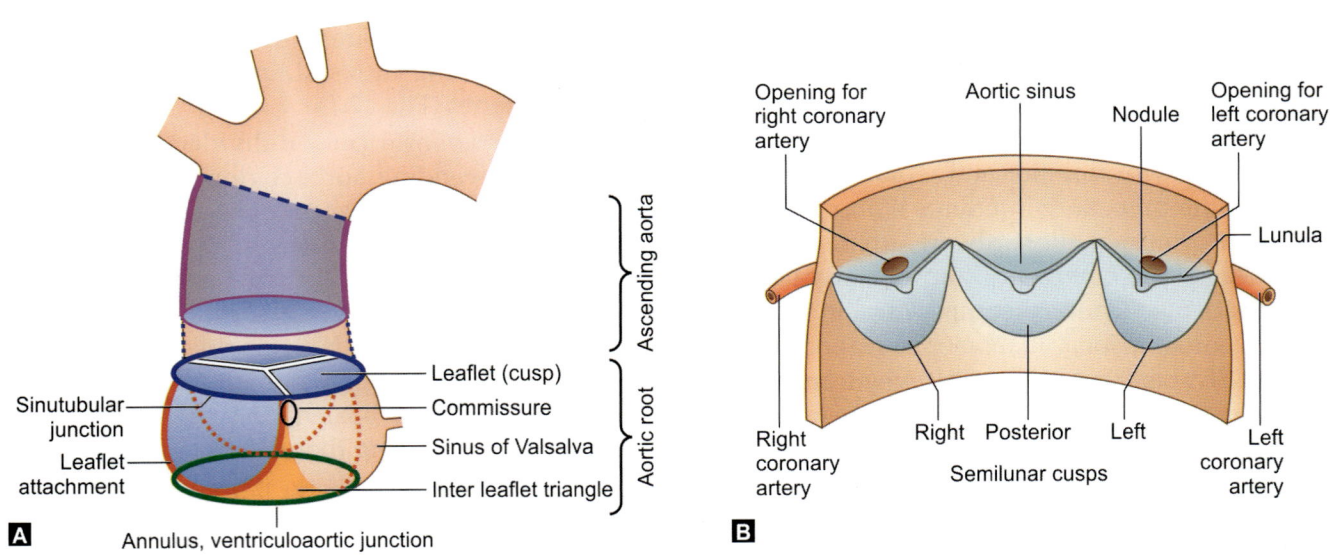

**Figs 12.2A and B:** (A) Anatomy of the aortic root, (B) cut section of aortic root showing the three cusps of aortic valve

and 5 within the arch and zone 6 corresponding to the descending aorta. Zone 1 is closest to the aortic root, zone 2 corresponding to the site for proximal anastomosis of coronary graft and zone 3 being the site for aortic cross clamping during cardiopulmonary bypass (CPB). Zone 4 is the proximal arch and zone 5 corresponding to the distal half of the arch. The aortic cannula is placed in the distal region of zone 3 and proximal region of zone 4 (Fig. 12.3).

Thus from the point of view of TEE assessment it is important to note the position of aorta in relation to esophagus as our probe lies in the esophagus. The ascending aorta initially lies directly anterior to the esophagus, but as it ascends it comes slightly to right of the esophagus. The arch is immediately anterior to the esophagus. The upper descending thoracic aorta is anterior and to the left of esophagus, the mid DTA is just lateral and the lower DTA is although posterior to the esophagus is slightly on the left side. The aorta below the diaphragm is immediately posterior to the

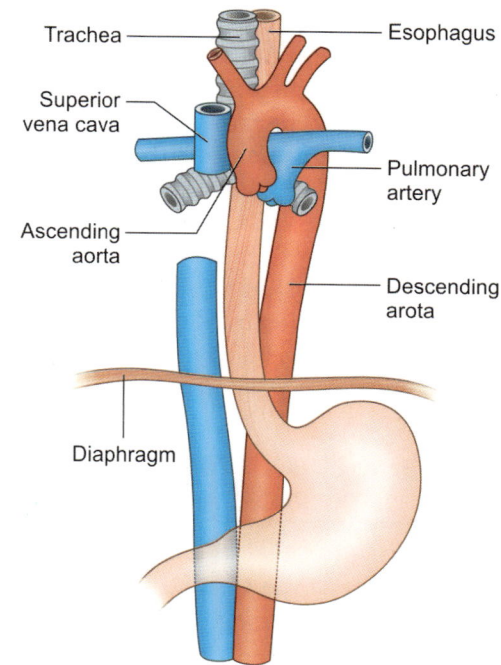

**Fig. 12.4:** Anatomic relationship between thoracic aorta and esophagus: The ascending aorta, arch and descending thoracic aorta (DTA) near the arch are anterior to esophagus. DTA is lateral to esophagus in mid thorax and posterior to esophagus at diapragmatic hiatus

esophagus. The right pulmonary artery courses between the esophagus and the ascending aorta (Fig. 12.4). So, accordingly the echocardiographer should orient the probe for the assessment of aorta (Fig. 12.4).

## NORMAL DIMENSIONS OF AORTA

Before proceeding for echocardiographic assessment and interpretation it would be worthwhile to have knowledge of normal dimensions as well as norms set up for dimensions measurements. The normal values of the aortic segment dimensions vary with the age, gender and body size.[3-5] The aortic diameter increases with age, and are larger for men than women (Table 12.1). But when the aortic root diameter is indexed to the body

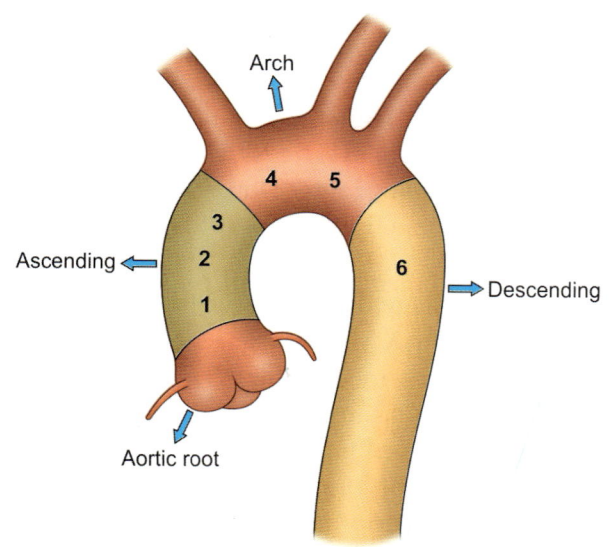

**Fig. 12.3:** Basic anatomy of thoracic aorta showing division into six zones for the purpose of TEE evaluation

| Table 12.1: Normal adults throacic aortic dimensions[4-5] | | | |
|---|---|---|---|
| Aortic Segment | Men: Mean ± SD (cm) | Women: Mean ± SD (cm) | Imaging Technique |
| Aortic valve annulus | 2.6 ± 0.3 | 2.3 ± 0.2 | Echo |
| Sinuses of Valsalva | 3.4 ± 0.3 | 3.0 ± 0.3 | Echo |
| Sinotubular Junction | 2.9 ± 0.3 | 2.6 ± 0.3 | Echo |
| Proximal ascending aorta | 3.0 ± 0.4 | 2.7 ± 0.4 | Echo |
| Mid-descending aorta | 2.7 ± 0.3 | 2.5 ± 0.3 | CT |
| Distal descending aorta | 2.6 ± 0.3 | 2.4 ± 0.3 | CT |

CT—computed tomography; Echo—echocardiography; SD—standard deviation surface area, the influence of sex is neutralized. The aortic diameter is largest at the mid sinus segment of the aortic root, and thereafter it tapers gradually beyond sinotubular junction. As per recent guidelines, echocardiographic measurement should be from intima to intima and perpendicular to the axis of blood flow (Class I Recommendation, Level C Evidence).[3] The aortic dimensions measured by CT are adventitia to adventitia at perpendicular axis to blood flow. Thus CT dimensions are larger than the echocardiographic dimensions. Normally, in the ascending aorta, diameter is largest at the sinus level (Table 12.1).

## TRANSESOPHAGEAL ECHOCARDIOGRAPHY (TEE) IMAGING OF THORACIC AORTA

Almost the entire thoracic aorta can be imaged by multiplane TEE except the distal ascending aorta and the proximal arch[6] as here trachea and the left main stem bronchus intervene between the oesophagus and the aorta.

A stepwise systematic assessment of thoracic aorta includes firstly, the assessment of aortic root in the mid-esophageal aortic valve short axis view (ME AV SAX view) and mid esophageal aortic valve long axis view (ME AV LAX view). This is followed by assessment of ascending aorta in mid-esophageal ascending aorta long axis view (ME ascending aorta LAX view), and mid-esophageal ascending aorta short axis view (ME ascending aorta SAX view); the descending aorta in descending aorta short-axis view (descending aorta SAX view) and descending aorta long-axis view (descending aorta LAX view); and lastly the aortic arch in upper oesophageal aortic arch long-axis view (UE aortic arch LAX view) and upper esophageal aortic arch short axis view (UE aortic arch SAX view).[7–9]

### Assessment of Aortic Root

The aortic root assessment should be done in **mid-esophageal aortic valve short axis view 40 degree (ME AV SAX view)** (Fig. 12.5). In this view, the aortic valve cusps are identified. A normal aortic valve is a trileaflet valve with left coronary cusp imaged posteriorly (in near field) and to the right of display. The noncoronary cusp will be on the left of display and adjacent to interatrial septum. The right coronary cusp is on the anterior (far field) adjacent to right ventricular outflow tract (RVOT). The aortic valve should be assessed for the presence of any congenital anomaly like bicuspid aortic valve, the

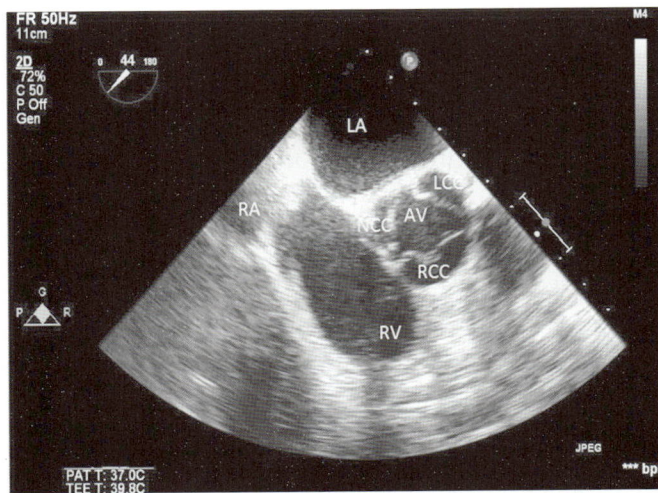

**Fig. 12.5:** Midesophageal (ME) aortic valve short-axis view showing tricuspid AV. AV: Aortic valve, LCC: Left coronary cusp, RCC: Right coronary cusp NCC: Noncoronary cusp, LA: Left atrium, RA: Right atrium, RV: Right ventricle

mobility, calcification and for any dissection flap. Measurement of valve area can be done by planimetry of the area between the leaflets during systole. Thereafter, assessment of regurgitation in relation to any of the cusps can be done with colour flow Doppler. Further, assessment of the origin of right and left coronary arteries is performed. The TEE probe is slightly withdrawn with colour flow Doppler to assess for the early bifurcation or dissection flap if any into the left coronary artery.

**The mid esophageal aortic valve long axis view 120 degree (ME AV LAX View)** (Fig. 12.6) is useful for the measurement of diameter of left ventricular outflow tract (LVOT), aortic annulus, aortic root, the sinotubular junction and the ascending aorta. The aortic cusps can be analysed. The right coronary cusp is placed anteriorly (far field). The posterior cusp in the near field can be either noncoronary cusp or the left coronary cusp depending on the imaging window. The aortic valve cusps should be assessed for the mobility and calcification. With the colour Doppler the aortic valve can be assessed for the severity of regurgitation and flow to the right coronary ostium.

The aortic annular diameter may be measured in diastole between hinge points of aortic valve leaflets (inner edge to inner edge) in the ME AV LAX View that reveals largest aortic annular diameter.[5] But for valve sizing prior to transcatheter and surgical valve replacement the measurement should be made during systole.[10, 11]

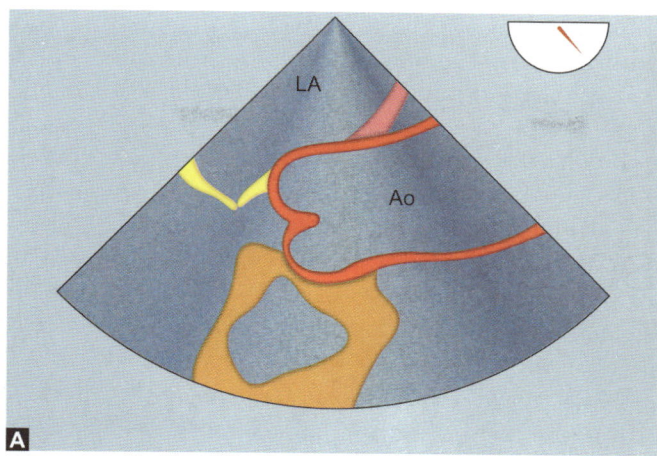
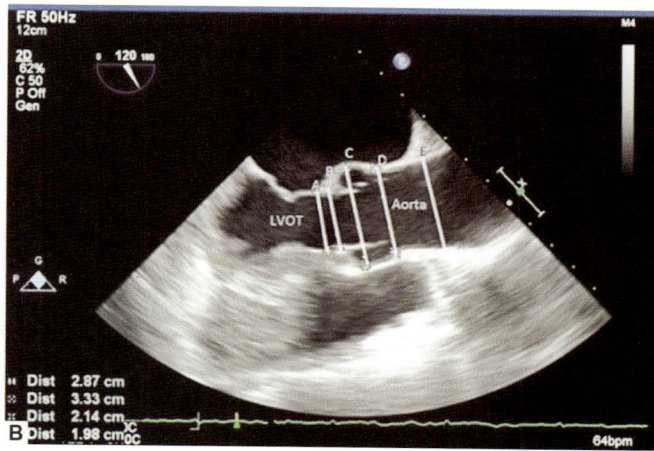

**Figs 12.6A and B:** Midesophageal (ME) aortic valve long-axis view showing aortic root in cross-section and is ideal for quantifying diameters of (A) left ventricular outflow tract (LVOT), (B) aortic valve annulus. C: Aortic root, D: Sinotubular junction, E: Tubular part of ascending aorta, Ao: Aorta, LA: Left atrium

## Assessment of Ascending Aorta

**The ME ascending aorta LAX view** (Fig. 12.7) is obtained by the slight withdrawal of the probe from ME AV LAX view (120°–140°) along with the backward rotation of the probe to approximately 90° to 110°. The view allows the assessment of the proximal ascending aorta. The right pulmonary artery is seen in short axis posterior to the ascending aorta. In this view evaluation of ascending aortic diameter, aortic wall for signs of aortic atheroma, calcification and dissection can be done. It is to be noted that only the proximal ascending aorta is visualized and the distal ascending aorta and the proximal aortic arch lies in the blind spot of TEE.[6] **The ME ascending aorta SAX view** (Fig. 12.8) can be visualized by further backward rotation of the probe to

approximately 0° to 30°. Alternately this view can be obtained by slight withdrawal and antiflexion of probe from ME AV SAX view. In this view ascending aorta is visualized in the short axis. The diameter of ascending aorta can be determined. In addition superior vena cava (SVC) can also be visualized in short axis. The main pulmonary artery (on right display) and the right lobar pulmonary artery (near field) can be seen.

## Assessment of Descending Aorta

The examination of the descending aorta can begin after obtaining transgastric mid-papillary short-axis view of the ventricle and turning the probe to the left until the descending aorta is seen in the short-axis between 0° and 10° rotation as circular image. This is the **descending aorta SAX view** (Fig. 12.9). This view enables to measure

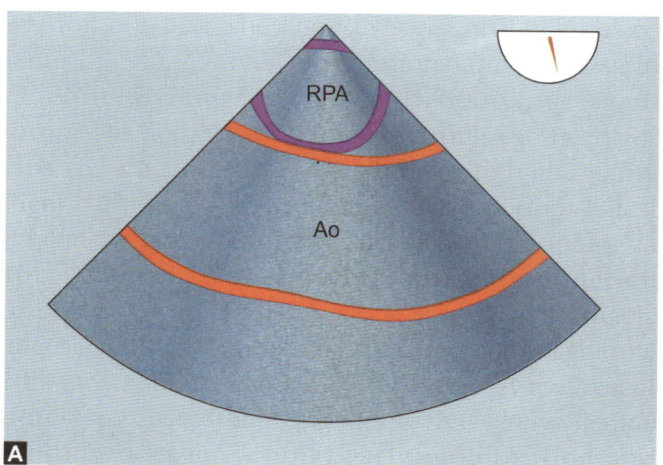
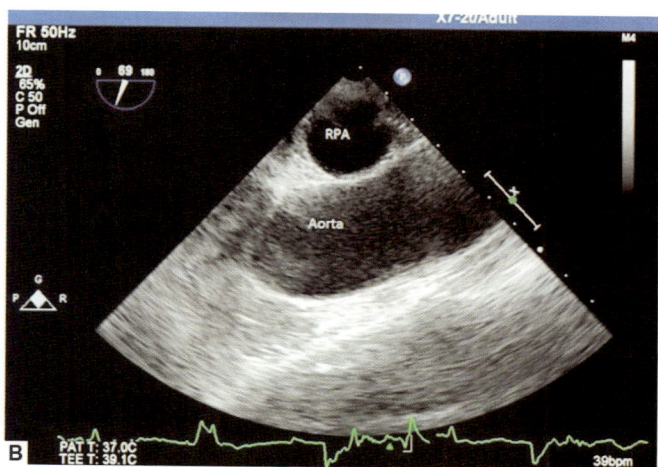

**Figs 12.7A and B:** Midesophageal (ME) ascending aortic long-axis view at multiplane angle of 69°. The view facilitates assessment of ascending aorta at level of right pulmonary artery with regard of dimensions, dissection, aneurysm, atheroma, calcification, and rupture. Ao: Aorta; RPA: Right pulmonary artery

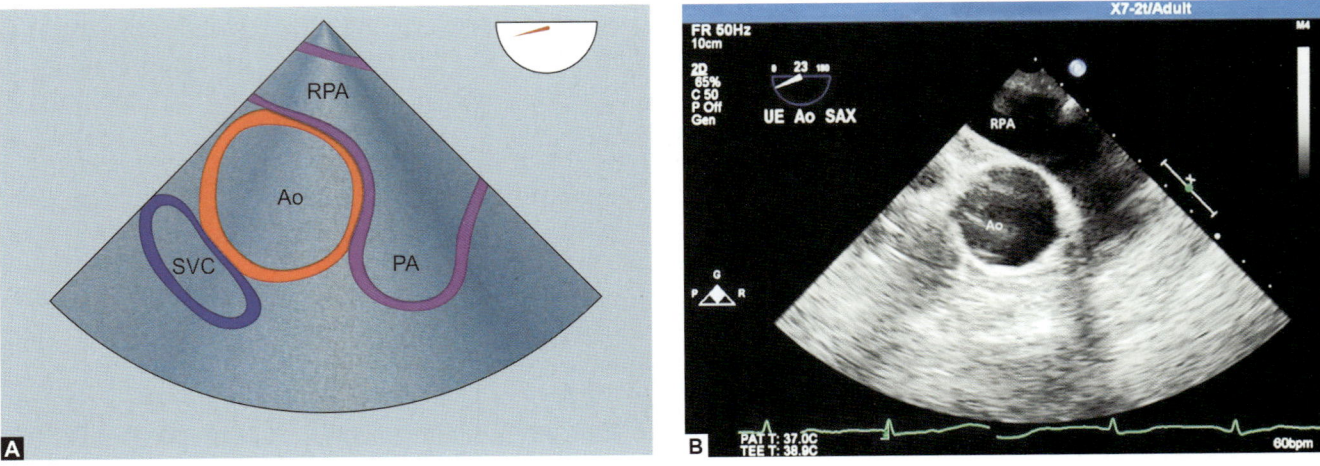

**Figs 12.8A and B:** Midesophageal (ME) ascending aortic short-axis view with a multiplane angle at 23°. Ascending aortic diameter at level of RPA can be measured; and assessment for dissection and aneurysm can be done. Ao: Aorta, PA: Pulmonary artery, RPA: Right pulmonary artery, SVC: Superior vena cava

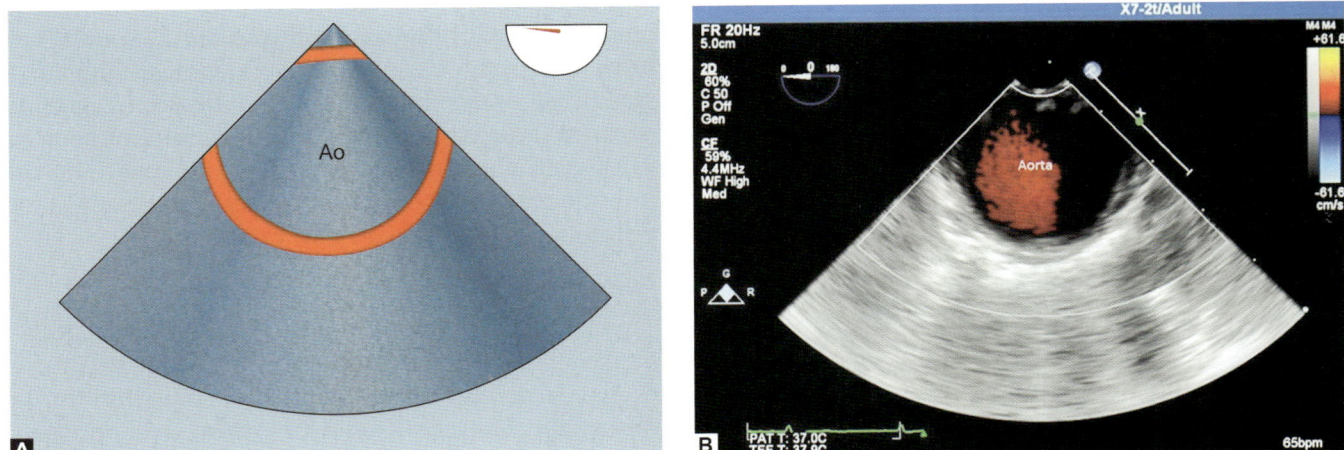

**Figs 12.9A and B:** Midesophageal (ME) descending aortic short-axis view at a multiplane angle of 0. Descending aortic diameter can be measured and entire length of aorta can be evaluated for dissection and aneurysm by manipulating TEE probe. Ao: Aorta

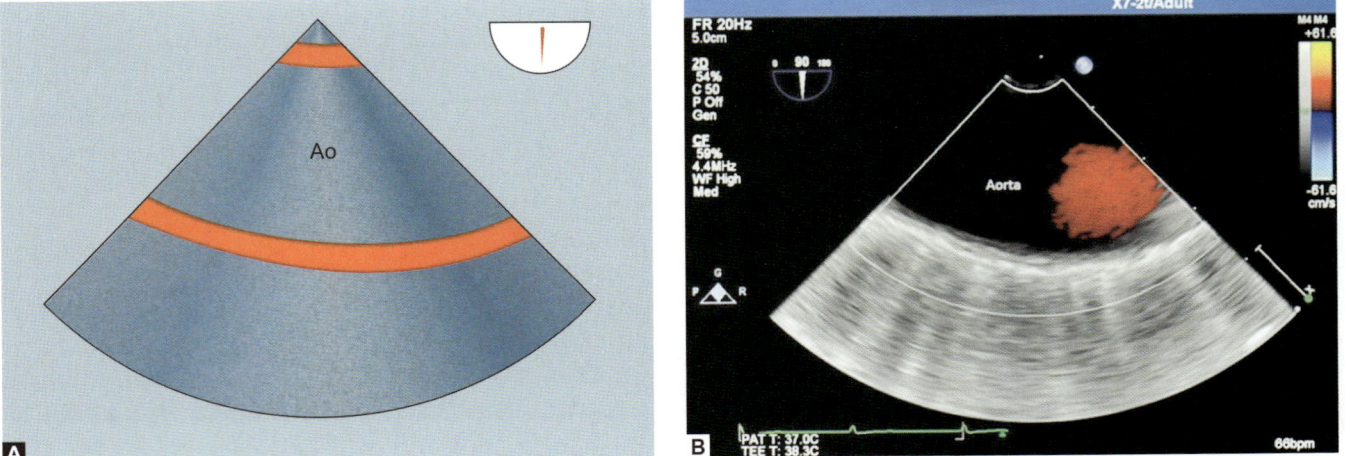

**Figs 12.10A and B:** Midesophageal (ME) descending aortic long-axis view at a multiplane angle of 90. Detailed evaluation for any dissection, aneurysm, atheroma can be done. Ao:Aorta

dimensions of DTA; and in assessment for aneurysm, dissection, atherosclerosis and pleural effusion. From the descending aorta SAX view the **descending aorta LAX view** (Fig. 12.10) can be obtained at angle rotation between 90° and 100°. The image depth is decreased between 6 and 8 to enlarge the image. Focus is moved to the near field. To optimize the image of aorta in the near field gain should be adjusted. To image the entire descending aorta the probe is advanced and withdrawn. It is to be noted that as lower descending thoracic aorta (DTA) is located posterior and to the left of oesophagus, the TEE probe should face the left thoracic cavity while imaging. The intercostals arteries arising from the descending aorta can be seen on the right of the display. The hemiagygous vein that drains the left posterior thorax may at times be seen in the far field. In the mid to upper thorax the hemiagygous vein joins the agygous vein (that drains the right posterior thorax). The agygous vein runs typically parallel to the ascending aorta and aortic arch and eventually drains into the SVC. As their walls are contiguous the two structures can be mistaken from dissection flap within the aorta.[7] Differentiation between the arterial and venous flow can be done with colour flow or pulsed Doppler.[7] Apart from dissection, DTA should be assessed for atherosclerosis, aneurysm and calcification. DTA can interrogated distally below the diaphragm typically beginning at the celiac artery, but the abdominal gas and variable aortic position prevents adequate imaging. The proximal DTA can be interrogated as TEE probe is rotated and gradually withdrawn. It is difficult to define the exact location of a particular lesion. The distance from the incisors to the distal arch is at 20–25 cm, mid DTA at 30–35 cm and diaphragm at 40–45 cm.

### Assessment of Aortic Arch

The distal aortic arch can be imaged as the probe is withdrawn gradually from DTA at multiplane of 0° to 10° until the circular view of descending aorta in descending aorta SAX view becomes tubular view of the arch in LAX view. This is called the **UE aortic arch LAX view** (Fig. 12.11) with distal arch to the right of the image display and proximal arch to the left of the display. As the aorta is anterior to the oesophagus at this location complete visualization of aortic arch with posterior wall at top and anterior wall at the bottom of image can be done by turning the probe to right and left. From the UE aortic arch LAX view a multiplane rotation to 70°–90° displays aortic arch in short axis. This is called **UE aortic arch SAX view** (Fig. 12.12). In this view aorta is seen in the near field. In addition the main pulmonary artery and the pulmonary valve can be imaged in long axis in the far field. But their visualization requires adjusting the imaging depth, frequency of probe and focal zone. Because of the curvature of the aorta, the right brachiocephalic, left common carotid artery and left subclavian artery may be seen arising from the aorta between the SAX and LAX view of the aortic arch typically in to the right of the display in the near field. In some individuals withdrawal of the transducer from the UE aortic arch LAX view can image the left subclavian artery and left carotid artery.[7] During TEE evaluation of the arch, in addition left innominate vein can be frequently imaged with venous flow by color flow Doppler.[7]

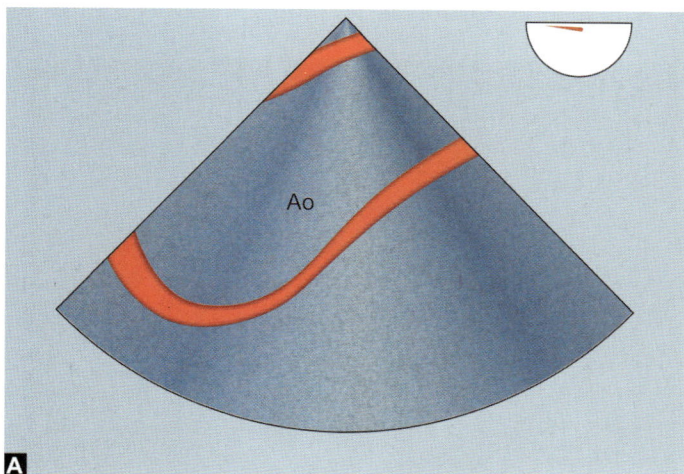
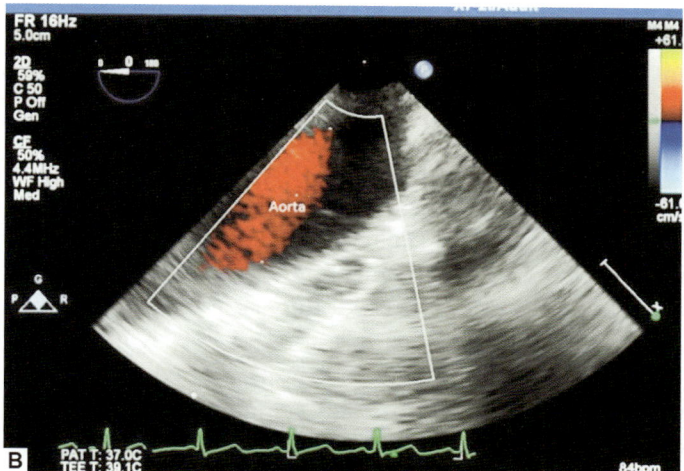

**Figs 12.11A and B:** Upper esophageal (UE) aortic arch long-axis view at a multiple angle of 0 . Distal aortic arch can be interrogated for any dissection and/or aneurysm. Ao: Aorta

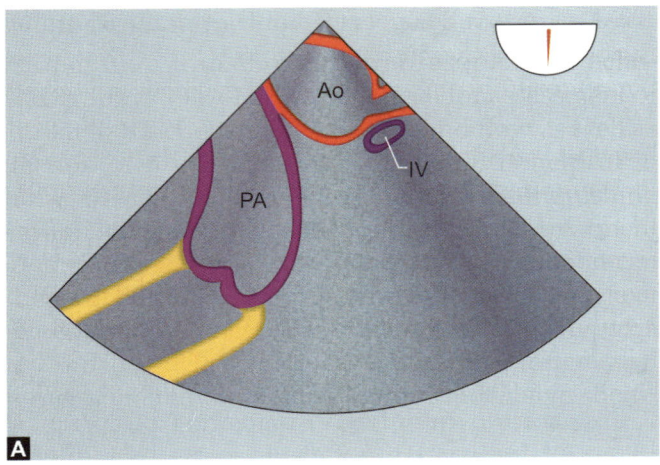

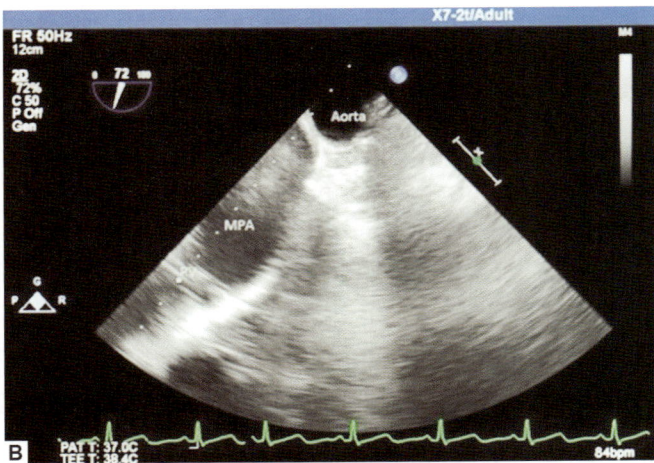

**Figs 12.12A and B:** UE aortic arch short-axis view at a multiplane angle of 72°. Distal aortic arch can be evaluated for dissection or aneurysm. Pulmonary artery and pulmonary valve can also be seen. Innominate vein, subclavian artery origin, and left carotid artery origin may also be seen. Ao: Aorta, PA: Pulmonary artery, IV: Innominate vein, MPA: Main pulmonary artery

## PERIOPERATIVE TEE ASSESSMENT OF THORACIC AORTIC DISEASES

### Aneurysms

An aortic aneurysm is the dilatation of aorta more than 50% of the normal aortic diameter. Ectasia denotes dilatation of aorta which is less than 50% of normal aortic dimensions. Age and overall body surface area affects the normal diameter of aorta.[12] Morphologically aneurysm can be classified as saccular (focal out pouching), fusiform (cylindrical dilatation affecting the entire circumference of aorta) and diffuse.

Aneurysm of ascending aorta is typically fusiform. The dilatation of aorta between the aortic valve annulus and sino-tubular junction (STJ) is known as 'root' aneurysm. If the dilatation of aorta starts distal to STJ it is known as tubular or supra-coronary aneurysm.[13] The root type aneurysm requires coronary artery re-implantation and possibility aortic value (AV) repair/replacement, while the tube type mostly does not require AV repair/replacement. Dilatation involving both root and ascending aorta are referred to as "diffuse" and typically result in obliteration of STJ.

With the ascending aortic diameters ≥6 cm, the risk of rupture increases (Fig. 12.13). So surgical treatment is recommended for asymptomatic patients with aortic dimensions ≥5.5 cm. But etiology of aneurysm should also be taken into consideration, and is an important risk factor for prediction of complications. Aneurysm may congenital or acquired. Congenital are caused by connective tissue disorders such as Marfans and Ehlers-Danlos syndrome. In patients with known connective tissue disorders surgical treatment is required at aortic dilatation of 4.2 to 5 cm.[14] The acquired aneurysm may

be due pathologic effects of advanced age, smoking, hypertension and hypercholesterolemia. As pseudo-aneurysms and saccular aneurysms are less predictable, surgical repair is indicated whenever feasible, regardless of size. Recent guidelines suggests, that patient undergoing cardiac surgery, and incidental finding of either root or ascending aorta dilatation ≥4.5 cm, should be considered for concomant aortic repair.[3]

So, TEE measurement of annulus, root, STJ and tubular part of ascending aorta is essential in surgical decision making (Fig. 12.13). Knowledge of normal dimensions for age and sex and cut offs for surgical decision making is important. Also it is important to realize that diameter measurements on CT angiography are from vessel adventitia to adventitia, but on echocardiography the measurements are from vessel intima to intima. A detailed description about the dimensions at which intervention is recommended according to

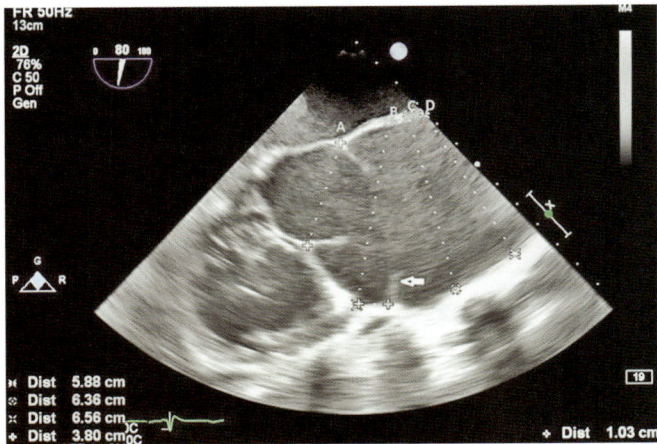

**Fig. 12.13:** Midesophageal ascending aortic LAX View showing dilated aortic root and tubular part of the ascending aorta

pathology is discussed in detail in chapter on anesthesia for ascending aortic aneurysm.

Thoracoabdominal aneurysm is categorized according to Crawford classification. Type I originate in proximal descending thoracic aorta and ends above the renal artery, Type II begins from proximal descending thoracic aorta and ends below renal arteries. Type III originate in the mid descending thoracic aorta and terminates below the renal arteries, Type IV originates at the diaphragm and is limited to abdominal aorta. There is an increased risk of rupture with aortic diameters >7 cm.[14] Therefore, surgical repair or stent placement is recommended at size of ≥6 cm or ≥5.5 cm if chronic dissection or connective tissue disorder are present.[3] TEE helps in the measurement of aortic dimensions as well as guide for placement of arterial cannula/guide wire from femoral artery into the aorta (Figs 12.14 and 12.15).

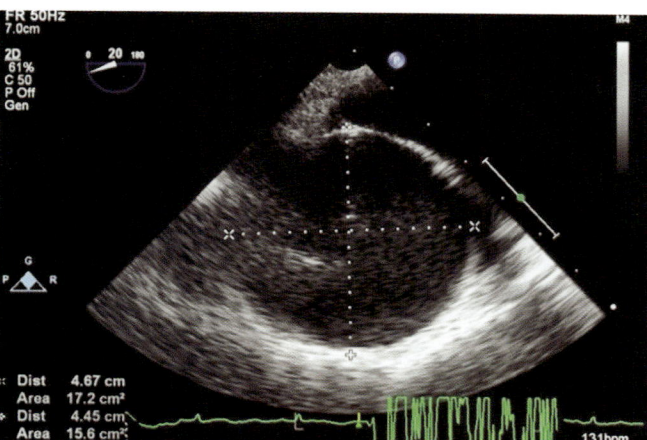

**Fig. 12.14:** Measurement of dimensions of descending thoracic aorta in midesophageal descending aortic short-axis view at a multiplane angle of 20°

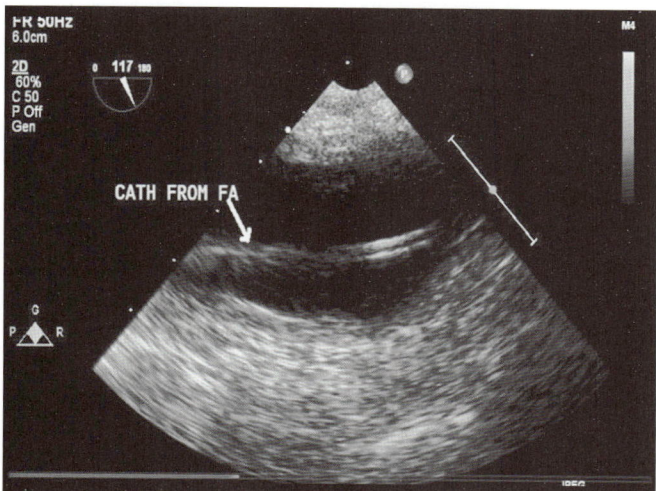

**Fig. 12.15:** Arterial cannula in midesophageal descending aortic long-axis view at a multiplane angle of 117°. FA: Femoral artery, Cath: Catheter

TEE is less useful for assessment below the diaphragm as mentioned above. Also, use of TEE is limited in torturous aorta, since in such a situation, aorta may be separated from the esophagus resulting in difficulty in imaging these resulting segments.[15]

To conclude, with the use of TEE, an echocardiographer should be able to decide whether AV is diseased and requires either repair or replacement? Is the aortic root diseased and needs replacement? Whether ascending aorta, arch or DTA needs to be replaced? Further, TEE can help intraoperatively as well as in post-repair assessment.

## ACUTE AORTIC SYNDROMES

Acute aortic syndromes includes a group of life threatening conditions including aortic dissections, intramural hematoma and penetrating aortic ulcers. There may be fluid extravasations into the pericardium or a periaortic hematoma may develop which have poor prognosis.[16] Amongst these, aortic dissection is the most common and widely studied. Aortic dissection may be associated with complications like aortic regurgitation, hemopericardium, cardiac temponade, myocardial ischemia by dissection into the coronary ostia or stroke from occlusion of aortic arch vessels.

### Aortic Dissections

A dissection is a breach or tear in the intima of the aortic wall allowing blood from the true lumen of the aorta to percolate below the intima into the media/or adventitia, thus resulting in a flap of tissue known as the 'dissection flap'. Dissection may be initiated by predisposing factors such as hypertension, advanced age, connective tissue disorders (Marfan and Erlos-Danlos syndromes) and thoracic trauma. As more blood escapes between the layers of the media a false lumen is created. The blood from this lumen can extend both proximally and distally leading to compromise of branch vessels, detach the aortic valve leaflets from the valve, thereby causing aortic insufficiency, or can even rupture into the peri-cardial or thoracic cavity.

Two classification systems used to describe the aortic dissections, namely the DeBakey and the Stanford system, are described in detail in chapter on aortic dissection. Acute dissections of ascending aorta (DeBakey Types I and II, or Stanford Type A) are surgical emergencies with high mortality if not surgically treated in time, whereas dissection involving descending aorta (DeBakey Types III, or Stanford Type B) are relatively less lethal.[17,18]

Aortography was once considered as the gold standard for the diagnosis of dissections. But presently, surgical intervention is usually based on CT findings, as CT can be performed quickly and safely in patients of aortic dissections. CT, MRI and TEE have comparative diagnostic accuracy in suspected aortic dissection. The sensitivity and specificity with TEE is more than 90%.[3,19–22] Several studies have demonstrated the accuracy of TEE in the diagnosis of aortic dissection with sensitivity of 86–100%, specificity 90–100%, and a negative predictive value of 86–100%.[23–26]

Intraoperative TEE in aortic dissection has a role in confirmation of diagnosis, in guidance and assessment of surgical repair. It thus helps the surgeon to consider different cannulation sites, decide for aortic root or valve replacement, coronary bypass grafting, arch replacement or a simple ascending aortic tubular graft replacement. A brief summary is outlined in Table 12.2.

The goals of intraoperative TEE include:

1. Confirmation of the diagnosis. The presence of intimal flap is the hall mark of diagnosis of dissection. An undulating linear density of intimal flap, which is seen within the aortic lumen, and separating the true from false lumen is diagnostic of dissection. Thus the normally seen single aortic wall appearance is replaced by two separate echo densities. The intimal flap is irregular, and at times highly mobile. But the intimal flap has to be confirmed in at least two views, as various artifacts can be misinterpreted as intimal flap (Figs 12.16A to C). The possible artifacts may be calcifications on the AV or root or an atheroma on the aortic wall.[27] Also a pulmonary artery (PA) catheter can cause reverberation artifact and mimic a dissection flap. In such a situation the PA catheter can, however, be pulled back to confirm the presence or absence of dissection flap.[28]

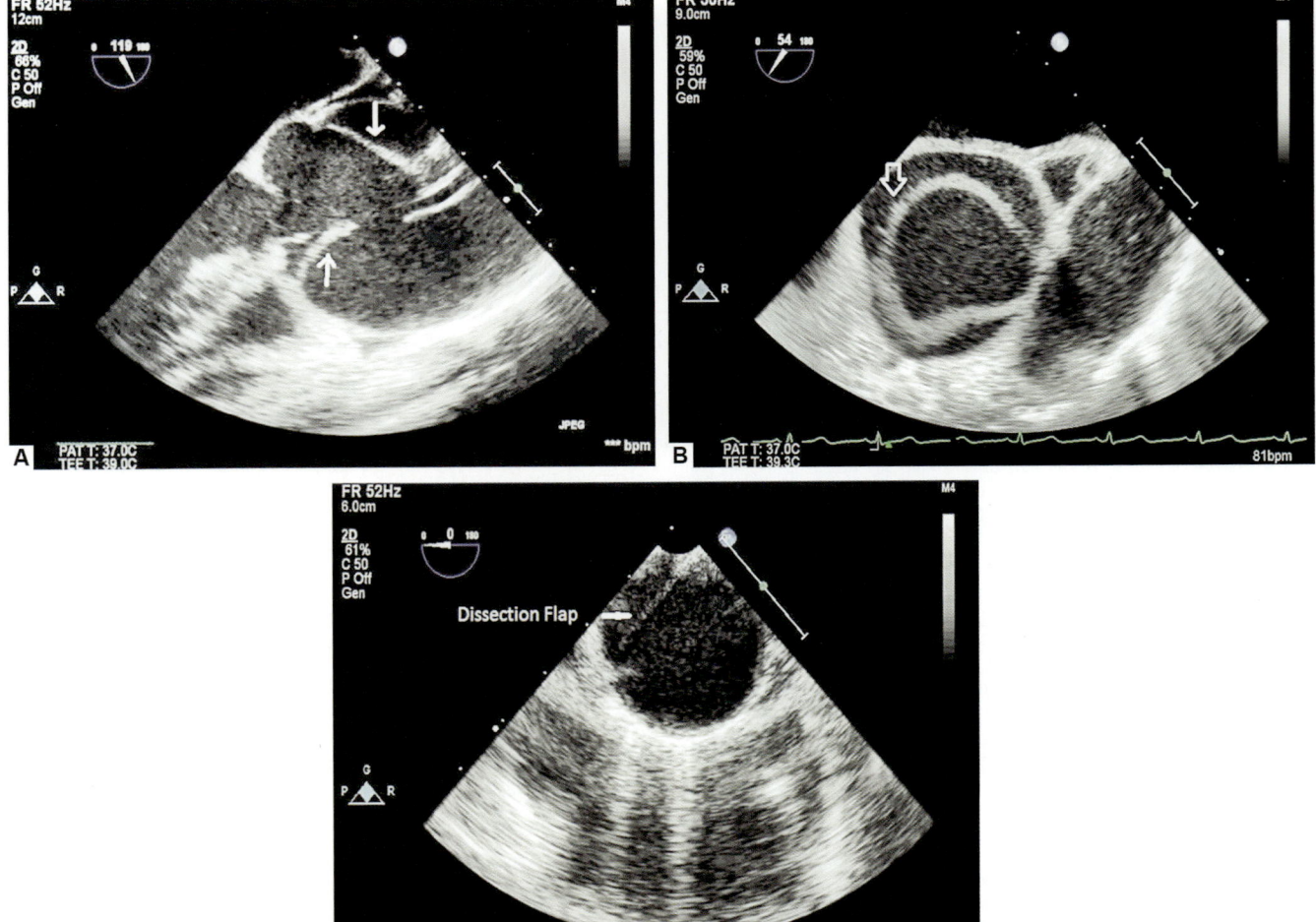

Figs 12.16A to C: Dissection flap in (A) Midesophageal aortic valve long-axis view at multiplane angle of 119 , (B) Midesophageal aortic valve short-axis view at multiplane angle of 54 , (C) Midesophageal descending aortic short-axis view at multiplane angle of 0

2. Identification of the entry point is important from the surgical view point. TEE provides identification of the tear in 78–100% of cases, and measurements can also be taken.[29]

3. True lumen identification. The surgeon wants to know whether the branch arteries originate from the false or true lumen of the aorta. Also it is important to differentiate between true and false lumen in endovascular stent-grafting. The true lumen can be differentiated from the false lumen (Fig. 12.17). The true lumen is often smaller than the false lumen, expands during systole, there is systolic antegrade flow, there is flow from the true lumen to the false lumen in systole, and on contrast echocardiography, the contrast echo flow is seen early and fast to appear as compared to the false lumen. Whereas, the false lumen is commonly larger than the true lumen, gets compressed during systole, systolic antegrade flow is reduced or absent, rather there may be retrograde flow and on contrast echocardiography, the contrast flow is delayed and slow. The false lumen often has a thrombus within it, particularly in the descending aorta.[15, 24] Color flow Doppler is also used to visualize flow from true to false lumen; color flow Doppler can also reveal the presence of multiple communications between two lumina especially in descending aorta corresponding to intercostals and visceral arteries (Fig. 12.18). Using pulse Doppler imaging of the flow

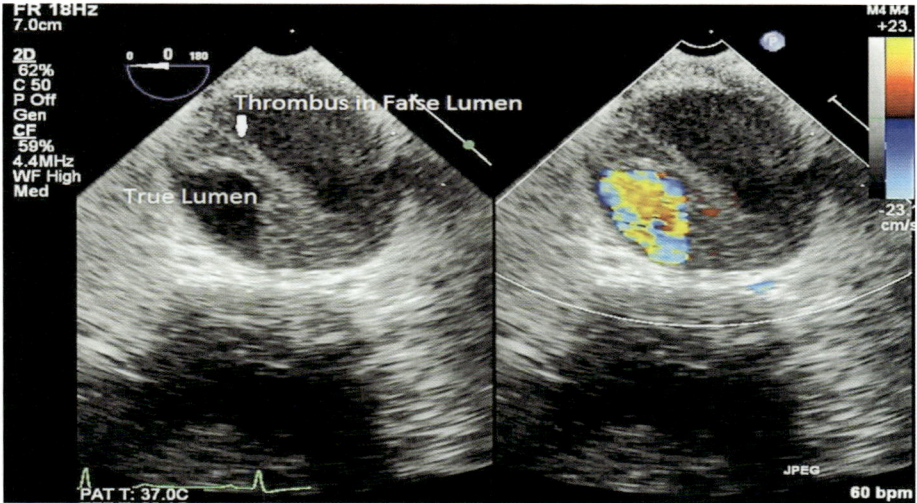

**Fig. 12.17:** Midesophageal descending aortic short-axis view at multiplane angle of 0 showing dissection with small true lumen with blood flow and a large false lumen with a thrombus

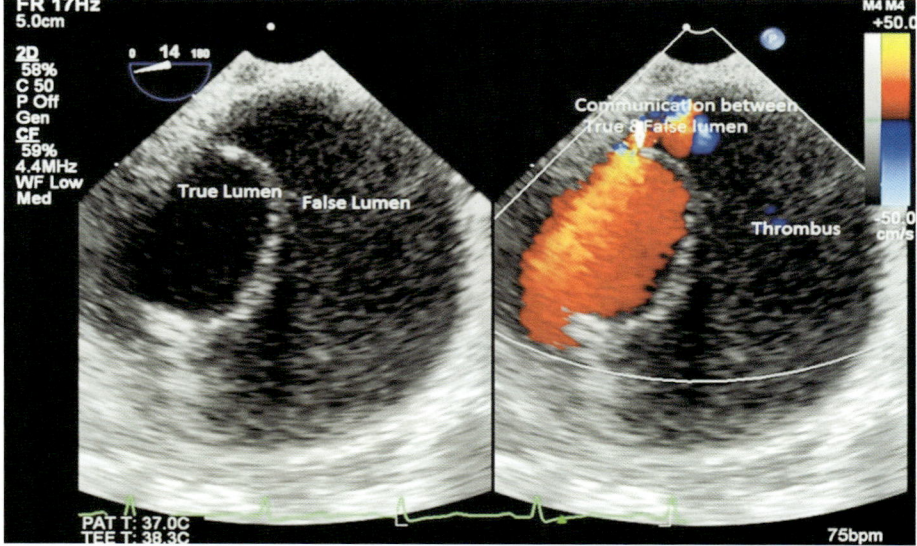

**Fig. 12.18:** Midesophageal descending aortic short-axis view at multiplane angle of 0 with color flow Doppler showing blood flow from true into the false lumen

through the intimal tear the pressure gradients between the true and the false lumens can be estimated.

4. Assessment of AV, aortic root and coronary ostia. Evaluation of AV is crucial in aortic dissection surgical decision making. Aortic regurgitation (AR) may be present in nearly 40–76% of patients[15] (Fig. 12.19). The possible mechanisms influencing AR includes—(a) aortic root dilatation alone without commissural detachment which could be secondary to dilatation of the ascending aorta, (b) destruction of commissural support, (c) dissection flap prolapsed into the left ventricular outflow tract, (d) rupture of annular support or tear in the implantation of one of the valvular leaflets, (e) in asymmetric dissections, the hematoma itself may displace a sigmoid below the coaptation level, (f) pre-existing AV disease.[30,31]

Dissection may involve the coronary arteries in up to 20% of cases, the right coronary artery being commonly involved (Fig. 12.20). Using TEE it can be verified whether coronary dissection is present or the coronary ostium is arising from the false lumen. Early detection of coronary artery involvement along with regional wall motion abnormality can alert the surgical team for early harvesting of saphenous vein graft.[30]

5. Assessment of Global and Regional Myocardial Function. Global dysfunction can occur due to severe AR, coronary artery involvement, pericardial temponade, or pre-existing cardiomyopathy. Regional wall motion abnormality should alert the team as to the need of coronary artery bypass grafting of the affected region as these patients are usually not subjected to preoperative coronary angiography.

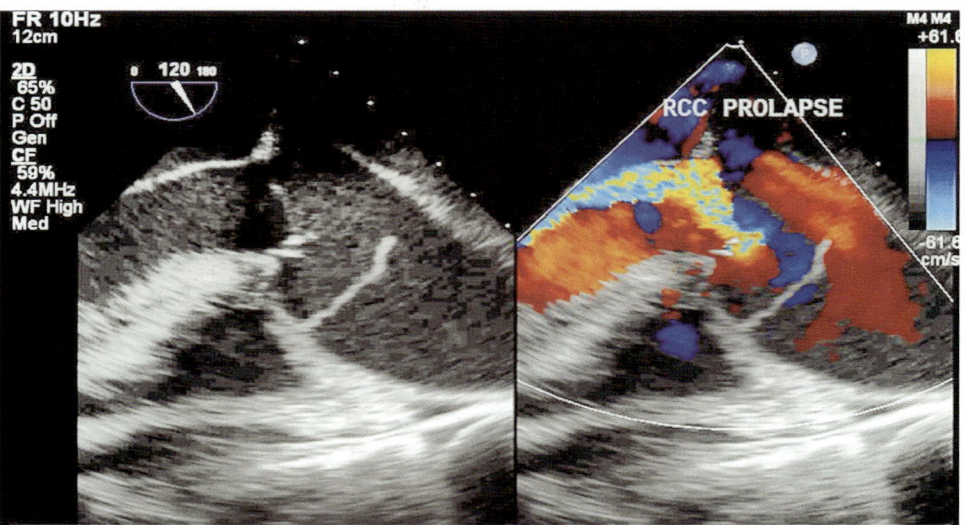

**Fig. 12.19:** Midesophageal aortic valve long-axis view at multiplane angle of 120 showing dissection flap, right coronary cusp (RCC) prolapse and aortic regurgitation

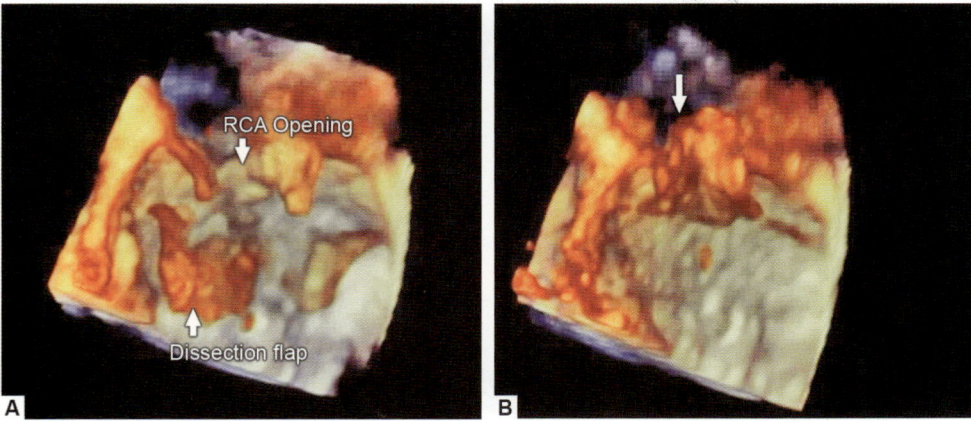

**Figs 12.20A and B:** (A) 3D image showing RCA opening above and a dissection flap below. (B) showing dissection flap obstructing the RCA opening. RCA: Right coronary artery

6. Assessment for other complications of aortic dissection. (a) Dissection of branches of aorta. The color Doppler can help detect any arterial vessel involvement. TEE is not a choice of technique for assessment of supra-aortic branch vessels involvement. The origin of left subclavian artery is easily observed as compared to that of innominate and left carotid arteries which are not always detected on TEE. Using TEE involvement of celiac trunk can be appreciated where as renal and iliac arteries are better detected by CT. (b) Pericardial effusion and periaortic bleeding. Pericardial effusion may result from extravasations of blood from aorta or secondary to irritation of adventitia produced by aortic hematoma (Fig. 12.21). TEE plays an important role for diagnosing the presence and quantifying severity of temponade. Periaortic hematoma and pleural effusion are best diagnosed by CT and are indicators of increased mortality.[23,29]

7. Rule out additional cardiac pathology. Many a times due to urgency of the surgery a complete investigative workup may not be possible. A complete TEE evaluation intraoperatively helps to rule out any other cardiac pathology.

8. Monitoring for left ventricular distension. (a) Repair of the dissection commonly requires cooling. During cooling ventricular fibrillation may occur. In the presence of AR, the ventricle may distend resulting in poor myocardial protection. Intraoperative TEE monitoring is useful in monitoring left ventricular distension and can alert the surgical team about the need of left ventricular venting or cross clamp application with cardioplegic arrest. The utility of TEE monitoring is even greater in type B aortic dissection when the patient is being operated in thoracotomy position and the heart cannot be directly visualized for detection of left ventricular distension.

(b) TEE is also helpful in guiding the placement of the guide wire/arterial cannula via the femoral artery into the true lumen of aorta.

9. Post Repair Assessment. Post repair TEE assessment should be done for de-airing, degree of residual AR, any paravalvular leak and, ventricular function. The proximal and distal ends of the graft should be identified. The grafts used for aortic repair are usually of polytetrafluoroethylene (PTFE) or polyester fibre (Dacron) and have a serrated appearance on TEE.[28] Gradients across the valved conduit can be measured. Thus it helps the surgeon to decide for the need of any further intervention. When a two-staged procedure of aortic repair is planned and an "elephant trunk" is placed, then using TEE, elephant trunk can be visualized floating in the DTA and a colour flow Doppler can help confirm the flow.[28] A grade >2+ AR would prompt the surgeon to replace the valve, a regional wall motion abnormality would suggest a coronary bypass grafting and increased gradients across the valved conduit may suggest a re-do repair.

## Intramural Hematoma

Intramural hematoma (IH) is primarily a result of hemorrhage of small vessels (vasa vasorum) in the medial layers of the aorta.[32] The accumulated blood causes a thickening of the medial layer of the aorta. Progressive increase in the accumulated blood, may later lead to either intimal tear or flap formation similar to aortic dissection, or outward rupture of aortic wall. IH typically develops in old hypertensive patients. However, blunt chest trauma resulting in aortic injury or a penetrating atherosclerotic ulcer can also result in IH.

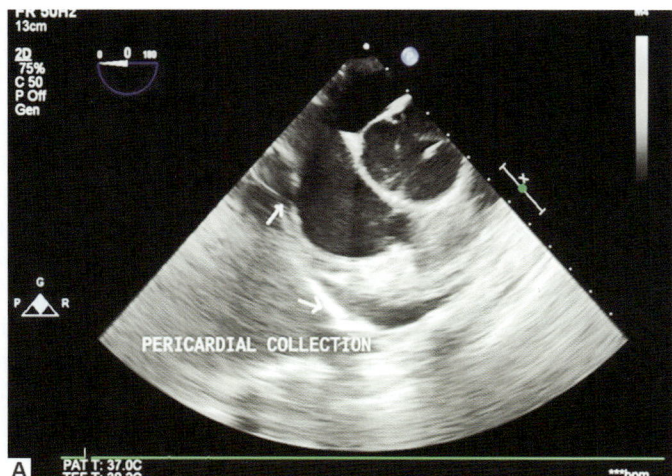
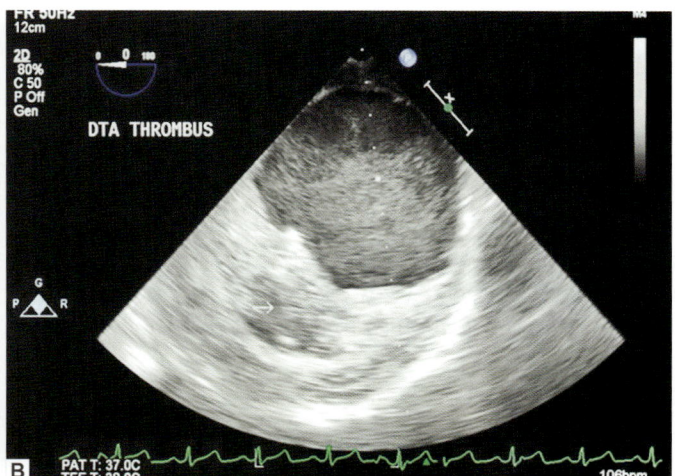

**Figs 12.21A and B:** Midesophageal four chamber view showing (A)pericardial collection in a patient with descending thoracic aortic aneurysm with a thrombus, (B) Midesophageal descending aortic short-axis view of the same patient showing a thrombus

**Table 12.2:** Role of Intraoperative TEE in aortic dissection

| | |
|---|---|
| 1. Confirmation of diagnosis | • Presence of intimal flap in two separate views<br>• Exclude artifacts like calcification on AV/root, atheroma, PA catheter |
| 2. Identification of entry point | • Determine the proximal extent of the flap<br>• Measurements of aortic dimensions |
| 3. Differentiation of true and false lumen | • True lumen is often smaller than false lumen<br>• True lumen expands during systole and there is systolic compression in the false lumen.<br>• There is systolic antegrade flow in true lumen while in the false lumen systolic antegrade flow is reduced or absent or there may be retrograde flow<br>• On contrast echocardiography echo flow is early and fast in true lumen as compared to false lumen<br>• Color flow Doppler to show flow from true to false lumen in systole<br>• The false lumen often has thrombus |
| 4. Determination of AV/root, coronary involvement | • Look for AV disease, any aortic root dilatation, mechanism of AR if any<br>• Grade severity of any AR<br>• Determine if AV may be repairable<br>• Look for flap extending into aortic root and coronary ostia |
| 5. Assessment of global and regional myocardial function | • Look for regional wall motion abnormalities<br>• Assess ventricular function |
| 6. Assessment for complications of aortic dissection | • Look for dissection involving any branch of the aorta<br>• Pericardial and pleural effusions are common |
| 7. Rule out additional cardiac pathology | • Preoperative workup is often minimal due to the urgency of surgery<br>• A complete examination is essential for any other pathology |
| 8. Intraoperative monitoring | • In the presence of AR monitoring for left ventricular distension helps in decision regarding ventricular venting/need of cross clamp application with cardioplegic arrest<br>• Placement of the guide wire/arterial cannula via the femoral artery into the true lumen of aorta |
| 9. Post-repair assessment | • Helps in de-airing<br>• Assessment of residual AR, paravalvular leak, ventricular function<br>• Proximal and distal ends of the graft identified and gradients across the valve/conduit measured |

AV: Aortic valve, AR: Aortic regurgitation

On TEE, IH is seen as cresenteric or circular thickening in the medial wall of aorta measuring greater than 5 mm with no flow within.[33-35] Areas of echolucency may be seen within the medial layers of aorta. Intramural hematoma has to be differentiated, from a dissection with a thrombosed false lumen and an intraluminal thrombus. In the IH, accumulation of blood in the medial layer causes medial displacement of intimal calcification. Therefore, it appears as aortic thickening with a smooth inner margin. Thus the intima appears as a bright smooth echo-dense with aortic thickening. Whereas in classical aortic dissection flow is commonly observed in lumina. In aneurysmal diltation with mural thrombi intimal margin are irregular. However, it is difficult to confirm diagnosis if false lumen of dissection is totally thrombosed.[29,36]

### Penetrating Atherosclerotic Ulcer

The common presentation of the atherosclerotic disease is the protrusion of atherosclerotic plaque above the aortic intimal layer into the aortic lumen. Less commonly, there occurs penetrating atherosclerotic ulcers (PAU),

which are the plaques that erode through the internal elastic lamina into the aortic media.[37]The erosion of the medial wall can thus lead to aneurysm formation or aortic rupture. There is usually no dissection flap.

On echocardiography, there is a crater-like out pouching of the aortic wall with associated extensive athermatous plaques.[38] There may be areas of echolucency with no flow into these areas seen within the plaques. The exact borders of the aortic lumen cannot be visualized due to erosion of plaque into the medial layer. Apart from extensive areas of atherosclerotic disease, sometimes effusions or fluid collections are also seen[28]. TEE helps to differentiate between ulcerated plaques, PAU, and ulcer like images formed due to intimal tear secondary to intramural hematomas.[15] Intramural hematoma can be diagnosed by the aortic wall thickening with inward displacement of intimal calcification and associated inner smooth margins.

### TRAUMATIC INJURIES

Common survivable aortic injuries result from blunt chest trauma/rapid deceleration. These involve the aortic isthmus between the aortic arch and the DTA. Although CT is the most common diagnostic tool, but TEE has certain advantages. It is portable, can be performed along bedside and operating room with immediate diagnosis, can detect any cardiac temponade or hypovolemia. The echocardiographic features that may be present in traumatic aortic injury includes intimal tear, intimal flap, pseudoaneurysm and aortic rupture.[39] As the most common suspected site of injury among patients who survive up to the hospital is isthmus, the proximal DTA should be examined carefully with TEE. But a comprehensive echocardiographic examination of all the segments is required as other sites may also be injured.

## ENDOVASCULAR PROCEDURE

With the advancements in technology more and more patients with aortic pathology, are now being treated with endovascular aortic stent grafts. This procedure of thoracic endovascular aortic repair (TEVAR) is commonly performed in aneurysm or dissection. TEVAR aims at deployment of stent graft that seals the normal diameter of aorta above as well as below the aneurysm or dissection, thus excluding the pathology from the systemic blood flow, distending arterial pressure, and thus eliminating the risk of rupture. These aortic stent grafts are usually deployed under general anesthesia using fluoroscopy. TEE plays an important role in confirming the accuracy of deployment and in detection of endoleaks if any[30, 40–42] (Fig. 12.22). Studies have shown TEE to be more sensitive and specific for detection of endoleaks as compared to angiography.[43–45] It is to be noted that TEE probe has to be pulled proximally during angiographic imaging of the aorta.

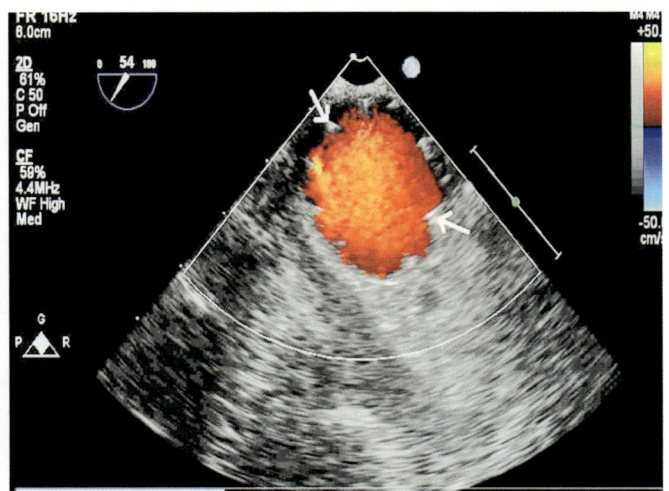

**Fig. 12.22:** Midesophageal descending aortic short-axis view with color flow Doppler showing a bright echogenic shadows of deployed endovascular stent

Endoleak is the continuation of blood flow out from the lumen of the stent graft into the surrounding aneurysmal sac or adjacent vascular segment being treated by the graft.[46,47] Type I endoleak is persistence of flow around the attachment site either at proximal or distal end of the stent graft due to ineffective seal at the graft end. Type II endoleak occurs due to retrograde flow into the aneurysmal sac from the collaterals. Type III endoleak is due to defect or tear in the fabric of the stent-graft or leakage between modular segments of stent-graft. This is more common in thoracic region because of greater hemodynamic stress in this region resulting in either early or late stent-graft leakage. Type IV endoleak is difficult to differentiate from other types of graft leakage and is termed as "endoleak of undefined origin". This could be due to porous material of the stent-graft. Endoleaks are termed as "Primary" if they are detected within 30 days of deployment. Beyond 30 days they are termed as "Secondary". Type I and type III endoleaks should be treated.

Although angiography is the gold standard, TEE can add significant information during endovascular repair. The TEE probe is useful marker of aortic level on fluoroscopy without contrast injection.

Prior to stent graft deployment, TEE can provide information about the cardiac functions, valvular competency, sizing and positioning of the stent-grafts. In dissections, TEE is useful in guidewire positioning into the true lumen rather than false lumen which is not possible with fluoroscopy. The differential flow between the true and the false lumen can be appreciated. On TEE image, the guide wire appears as bright echodense structure in the aorta. In patients with previous aortic arch surgery TEE is useful for the correct guidewire entrance into the elephant trunk prosthesis. In atherosclerotic aortic aneurysm, plaques are detected by TEE and not by angiography/fluoroscopy. The protruding plaque at the proximal neck can prevent tight adhesion between the stent-graft and the aortic wall leading to dangerous leaks. Thus, prior to stent-graft placement, TEE can help selection of aortic wall segment without protruding plaques and in selection of stent-graft diameter.

During stent-graft deployment and ballooning to enable fixation of stent-graft to the wall, transient acute hemodynamic disturbances occur due to occlusion of aorta. Using TEE cardiac performance can be monitored and appropriate action taken.[48]

At times, diastolic dysfunction may be the only manifestation of myocardial injury perioperatively being undetected by other monitoring modality.[48]

After stent-graft deployment, TEE is useful for the detection of peri-stent leaks by using colour Doppler. Endoleaks may also be indicated by development of spontaneous echocontrast, or echocardiographic "smoke" within aneurysm sac.[49] The contrast that swirls around the sac suggests continued flow into the sac suggesting an endoleak. This can be promptly treated by balloon dilatation or further stent-graft deployment. It is important to note that most of these leaks are not visible on angiography. In aortic dissection, TEE is beneficial for detection of small distal re-entry tears which are not visible on angiography. These can also be promptly treated by deploying additional stent-graft.

TEE for aortic endovascular stent grafting is not without limitations. Firstly, TEE is not able to guide the abdominal endovascular stenting. Secondly, visualization of the innominate and the left carotid artery ostia is not always possible with TEE, the proximal positioning of the of the stent graft in this region is hampered. Thirdly, as PTFE, acts as a barrier to ultrasound, the TEE modality is beneficial with Dacron stent graft and not the PTFE (Gortex) graft. The course of aorta may be tortuous, and so imaging may become difficult with inaccurate interpretation as aorta may disappear at crucial points.[48] Imaging of the aneurysm may be difficult due to high echo-density of the stent-graft hardware into the aorta.

## INTRAVASCULAR ULTRASOUND

In abdominal endovascular procedures, where TEE is not able to guide, intravascular ultrasound (IVUS) or intraluminal phased array ultrasound imaging (IPAI) plays an important role. IPAI has proved superior to TEE and IVUS in detection of communication between true and false lumen of aortic dissection.[50] But both these are disposables and costlier than TEE.

Dissection and malperfusion of carotid arteries can be detected by Ultrasound Vascular Duplex imaging.

## AORTIC ATHEROMA

Presence of aortic atheroma is a marker of coronary artery disease and is a source of embolism.[51,52] Presence of aortic atheroma increases with age, smoking and pulse pressure.[15] Basic characteristic of aortic atheroma is an irregular thickening of minimum 2 mm of aortic intima on TEE with additional thrombi seen as mobile component.[53] TEE is the better modality than TTE for diagnosing aortic atheroma. So quite often atheroma is first detected on operation table when patient is to undergocardiac surgery, as TEE provides higher resolution image as compared to TTE.[54] It is important

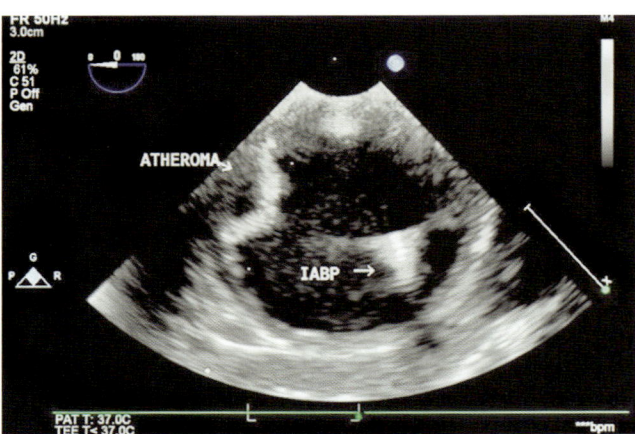

Fig. 12.23: Midesophageal descending aortic short-axis view showing large atheromatous plague (which was highly mobile) seen close to intra-aortic balloon pump (IABP) tip

to know the location of aortic atheroma, as it can help surgeon to avoid manipulation of these areas and thus prevent embolic episodes. The surgeon can thus avoid aortic cross clamping, aortic cannulation at a particular site and also undergo epiaortic scanning.[55]

Using TEE, the thickness of plagues, ulceration, calcification and presence of any superimposed mobile thrombi to determine the embolic potential can be detected. TEE provides real time accuracy of size, and mobility of atheroma (Fig. 12.23). The commonly used classification scale for assessment of atheromatous plague is by Katz et al which has classified aortic atheroma into five grades.[56] Grade I is normal intimal thickness, Grade II when an intimal thickening is present without protrusion into lumen, Grade III is when plaque protrudes <5 mm into aortic lumen, Grade IV is when plaque protrudes $\geq$ 5 mm into aortic lumen, Grade V is any plaque with a mobile component.[56]

## EPIAORTIC IMAGING

TEE is an important intraoperative diagnostic tool for aortic pathologies, but its use is limited by its inability to image the distal ascending aorta and the proximal aortic arch. Direct epivascular or epiaortic ultrasonographic (EAU) imaging has recently gained importance as a strategy to reduce the embolic load in patients with atherosclerotic disease. A few studies show a lower stroke rate in patients where surgical technique was modified based on EAU guidance.[57–59] Various guidelines have been published for the use of intraoperative epiaortic ultrasonography.[60] EAU imaging is indicated in patients with the increased perioperative stroke like history of cerebrovascular or peripheral vascular disease and evidence of aortic atherosclerosis or calcification on various imaging modalities. The guidelines recommend the use of high frequency probe ($\geq$7 MHz) which can be

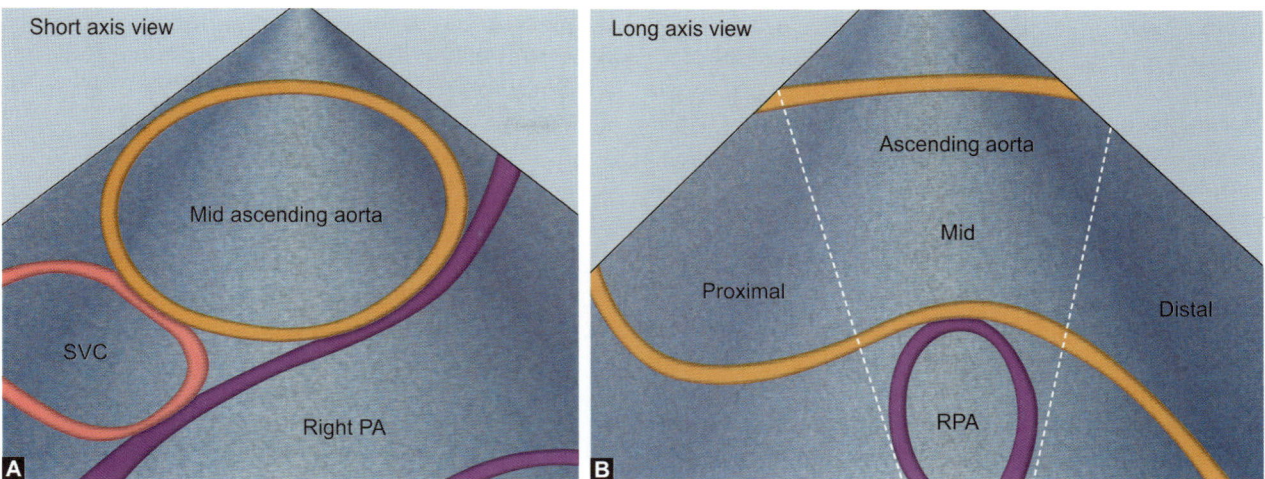

**Figs 12.24A and B:** Epiaortic imaging of ascending aorta in short axis (A) and long axis (B). RPA: Right pulmonary artery, PA: Pulmonary artery SVC: Superior vena cava. Proximal, mid and distal is in relation to RPA. The walls of ascending aorta are designated as anterior, posterior, right lateral and left lateral

either a Linear Sequential array transducers, a Standard Phased-array adult or pediatric transthoracic transducer or a Matrix-array transducer. These transducers are placed in a sterile sheath, which is filled with either sterile saline or a ultrasound transmission gel. A few echocardiographers suggest the use of two sheaths to confirm sterility. To enhance acoustic transmission the mediastinal cavity is filled with warm sterile saline. The linear transducers can be placed directly on the aorta but does not include all the walls in single image. The Phased-array probe can visualized all the walls in one image but has to be placed 1 cm above the aorta. The entire aorta can be imaged in a single long axis (LAX) imaging plane. Matrix-array transducer enables 3D image or a 2D image with two orthogonal planes eliminating the need to acquire both short-axis (SAX) and long-axis (LAX) views (Fig. 12.24). The comprehensive EAU examination include minimum five views for the ascending aorta from the sinotubular junction to the origin of innominate artery and aortic arch. These include 3 SAX views of the ascending aorta (proximal, mid, and distal) one LAX view of the ascending aorta and one LAX of the proximal aortic arch. As indicated by the disease additional views within each segment may be acquired. If the atheromatous plaque is detected then three measurements should be recorded, including the maximum plaque height/width, location of the maximal plaque within the ascending aorta and presence of any mobile component.

## SAFETY ISSUES

Care must be taken while inserting the probe in a patient with known case of aneurysmal dilatation of the thoracic aorta or in patients with preoperative history of dysphagia, hoarseness or stridor. At times it may be impossible to pass the probe. An echocardiographer should be aware of the contraindications of TEE probe insertion due to patients anatomy, esophageal pathology like Zenker's diverticulum, stricture, cancer, recent gastroesophageal surgery, significant dysphagia or odynophagia.

### Key Notes

1. With the better diagnostic modalities increasing number of patients are being benefited by aortic surgery. Echocardiography as a diagnostic modality has a definite role in urgent situations when patients cannot be subjected to other investigations.

2. TEE has an advantage over TTE in the assessment of thoracic aorta, as being in close proximity to the probe, it provides a high resolution images. Intraoperatively, TEE helps not only in diagnosis, but also has an extensive role in important surgical decision making.

3. A knowledge of the normal aortic anatomy, aortic dimensions according to age and body surface area and the imaging views by the echocardiographers is essential for important decision making.

4. In aneurysmal dilatation of aorta important decisions have to be made as to need of aortic valve repair/replacement alone, or ascending aortic graft alone, or a combined aortic valve replacement with ascending aortic graft, or a Bentalls procedure or an aortic valve sparing root replacement.

5. Aortic dissection is the most common surgical emergency of aorta. TEE has the advantage over other diagnostic modalities of being rapid in diagnosis, absence of radiographic contrast agents and aortic valve and ventricular functions can be assessed. Complications of dissection like hemopericardium, temponade, myocardial ischemia due to dissection of coronary ostia can also be diagnosed.

*(contd.)*

6. During endovascular aortic stent-graft deployment TEE has a definitive role in guide-wire positioning and in detection of endoleaks.

7. TEE although a very useful modality, is not without disadvantages. It is semi-invasive, requires esophageal intubation, cannot image the distal ascending aorta and the proximal aortic arch. TEE may have various imaging artefacts. Moreover, the diagnostic capability depends on the learning curve of the echocadiographer.

8. Aortic atheroma is an important source of embolism and neurological sequel in patients undergoing cardiac surgery. TEE is an important modality for diagnosing the atheroma and helps to guide surgeon to avoid manipulation of these areas. But TEE cannot visualize distal ascending aorta and the proximal aortic arch. Use of epiaortic ultrasonography can help detection of atheroma in these areas.

## REFERENCES

1. Jakanani GC, Adair W. Frequency of variations in aortic arch anatomy depicted on multidetector CT. Clin Radiol 2010;65: 481–7.

2. Royse C, Royse A, Blake D, Grigg L. Assessment of thoracic atheroma by echocardiography: A new classification and estimation of risk of dislodging atheroma during three surgical techniques. Ann Thorac Cardivasc Surg 1998;4: 72–7.

3. Hiratzka LF, Bakris GL, Beckman JA, et al. ACCF/AHA/ AATS/ACR/ASA/SCA/ SCAI/SIR/STS/SVM guidelines for the diagnosis and management of patients with thoracic aortic disease. A report of the American College of Cardiology Foundation/American Heart Association Task Force on Practice Guidelines, American Association for Thoracic Surgery, American College of Radiology, American Stroke Association, Society of Cardiovascular Anaesthesiologists, Society for Cardiovascuiar Angiography and Interventions, Society of Interventional Radiology, Society for Thoracic Surgeons, and Society for Vascular Medicine. J Am Coll Cardiol 2010;55(14):e27–e129.

4. Johnston KW, Rutherford RB, Tilson MD, et al. Suggested standards for reporting on arterial aneurysms. Subcommittee on Reporting Standards for Arterial Aneurysms, Ad Hoc Committee on Reporting Standards, Society for Vascular Surgery and North American Chapter, International Society for Cardiovascular Surgery. J Vasc Surg 1991;13(3):452–8.

5. Roman MJ, Devereux RB, Kramer-Fox R, et al. Two-dimensional echocardiographic aortic root dimensions in normal children and adults. Am J Cardiol 1989;64(8):507–12.

6. Konstadt SN, Reich DL, Quintana C, Levy M. The ascending aorta: how much does transesophageal echocardiography see? Anesth Analg 1994;78(2):240–4.

7. Hahn RT, Abraham T, Adams MS, et al. Guidelines for performing a comprehensive Transesophageal echocardiographic examination: recommendations from the American Society of Echocardiography and the Society of Cardiovascular Anesthesiologists. J Am Soc Echocardiogr 2013; 26:921–64.

8. Soltesz EG, Svensson LG. Surgical Considerations and Assessment in Aortic Surgery. In: Savage RM, Aronson S, Shernan SK (Eds). Comprehensive Textbook of Intraoperative Transesophageal Echocardiography, 2nd edn. Philadelphia: Lippincott William & Wilkins, 2011;590–8.

9. Augoustides JG, Cheung AT. Aneurysms and Dissections. In: Perioperatve Transesophageal echocardiography. A companion to Kaplan Cardiac Anesthesia. 1st edn. Reich DL, Fischer GW. Elsevier Saunders, Philedelphia. 2014;191–217.

10. Zamorano JL, Badano LP, Bruce C, Chan KL, Goncalves A, Hahn RT, et al. EAE/ASE recommendations for the use of echocardiography in new transcatheter interventions for valvular heart disease. J Am Soc Echocardiogr 2011;24: 937–65.

11. Bloomfield GS, Gillam LD, Hahn RT, Kapadia S, Leipsic J, Lerakis S, et al. A practical guide to multimodality imaging of transcatheter aortic valve replacement, JACC Cardiovasc Imaging 2012;5:441–55.

12. Lang RM, Bierig M, Devereux RB, et al. Recommendations for chamber quantification: A report from the American Society of Echocardiography's Guidelines and Standards Committee and the Chamber Quantification Writing Group, developed in conjunction with the European Association of Echocardiography, a branch of the European Society of Cardiology. J Am Soc Echocardiogr 2005;18:1440–63.

13. Elefteriades JA. Thoracic aortic aneurysm: reading the enemy's playbook. Curr Probl Cardiol 2008;33:203–77.

14. Coady MA, Rizzo JA, Hammond GL, et al. What is the appropriate size criterion for resection of thoracic aortic aneurysms? J Thorac Cardiovasc Surg 1997;113:476–91; discussion 489–91.

15. Evangelista A, Flachskampf FA, Erbel R, Antonini- Canterin F, Viachopoulos C, Rocchi G, Sicari R, Nihoyannopoulos P, Zamorano J. European Association of Echocardiography; Document Reviewers; Pepi M, Breithardt OA, Plonska-Gosciniak E. Echocardiography in aortic diseases: EAE recommendations for clinical practice. European Journal of Echocardiogr 2010;11:645–58.

16. Tsai TT, Nienaber CA, Eagle KA. Acute aortic syndromes. Circulation 2005;112:3802–13.

17. Harris KM, Strauss CE, Eagle KA, et al. Correlates of delayed recognition and treatment of acute type aortic dissection: the International Registry of Acute Aortic dissection (IRAD). Circulation 2011;124(18):1911–8.

18. Bonser RS, Ranasinghe AM, Loubani M, et al. Evidence, lack of evidence, controversy and debate in the provision and performance of the surgery of acute type A dissection. J Am Coll Cardiol, 2011;58(24):2455–74.

19. Golledge J, Eagle KA. Acute aortic dissection. Lancet. 2008;372(9632):55–66.

20. Nienaber CA, Powell JT. Management of acute aortic syndromes. Eur Heart J 2012;33(1):26–35.

21. Shiga T, Wajima Z, Apfel CC, et al. Diagnostic accuracy of Transesophageal echocardiography, helical computed tomography, and magnetic resonance imaging for suspected thoracic aortic dissection: systematic review and meta-analysis. Arch Intern Med 2006;166(13):1350–6.

22. Moore AG, Eagle KA, Bruckman D, et al. Choice of computed tomography, transesophageal echocardiography, magnetic resonance imaging, and aortography in acute aortic dissection: International Registry of Acute Aortic Dissection (IRAD). Am J Cardiol 2002;89(10):1235–8.

23. Erbel R, Engberding R, Daniel W, Roelandt J, Visser C, Rennollet H. Echocardiography in diagnosis of aortic dissection. Lancet 1989;(8636)1:457–61.

24. Evangelista A, Avegliano G, Aguilar R, Cuellar H, lgual A, Gonzalez-Alujas T, et al. Impact of contrast-enhanced echocardiography on the diagnostic algorithm of acute aortic dissection. Eur Heart J 2010;31:472–79ü.

25. Meredith EL, Masani ND. Echocardiography in the emergency assessment of acute aortic syndromes. Eur J Echocardiogr 2009;10:131–9.

26. Pepi M, Campodonico J, Galli C, Tamborini G, Barbier P, Doria E. Rapid diagnosis and management of thoracic aortic dissection and intramural haematoma: A prospective study of advantages of multiplane vs biplane transoesophageal echocardiography. Eur J Echocardiogr 2000;1:72–9.

27. Appelbe AF, Walker PG, Yeoh JK, et al. Clinical significance and origin of artifacts in Transesophageal echocardiography of the thoracic aorta. J Am Coll Cardiol 1993;21:754–60.

28. Sniecinski RM. Transesophageal Echocardiography of the Thoracic Aorta. In: A Practical Approach to Transesophageal Echocardiography. Perino AC, Reeves ST (Ed.) III, Lippincott & Wilkins 347–63.

29. Erbel R, Oelert H, Meyer J, Puth M, Mohr-Katoly S, Hausmann D, et al. Effect of medical and surgical therapy on aortic dissection evaluated by transesophageal echocardiography. Implications for prognosis and therapy. The European Cooperative Study Group on Echocardiography. Circulation 1993;87:1604-15

30. Schütz W, Gauss A, Meierhenrich R, et al. Transesophageal echocardiographic guidance of thoracic aortic stent-graft implantation. J Endovasc Ther 2002;9(Suppl 2):II14–II19.

31. Movsowitz HD, Levine RA, Hilgenberg AD, Isselbacher EM. Transesophageal echocardiographic description of the mechanisms of aortic regurgitation in acute type A aortic dissection: implications for aortic valve repair. J Am Coll Cardiol 2000;36:884–90.

32. Song JK, Kim HS, Kang DH, et al. Different clinical features of aortic intramural haematoma versus dissection involving the ascending aorta. J Am Coll Cardiol 2001;37:1604–10.

33. Mohr-Kahaly S, Erbel R, Kearney P, et al. Aortic intramural hemorrhage visualized by transesophageal echocardiography: findings and prognostic implications. J Am Coll Cardiol 1994;23:658–64.

34. Harris KM, Braverman AC, Gutierrez FR, Barzilai B, et al. Transesophageal echocardiographic and clinical features of aortic intramural hematoma. J Thorac Cardiovasc Surg 1997; 114:619–26.

35. Song JM, Kang DH, Song JK, Kim HS, et al. Clinical significance of echo-free space detected by transesophageal echocardiography in patients with type B aortic intramural hematoma. Am J Cardiol 2002:89:548–51.

36. Evangelista A, Avegliano G, Elorz C, et al. Transesophageal echocardiography in the diagnosis of acute aortic syndrome. J Card Surg 2002;17:95–106.

37. Nathan DP, Boonn W, Lai E, et al. Presentation, complications, and natural history of penetrating atherosclerotic ulcer disease. J Vasc Surg 2012;55:10–15.

38. Vilacosta I, San Román JA, Aragoncillo P, et al. Penetrating atherosclerotic aortic ulcer: Documentation by transesophageal echo cardiography. J Am Coll Cardiol 1998;32:83–9.

39. Starnes BW, Lundgren RS, Gunn M, et al. A new classification scheme for treating blunt aortic injury. J Vasc Surg 2012;55(1):47–54.

40. Koschyk DH, Nienaber CA, Knap M, et al. How to guide stent-graft implantation in type B aortic dissection? Comparison of angiography, transesophageal echocardiography, and intravascular ultrasound. Circulation 2005;112 (Suppl 9):1260–4.

41. Rocchi G, Lofiego C, Biagini E, et al. Transesophageal echocardiography-guided algorithm for stent-graft implantation in aortic dissection. J Vasc Surg 2004;40(5):880–5.

42. Rapezzi C, Rocchi G, Fattori R, et al. Usefulness of transesophageal echocardiographic monitoring to improve the outcome of stent-graft treatment of thoracic aortic aneurysms. Am J Cardiol 2001;87(3):315–9.

43. Fattori R, Caldarera I, Rapezzi C, et al. Primary endoleakage in endovascular treatment of the thoracic aorta: importance of intraoperative transesophageal echocardiography. J Thorac Cardiovasc Surg 2000;120(3):490–5.

44. Gonzalez-Fajardo JA, Gutierrez V, San Roman JA, et al. Utility of intraoperative transesophageal echocardiography during endovascular stent-graft repair of acute thoracic aortic dissection. Ann Vasc Surg 2002;16(3):297–303.

45. Swaminathan M, Lineberger CK, McCann RL, et al. The importance of intraoperative transesophageal echocardiography in endovascular repair of thoracic aortic aneurysms. Anesth Analg 2003;97(6):1566–72.

46. White GH, Yu W, May J, et al. Endoleak as a complication of endoluminal grafting of abdominal aortic aneurysms: classification, incidence, diagnosis and management. J Endovasc Surg 1997;4(2):152–68.

47. White GH, Yu W, May J. Endoleak—a proposed new terminology to describe incomplete aneurysm exclusion by an endoluminal graft. J Endovasc Surg 1996;3(1):124–5.

48. Lee TC, Swaminathan M, Hughes GC. Surgical Considerations and Assessment of Endovascular Management of Thoracic Vascular Disease In: Savage RM, Aronson S, Shernan SK eds. Comprehensive Textbook of Intraoperative Transesophageal Echocardiography, 2nd edn. Philadelphia: Lippincott William & Wilkins, 2011;599–610.

49. Swaminathan M, Mackensen GB, Podgoreanu MV, et al. Spontaneous echocardiographic contrast indicating successful endoleak management. Anesth Analg 2007;104(5): 1037–9.

50. Bartel T, Eggebrecht H, Müller S, Gutersohn A, et al. Comparison of diagnostic and therapeutic value of transesophageal echocardiography, intravascular ultrasonic imaging, and intraluminal phased-array imaging in aortic dissection with tear in the descending thoracic aorta (type B). Am J Cardiol 2007;99:270–4.

51. Fazio GP, Redberg RF, Winslow T, et al. Transesophageal echocardiographically detected atherosclerotic aortic plaque is a marker for coronary artery disease. J Am Coll Cardiol. 1993;21:144–150.

52. Tunick PA, Kronzon I. Atheromas of the thoracic aorta: Clinical and therapeutic update. J Am Coll Cardiol 2000;35:545–54.

53. Montgomery DH, Ververis JJ, McGorisk G, Frohwein S, Martin RP, Taylor WR. Natural history of severe atheromatous disease of the thoracic aorta: a Transesophageal echocardiographic study. J Am Coll Cardiol 1996;27:95–101.

54. Zaidat OO, Suarez JI, Hedrick D, Redline S, Schluchter M, Landis DM, et al. Reproducibility of Transesophageal echocardiography in evaluating aortic atheroma in stroke patients. Echocardiography 2005;22:326–30.

55. Konstadt SN, Reich DL, Kahn R, et al. Transesophageal echocardiography can be used to screen for ascending aortic atherosclerosis. Anesth Analg 1995;81:225–8.

56. Katz ES, Tunick PA, Rusinek H, et al. Protruding aortic atheromas predict stroke in elderly patients undergoing cardiopulmonary bypass: Experience with intraoperative transesophageal echocardiography. J Am Coll Cardiol 1992; 20:70-77

57. Rosenberger P, Shernan SK, Löffler M, et al. The influence of epiaortic ultrasonography on intraoperative surgical management in 6051 cardiac surgical patients. Ann Thorac Surg 2008;85:548–53.

58. Djaiani G, Ali M, Borger MA, et al. Epiaortic scanning modifies planned intraoperative surgical management but not cerebral embolic load during coronary artery bypass surgery. Anesth Analg 2008;106:1611–8.

59. Hangler HB, Nagele G, Danzmayr M, et al. Modification of surgical technique for ascending aortic atherosclerosis: impact on stroke reduction in coronary artery bypass grafting. J Thorac Cardiovasc Surg. 2003:126:391-400.

60. Glas KE, Swaminathan M, Reeves ST, et al. Guidelines for the performance of a comprehensive intraoperative epiaortic ultrasonographic examination: Recommendations of the American Society of Echocardiography and the Society of Cardiovascular Anesthesiologists; endorsed by the Society of Thoracic Surgeons. J Am Soc Echocardiogr 2007;20: 1227–35.

# CHAPTER 13

# Postoperative Management

Minati Choudhury

In the past decade, postoperative management of the patients undergoing vascular surgery has been one of the main end points of several research studies. Despite the fact that success in vascular surgery depends upon careful patient selection, expert technical execution of the operations, and anticipation of complications, optimization of postoperative care is one of the major keys to successful recovery of the patient. Most of the patients undergoing vascular surgery are elderly with worse comorbidities. Severe complications such as myocardial infarction, pneumonia and acute renal failure are observed in about 60% of the patients undergoing open surgical repair of the lesion.[1,2] It is necessary to identify the most appropriate environment for early recognition and management of postoperative complications. The commonly used scoring systems such as American Society of Anesthesiologist (ASA) classifications and The Lee Revised Cardiac Index to quantify postoperative complications are most useful in identifying the low risk patients only.[3] Again appropriate decision making regarding the need for intensive care after surgery are the key to high quality patient care during their postoperative period. Latest data conclude that epidural anesthesia and analgesia improve the postoperative respiratory function compared to general anesthesia and systematic analgesia, with physiotherapy playing a significant role for the postoperative course of recovery.[4] A few recent studies suggested that perioperative *physiotherapy* including deep breathing, early mobilization and endurance training helps preventing postoperative complications such as respiratory dysfunction, ileus or delirium.[5]

## GENERAL PRINCIPLES

a. Intrahospital transport
b. Preparatory phase
c. The transport phase
d. The post-transport stabilization phase

Once surgery is completed patient has to be shifted to the intensive care unit (ICU) or high dependency unit (HDU), a process that inevitably put the critically ill patients at an increased risk of morbidity and mortality, despite the relatively short distance involved. This risk has to be minimized by careful planning, proper team involvement and selection of appropriate equipment for monitoring and maintenance of patients' vital function.

### Preparatory Phase

The ICU/HDU team should be informed in advance about when the patient will be leaving the OR, all necessary drugs, equipment and staff should be ready before moving the patient from the operating room. It is important to ensure that, infusion pumps and transport ventilator batteries should be fully charged, and oxygen cylinder should be full. The anesthetic gases if on, should be discontinued at least 15 minutes before transport to ensure that any resultant hemodynamic changes have occurred before transport begins. It is better to change the infusion rates of intravenous anesthetic agents and opioids in advance, rather than during transport.

### Transport Phase

Shifting of the patient from operating table to the transport trolley is particularly dangerous and every care should be taken to prevent accidental disconnection of drugs, infusion lines and catheters. Once the patient is on the transport trolley adequacy of ventilation, oxygenation and perfusion must be confirmed. Continuous drift of tissue temperature and continued bleeding during post-CPB period may lead to hypotension. Hence, it is imperative that there should be easy access to appropriate intravascular volume and the means to administer them. Chest tubes should be free of clamps and drain collection containers must be placed below the level of the patient.

### Post-Transport Stabilization Phase

On arrival to ICU, transducers should be connected to the monitor, zeroed and recalibrated; and hemodynamic stability to be confirmed. Infusion pumps to be connected to the main supply, and infusion rate of the drugs to be checked. The patient is then transported to ICU ventilator with appropriate ventilator settings made. Chest drains need to be milked and volume status to be reassessed. Finally a complete handover should be made to the ICU team.

### Admission to Intensive Care Unit versus High Dependency Step Down Unit

Transfer of a patient to ICU or HDU depends upon the risk stratification. Patients undergoing an extensive surgical repair, with significant COPD or at increased risk of postoperative myocardial ischemia/bleeding/dialysis are usually managed in ICUs. Patients undergoing less invasive vascular procedures associated with lesser fluid shifts and lower surgical morbidity and can be safely managed in HDU. This is the case with

patients undergoing peripheral arterial bypass, elective repair of infrarenal abdominal aortic aneurysm (AAA) and carotid endarterectomy. ICU is the area of optimal patient management by providing decreased myocardial oxygen demand through expeditious rewarming, elective fluid resuscitation, effective patient analgesia, meticulous control of hemodynamics, and careful monitoring to aid in the early diagnosis and treatment of complications.

### MONITORING DURING POSTOPERATIVE PERIOD

Postoperative vascular surgery patients are at risk of development of abnormal physiology and its consequences even if they have a normal hemodynamic parameter during the preoperative period. Optimal management of patients throughout the postoperative phase requires appropriate clinical assessment and monitoring. In contrast with assessment of emergencies, which focuses on the initial diagnosis and stabilization after the patient has developed a complaint, postoperative care requires pre-emptive management. Regular assessment, selective monitoring and timely documentation are keys to postoperative care. Postoperative distribution hypoxia is a common phenomenon after any major vascular surgery, results from inadequate oxygen delivery to tissues exacerbated by the increased metabolic demands of tissues with resultant multiorgan dysfunction. Indicators of organ perfusion to guide resuscitation includes blood pressure, heart rate, oxygen saturation, central venous pressure,

| Table 13.1: Factors influencing postoperative complications and postoperative care | |
|---|---|
| *Type and extent of surgery* | Major vascular surgeries (thoracoabdominal aneurysms) and patients with longer surgical, CPB and aortic cross clamp time or patients who has undergone deep hypothermic circulatory arrest needs special care and monitoring. This group of patients suffer from more morbidity and mortality compared to these who undergoes simple vascular procedures (e.g. surgery for peripheral vascular diseases) |
| *Age and co morbidities* | Obesity, sleep apnea, Chronic heart failure, chronic obstructive pulmonary disease (COPD), coronary artery disease (CAD) and chronic renal failure are all predictors of increased mortality in surgical vascular patients |
| *Cardiorespiratory functional capacity of the patient* | Perioperative hemodynamic stability have a significant impact on postoperate outcome. Preoperative cardiopulmonary exercise testing (CPET) can be used to triage patients' postoperative care facility, rationalizing the use of critical care beds. Patients with an anaerobic threshold (AT) of <11 ml/kg/minute may benefit from postoperative critical care. |
| *Emergency versus elective surgery* | Emergency operations independently increased perioperative morbidity and mortality risk. These patients may be physiologically and hemodynamically compromised, and therefore at higher risk and need special care and monitoring. |

pulmonary capillary wedge pressure, cardiac output, urine output, blood lactate level, tissue $CO_2$ level, base deficits, mixed venous oxygen level and mixed venous carbon dioxide level. During interpretation of these indicators the trend over time rather than individual measurements are of value.

## Peripheral Pulse

Approximately 25% of all patients after major vascular surgery suffer from limb occlusion either in early or late postoperative period. Limb occlusion appears to be greater in woman, patients with associated occlusive disease and in grafts extending to the femoral artery. In the immediate postoperative period patients may present with absent peripheral pulse/oxygen saturation in the affected limb to the local sign of ischemia.[6] A Doppler examination gives a better clue to the diagnosis. Immediate thrombectomy or lytic therapy with secondary endovascular or open surgical intervention is required in such cases.[7] Standard mechanical ballon thrombectomy is less likely to be successful with endovascular aneurysm repair (EVAR) grafts because of sharp edges produced by stents and concerns related to dislodging or disrupting the sealing zones.

## Electrocardiograph Monitoring (ECG)

Conventional ECG monitoring using five leads, of which one is precordial and most often placed at V5.[8] In a study of 185 patients undergoing vascular surgery, full 12 lead ECG with computerized ST segment analysis and routine measurements up to 72 hour postoperatively showed transient myocardial ischemia in 21% and MI in 6.5%.[9] Leads placed at V3 and V5 were more predictive and the combination of two precordial leads lead to greater than 95% sensitivity when compared to troponin level for postoperative ischemia monitoring. Patients at increased risk of adverse cardiac events following EAVR or open surgical procedure should be considered for measurement of postoperative troponin level even if there is no ECG evidence of ischemia.[10]

## Arterial Pressure Monitoring

Cannulation of peripheral artery provides the direct measurement of blood pressure and blood gas sampling during postoperative period. The most common site for cannulation is radial artery, followed by femoral artery, axillary artery, and less commonly dorsalis pedis and ulnar arteries. Most of the time the radial artery is preferred site because of ease of cannulation and very low incidence of complication. For arch aneurysms, usually left radial or brachial artery is accessed because of the increasingly common use of right axillary artery for cannulation for arterial return while on CPB. At times femoral arterial catheter is placed to compensate for the relatively high incidence of falsely low radial artery pressure during post-CPB period. Complications are common to all sites and include bleeding, hematoma, thrombosis and limb ischemia.[11] One should not forget that systolic and diastolic measurements are affected by the distance of the measuring catheter from the heart, the length and compliance of the tubing, and presence of air bubble in the system. These variables affect systolic and diastolic pressure proportionately in opposite direction and have no net effect on the measurement of (MAP). For this reason measurement of mean arterial pressure MAP is a more accurate reflection of mean aortic pressure.

## Central Venous Pressure (CVP) Monitoring

Central venous pressure evaluation puts light and sense to managing the postoperative patients with intermediate unwanted chest X-ray findings, elevated beta nitriuretic peptide (BNP) levels, to infuse fluids, administer vasoactive drugs and to assess intravascular volume. The most common sites for placement of these catheters in vascular surgery patients are the internal jugular vein (IJV)/subclavian vein and femoral veins.[13] To measure CVP, IJV/subclavian venous catheters must be positioned with catheter tip in the distal segment of SVC. Most distal placement in the RA is associated with potential risk of erosion and cardiac tamponade.

## Temperature Monitoring

Careful monitoring of body temperature is essential following vascular surgery as residual hypothermia during the early postoperative period is associated with an increase risk of myocardial ischemia and morbidity.[14] In comparison to normal surgical patients, vascular surgery cases have a two to three fold greater risk of myocardial ischemia when core temperature is less than 35°C. In a prospective randomized trial, the relative risk of postoperative cardiac morbidity was reduced by 55% when normothermia was achieved by forced air warming system. Even mild hypothermia is associated with a 200–700 percent increase in norepinephrine levels, with generalized vasoconstriction and increase in blood pressure in postoperative patients.[15] Warmed inhaled gases and infused liquids have shown some benefit in warming the patients. The benefit of forced air warming blankets applied to the lower extremities, as opposed to the upper trunk, during prolonged aortic cross clamping is not known.

## Echocardiography

Postoperative transthoracic/transesophageal echo-cardiography (TTE/TEE) is beneficial for assessment of ventricular function, valve function and flow as well as detection of myocardial ischemia. TEE is helpful in guiding hemodynamic management by distinguishing right and left ventricular function and adjusts treatment appropriately, e.g. patients with poor LV function can be benefited from inotropic agent; whereas presence of hyperdynamic ventricle and evidence of tissue hypoxia may indicate the need for fluid challenge and vasopressors.[16] In the presence of normotensive shock, adequate after load reduction with a vasodilator, e.g. nitroglycerine is required. Diagnosis of pericardial tamponade, calculation of ejection fraction and cardiac output is also possible by echocardiography. However, expertise is required for such measurements. Transeso-phageal Doppler has been used to measure the blood flow in descending thoracic aorta; for which a correct positioning is always essential for accurate measure-ment.[17]

## Pulmonary Artery Pressure

Pulmonary artery catheter (PAC) is a useful tool in some cases for cardiac output measurement during postoperative period; however it is generally regarded as inferior to TEE in volume assessment. Postoperative ventricular compromise patients are better managed by PAC by some authors. In patients undergoing arch repair there is a possibility that hypothermia will cause significant stiffening of the catheter which may in turn lead to increased tendency for distal migration and an increase risk of pulmonary artery perforation during the postoperative period. So in general, patients with multiple risk factors who undergo vascular surgery have some benefit from the used of pulmonary artery catheter during perioperative period. However, advancement in echocardiography and noninvasive cardiac output monitoring omitted the use of this invasive monitoring aid which has a higher rate of complication.[18,19]

## Intra-abdominal Pressure

Elevated intra-abdominal pressure (IAP) leading to intra-abdominal hypertension (IAH) and abdominal compartment syndrome (ACS) is one of the causes of mortality especially after surgery on thoraco-abdominal/abdominal aorta. In one of the study high IAH (>15 mmHg) following aneurysm repair was asso-ciated with impaired cardiac, renal and respiratory function during ICU stay.[20-22] Intra-abdominal pressure is a steady state of pressure concealed within the abdominal cavity. For most of the critically ill patients,

an IAP of 5–7 mmHg is considered to be normal. According to most of the authors it is directly related to body mass index. The normal range in most of the time is not applicable for all the patients with increased abdominal girth that develop slowly may have higher baseline IAPs, e.g. obese individuals can have IAP of 10–15 mmHg without any adverse sequel. Elevated IAP is poorly defined but as the pressure increases, a spectrum of physiological effects is observed. IAH may develop into ACS. The later has been identified as an independent predictor for multiorgan failure during the postoperative course. Therapeutic intervention based on IAP measurements, such as restoration of volume status and abdominal decompression, may be important in reversing ongoing organ failure and preventing further harm. Elevated abdominal perfusion pressure (APP) [calculated as mean arterial pressure (MAP) minus IAP] reduces blood flow to the abdominal viscera. A target of APP of atleast 60 mmHg is correlated with improved survival from IAH and ACS. IAH is defined as a sustained intra-abdominal pressure of ≥12 mmHg. Acute IAH (elevation of IAP over hours) usually occurs as the result of intra abdominal hemorrhage and needs immediate attention. ACS is defined as a sustained IAP > 20 mmHg (with or without an increase in APP) that is associated with new organ dysfunction. Patients with IAP below 10 mmHg generally do not have ACS, while patients with an IAP >25 mmHg usually have ACS. Patients with an IAP of 10–25 mmHg may or may not have ACS depending upon individual variables such as blood pressure and abdominal wall compliance. Higher systemic blood pressure may maintain organ perfusion when IAP is increased. A conscious patient may have light headedness malaise, weakness, dyspnea, abdominal bloating or abdominal pain; where as a patient on ventilator may have a tensely distended abdomen with progressive oliguria, hypotension, tachy-cardia, elevated jugular venous pressure, peripheral edema, acute pulmonary decompression. There may be evidence of hypotension including lactic acidosis. Once the diagnosis is confirmed management initially consists of careful observation and supportive care. In some cases surgical decompression is required.

## Monitoring Mesenteric Perfusion

It is especially done during the presence of risk factors those can enhance the incidence of myocardial ischemia, e.g. supracoeliac cross clamp, IAH, atheromatous disease of superior mesenteric artery, and massive vasopressures requirements. An elevated arterial lactate and liver enzymes can provide some clue regarding compromised mesenteric perfusion.

## Neurological Monitoring

CNS metabolism and function varies and influenced by many physiological and pathological factors during the postoperative period. Regarding CNS metabolism and function monitoring, a minimal subdivision has to be respected; means the cerebral cortex and deeper structures are independent entities, each with a high level of differentiation and complexity. Multimodality monitoring is more recommended in postoperative practice and includes the more judicious combination of parameters from different origins (electrical, oxygen consumption and supply, and blood perfusion) to give the best possible answer for the specific settings. Many times postoperative neurologic monitoring is a continuation of that of the intraoperative period.

Glasgow Comma Scale status and transcranial Doppler monitoring is essential after carotid end-arteriectomy.

### Monitoring of Cerebrospinal Fluid Pressure (CSF) and Volumes

Patients who undergone thoracic abdominal aortic aneurysm (TAAA) repair, TEVAR patients with previous abdominal aortic aneurysm (AAA) repair, extensive stent coverage below T9, occlusion of left subclavian artery or hypogastric artery have the risk of development of spinal cord ischemia during the postoperative period and the need for CSF pressure and volume monitoring.

Finally, regarding brain and spinal cord metabolism and function, continued developments in monitoring methods provides more valuable information about the potential problem. The development of a real effective neuromonitoring, combining one monitoring modality of each family (electrophysiological, microdialysis, brain oxygen and cerebral blood flow) could be the final solution to adequate postoperative neurologic monitoring of such group of patients.

### Functional Hemodynamic Monitoring for Fluid Optimization

In the postoperative period of vascular surgery static markers of preload (CVP and PAOP) are poor predictors of fluid responsiveness when the patient is on positive pressure ventilation. The magnitude of cyclical changes can occur in the right and left ventricular stroke volumes are the predictors of the circulation to the intravenous fluids. The fluid responsiveness can be determined by using stroke volume variation (SVV), systolic pressure variation (SPV) and pulse pressure variation (PPV).

## Monitoring of Biomarkers for Assessment of Tissue Injury

Cardiac troponin (cTn) and brain natriuretic peptide (BNP) are two commonly estimated biomarkers during the postoperative period. A close relationship between the magnitude of of changes in postoperative cTn, and duration of ischemia on continuous ECG monitoring and postoperative mortality is observed by many authors. An increased postoperative BNP concentrations

**Table 13.2:** Postoperative complications those need prophylaxis/special care and strict monitoring

| Surgery | Complications |
|---|---|
| **Peripheral vascular disease** | ■ Myocardial infarction<br>■ Infection<br>■ Stroke<br>■ Respiratory<br>■ Bleeding<br>■ Shock |
| **Open repair (aortic aneurysm)** | ■ Myocardial infarction<br>■ Arrhythmias<br>■ Bleeding<br>■ Injury to the bowel<br>■ Limb ischemia<br>■ Embolus to other parts of the body<br>■ Infection of the graft<br>■ Lung problems<br>■ Kidney damage<br>■ Spinal cord injury |
| **Endovascular repair (EAVR) (aortic aneurysm)** | ■ Damage to surrounding blood vessels, organs, or other structures by instruments<br>■ Kidney damage<br>■ Limb ischemia<br>■ Groin wound infection<br>■ Groin hematoma<br>■ Bleeding—endoleak (continual leaking of blood out of the graft and into the aneurysm sac with potential rupture)<br>■ Spinal cord injury |
| **Carotid artery surgery** | ■ Wound hematoma<br>■ Stroke<br>■ Myocardial infarction<br>■ Cranial nerve injury<br>■ Hypertension<br>■ Hypotension<br>■ Hyperperfusion syndrome<br>■ Intracerebral hemorrhage<br>■ Seizures<br>■ Recurrent stenosis |
| **Major amputation** | ■ Myocardial infarction<br>■ Infection<br>■ Stroke<br>■ Respiratory<br>■ Bleeding<br>■ Shock |

are associated with cardiac death, nonfatal MI and major cardiac events during postoperative period following major vascular surgery. The optimal threshold for postoperative cTn and BNP concentrations have not been identified, and false positive may occur with several conditions including ventricular failure, diastolic dysfunction, pulmonary embolism, pulmonary hypertension, arrhythmias and sepsis.

## GASTROINTESTINAL COMPLICATION

Intra abdominal complications are rare but potentially lethal especially after elective abdominal aortic aneurysm repair and carries an overall mortality of 40–45%. Ischemic injury to the gut is a major phenomenon and may lead to hemorrhagic infarction and gangrene of a variable extent of bowel following any major vascular surgery. Prolonged CPB and aortic cross clamp time along with intraoperative surgical complications can cause low cardiac output and hypo perfusion of mesenteric vascular bed and thereby ischemic injury to the gut. Ischemic reperfusion injury, postoperative persistent acidosis and microembolization too have an important role in the development of major abdominal complications after vascular surgery (Box 13.1).

### Ischemia of the Mesenteric Vasculature

Mesentric vascular ischemia leading to infarction of several parts of the gut can occur following both open repair as well as thoracic endovascular repair (TEVAR) of thoracic aortic aneurysm. Acute ischemia of the mesenteric vasculature is common in case of open repair where as TEVAR patients are more prone for chronic mesenteric ischemia.[24,25] Inspite of the fact that, this

| Box 13.1 | Gastrointestinal complications |
| --- | --- |

1. Mesenteric vascular ischemia and gangrene of the gut
2. Small bowel obstruction
3. Pancreatitis
4. Colonic ischemia
5. Intestinal ischemia
6. Aorto-esophageal fistula
7. Gastrointestinal bleeding secondary to aorto enteric fistula
8. Aorto-dudonal fistula
9. Acute cholecystitis
10. Mechanical obstruction of the gut
11. Chyloperitonium
12. Colonic infarction and necrosis
13. Upper gastrointestinal bleeding
14. Ascitis
15. Ischemic colititis
16. Liver dysfunction

situation is a consequence to low cardiac output; use of vasopressures in this condition increases splanchic ischemia especially in patients with pre-existing occlusive vascular disease of the mesenteric arteries. Prolonged CPB, intraoperative thrombo embolism, pre existing mesenteric vascular disease and reperfusion injury to the gut are the major contributing factors. Ischemic reperfusion injury during major vascular surgery has a significant relevance in producing ischemic injury to the gut by production of oxygen metabolites and activation of polymorphonuclear neutrophils. Ischemic reperfusion injury also diminishes the barrier function of the gut wall and causes an increase in intestinal permeability.[26] Gut ischemia may lead to hemorrhagic infarction and gangrene of the bowel to a large extent limited by the area supplied by the artery involved. Colonic infarction is difficult to diagnose at times because of patients poor physical status. Confirmatory diagnosis can be made by colonoscopy. The overall mortality is quite large and can be as high as 89% in one of the series. Even if the incidence of colonic ischemia is very high, there is no definite method available to predict the occurrence in advance.[27] Measurement of D-lactate level tried by a group of authors, was not found to be reliable. Use of T-stat device which is an optical real time sensor, found to be useful to measure colonic ischemia in a case report.[28] Conservative treatment with local vasodilatation often helps. Non-respondent may undergo specialized approach that considers surgical and endovascular options for better outcome.[29, 30]

### Early Small Bowel Obstruction

Small bowel obstruction after abdominal aortic aneurysm surgery is not as common as that during other intestinal surgeries. However, this can be more frequent than other gastrointestinal complications like intestinal ischemia and pancreatitis in patients undergoing surgery on thoracoabdominal aorta. The management principles for these patients are similar to those for early postoperative bowel obstruction after any gastrointestinal procedure. At times these patients need a reoperation to relieve the bowel obstruction if the symptom persists beyond two weeks.

### Acute Pancreatitis

Acute pancreatitis can develop after thoracoabdominal/ abdominal aortic aneurysm repair. Potential intra-abdominal infection, pancreatic injury during AAA repair and infection of the retroperitoneal graft materials are the potential causes.[31] The therapeutic options range from a restrictive regime to radical necrosectomy and multiviseral resection.

## Chylous Ascites and Chyloperitonium

*Chylous ascites and chyloperitonium* are rare and fatal complications following abdominal aortic surgery.[32] Due to their anatomical relation with the abdominal aorta, cistern chyli injury is common following abdominal aortic aneurysm surgery than the other surgeries. Paracentesis, improvement in total parenteral nutrition provides the possibility of an extended period of oral starvation that reduces the lymphatic flow from the leaking gut. Medium chain triglyceride is generally accepted as reducing the production of lymphatics. If all conservative measures fail, surgical exploration is indicated. Placements of a peritonevenous shunt/ transfixing the damaged lymph vessels, and omentumplasty are the few described options with considerable good results. Direct ligation of the leak should be reserved for the patients not responding to treatment. The incidence of *acute acalculus cholecystitis* after abdominal aortic aneurysm repair is 0.3–18% with mortality of 50% in one series.[33, 34]

## Aortoesophageal and Aortobronchial Fistula

*Aortoesophageal and aortobronchial fistula* can occur later in postoperative period following aneurysm repair.[35,36] Though rare; these are devastating complications and needs immediate attention once diagnosis is confirmed. Endoluminal repair of thoracic aortic disease is associated with more risk of development of these fistulae. In one series the authors noted that the occurrence of perioperative complications after endovascular repair, particularly renal dysfunction and respiratory failure are significant predictors of development of these complications. Endoleak in the residual aneurysmal sac, erosion of the stent graft through the aorta and ischemic necrosis of the esophageal/bronchial wall resulting from stent coverage of the feeding arteries are the possible causes. A closer follow-up of these patients during postoperative period may help to recognize aortoesophageal/aorto-duodenal/aorto-bronchial fistula early; although there is no evidence that early detection can improve the prognosis. Inspite of the fact that both surgical and endovascular treatment are associated with high mortality but conservative treatment is not a viable option for these complications. Oesophageal stent grafting/oesophageal reconstruction, mediastinal drainage or even endoscopic uses of fibrin glue at the level of the fistula are some proposed management protocol for these patients.

## Postoperative Liver Dysfunction

*Postoperative liver dysfunction* can occur following aortic aneurysm repair. Prolonged surgical time, preoperative hepatic injury and massive blood transfusion are the major contributors. The management protocol is routine as per any other patient having postoperative hepatic dysfunction.[37]

## CARDIOVASCULAR DYSFUNCTION AND PHARMACOLOGIC SUPPORT

### Hypertension

Hypertension is common after vascular surgery and mainly caused by pre-existing hypertension, residual hypothermia following CPB, gastric/bladder distension, hypervolemia, pain and agitation.[38] High blood pressure (BP) increases myocardial oxygen consumption and can cause myocardial ischemia. It may contribute to bleeding through vascular anastomosis. At times a common cause of hypertension is simply neglecting to restart postoperative antihypertensive agents. Sedation, analgesia and rewarming mostly resolve many cases of mildly elevated blood pressure. After all possible causes have been addressed, drug treatment may be considered. In general BP treatment targets should be centered on systolic BP (SBP) value 20 mm Hg above or below the preoperative pressure. Deviation in MAP >20% from the preoperative value should be also treated. Several agents may be used; however vasodilators like nitroglycerine and sodium nitroprusside are the most preferred one. Beta-blockers, angiotensin enzyme inhibitors and calcium channel blockers to be used once the patient is non respondent to routine vasodilators.[39] Postoperative hypertensive crisis is not uncommon in these patients which is defined by an elevation of systolic BP to >179 mmHg and diastolic BP >109 mmHg. As these patients are prone to end organ damage, the goal is to reduce the diastolic BP below 109 mmHg over a period of 30–60 minutes by ultra short acting/short acting anti-hypertensive agent. Esmolol, labetolol and amlodipine are the commonly used agents.[39] Hypertensive patients mostly develop natriuresis, which causes fluid depletion hence fluid should be administered along with antihypertensive agents. Post-aortic surgery systolic BP should be reduced below 120 mm Hg within 5–10 minutes to prevent rupture of suture line.

### Hypotension

Common causes of hypotension after vascular surgery are hypovolemia, bleeding, cardiac dysfunction and a diffuse vasodilatory state with/without sepsis.[40,41] Hypotension needs immediate attention as it is associated with an increased risk of multiorgan failure, possible renal failure and graft thrombosis. The two management strategies for hypovolemia include administration of fluid/blood depending upon the deficit and vasoactive agent. A surgical cause should always be excluded. It should be always suspected if the patient requires greater than expected volume of fluid resuscitation during the postoperative period. The benefit from the fluid challenge should always be noted. If the patient is on the flat portion of the Frank-Straling curve, fluid loading increase tissue edema and worsen the situation. A large pulse pressure-stroke volume ratio (>10–15%) is the indication of hypovolemia and should be addressed. In case patient is non responsive to fluid challenge cardiac output should be optimized by administration of vasopressors. Ultrashort acting vasopressures like phenylephrine, dopamine, adrenaline or non-adrenaline are commonly used. Dobutamine is reserved to enhance contractility. Non-respondant cases may be given vasopressin. Intra-aortic ballon counter pulsation may be a necessary aid when pharmacologic means fail.

## Arrhythmia

It occurs mainly in patients with structural heart disease.[42,43] Common triggers for postoperative arrhythmia are similar to any other surgical patients, e.g. hypoxia, hypercarbia, acidosis, electrolyte abnormalities and myocardial ischemia. Treatment must focus on predisposing factors, and goal should be hemodynamic stabilization, control of ventilator response and restoration of rhythm. Tachyarrhythmias are most common and the usual once are sinus tachycardia, trial fibrillation, ectopic tachycardia, junctional tachycardia and ventricular tachycardia. The incidence of supraventicular tachycardia is 4–10% after abdominal surgery. Tachyarrhythmia especially atrial fibrillation is associated with increased 30 days postoperative mortality, increased ICU stay and increased hospital stay. It is always important to correct the underlying cause. Tachyarrhythmia if sustained in a hemodynamically stable patient, beta blockers to be used. In monitored setting, intravenous amiodarone can be given. In hemodynamically stable patient, with nodal reentrant tachycardia, adenosine 6–12 mg intravenous can be effective. Hemodynamically unstable patients should be electrically cardioverted. Ventricular tachyarrhythmias are ominous especially in the presence of coronary artery disease and needs immediate attention. In addition to treating the predisposing factors, electrical cardioversion and intravenous xylocard/amiodarone are effective. Brady arrhythmia following vascular surgery is not diagnostic challenge and the management options are straightforward. Those associated with sinus node dysfunction are mostly due to increased vagal tone and myocardial ischemia. No treatment is required in the absence of hemodynamic stability. Unstable patients may need bolus of atropine. Non-respondent patients get benefit from temporary pacemaker.

## Myocardial Infarction

Postoperative cardiac ischemia is not uncommon following vascular surgery.[44] Chest pains of ischemic origin is difficult to diagnose because of due to incision and are influenced by the concomitant use of analgesia and anesthetics. Because one-third of the patients after vascular surgery have ST segment changes, it is again difficult to diagnose myocardial ischemia from ECG. Up to 48% of ischemic events occur in the first 48–72 hours after surgery. Regardless, the presence of such changes correlates with an approximately 9–16 fold increased the risk of MI and death. Elevated level of myocardial enzymes (CK-MB and Troponin-I) following vascular surgery associated with increased mortality at 6 months. ST–segment MI mostly occurs in patients with altheromatous coronary arteries.[45,46] Prevention of tachycardia and its related factors (hypoxia, hypovolemia, pain, etc.) is crucial in prevention of myocardial ischemia. Once diagnosed; rapid resuscitation of the patient is done with supplemental oxygen, timely use of beta blockers, after load reduction agents, antiplatelet drugs, anticoagulants and percutaneous coronary intervention. Postoperatively, fibrinolysis is a relative contraindication, but this decision must be individualized to the patients according to the extent of surgery and time after operation. In the presence of clinically significant ischemia or cardiogenic stock, urgent revascularization is indicated. Beta blockers should be continued/started unless patients are hypotensive or have bradycardia or the presence of congestive cardiac failure. Prompt treatment of ischemia reduces postoperative increase in cardiac troponin level and six month mortality.

**Non ST-Segment MI:** It is characterized by presence of cardiac biomarkers denoting the presence of myocardial injury in the absence of ST elevation in ECG. Mortality risk in these patients directly related to the cardiac troponin level. These patients are usually managed by optimizing myocardial oxygen delivery and demand and preventing reinfarction and death. Supplemental oxygen, and nitroglycerine infusion is essential to decrease cardiac preload and after load. Administration of ACE inhibitors, beta blockers and acetylsalicylic acid has a role. Use of unfractionated heparin is also associated with mortality benefit.

*Monitoring methods for identification of postoperative myocardial ischemia*

1. **ECG**
   a. Changes in ST segment is the most sensitive indicator of early diagnosis of myocardial ischemia.

b. Computerized ST segment trend analysis is better than visual interpretation for detection of postoperative myocardial ischemia. Accepted ST segment changes used to detect myocardial ischemia is >0.1 mV measured 80 ms from J point. Postoperative ST segment changes with a prolonged duration (>6 minutes per episode/> 2 hrs cumulative length) are independent predictors of postoperative cardiac events.

2. **TEE:** Provides direct assessment of changes in ventricular wall motion, which may be related to ischemia. Changes in endocardial wall motion occur very fast in the setting of ischemia and at times occur even before ischemic changes are seen on ECG. The transgastric mid papillary short axis and multiple mid esophageal views are considered to be the best for detection of abnormal ventricular wall motion and thickening due to myocardial ischemia.

3. **Cardiac enzymes:** Elevated preoperative cardiac troponin level is a major predictor of postoperative MI according to a few reports and needs more evidence to support. The role of elevated cardiac troponin during ongoing ischemia is well established and should not be forgotten.

4. **Pulmonary artery pressure:** If a PA catheter in situ, the changes in pulmonary artery wave form and pulmonary arterial occlusion pressure can be sensitive indicator of myocardial ischemia. An ischemic event leads to prominent A and C waves, increased LVEDP, and increase in pulmonary artery pressure.

In general, many questions relating to perioperative pharmacological therapy to prevent postoperative MI (PMI) following vascular surgery remain unanswered. Careful perioperative monitoring for ischemia, a low threshold for treating and preventing tachycardia while avoiding hypotension, decreased cardiac output, and/or cardiac decompensation help prevent PMI. Coronary intervention is rarely indicated as the first line of treatment, and antithrombotic therapy may exacerbate bleeding. Future studies are needed to determine which patients with require intensified postoperative surveillance, medical therapy, and/or coronary intervention to improve long-term survival following vascular surgery.

## POSTOPERATIVE BLEEDING AND TRANSFUSION MANAGEMENT

Fluid administration in the postoperative period is tailored to the individual patient. A balance should be made between adequate tissue perfusion by volume replacement at surgery and during postoperative period, and postoperative volume overload. The consequence of hypovolemia as well as hypervolemia has to be kept in mind during volume supplementation. The medical cause of postoperative bleeding following major vascular surgery has to be identified during volume infusion. Residual heparinization is common post-surgery and usually occurs when insufficient protamine is used or heparinized pump blood is transfused following surgery. Decrease coagulation factor can occur from activation and dilution in the CPB circuit. The most basic principles of management of transfusion due medical bleeding are:

- Rule out surgical bleeding
- Measure the hemoglobin and hematocrit
- Diagnose underlying medical cause by coagulation tests
- Identify the sign of adequate perfusion to the vital organs
- Restore clotting factors to normal by means of medications (tranexaminic acid, aminocaproic acid, recombinant factor VII), normothermia during the transfusion of blood and blood products.

### Blood Transfusion

Considerable variability has persisted regarding this subject when clinical practice is concerned.[47] A recent randomized controlled trial has already demonstrated that restrictive perioperative transfusion does not result in inferior clinical outcome after cardiac surgery. However, the universal rule is blood has to be replaced with blood to prevent anemia related injury to vital organs is no longer validated. Liberal blood transfusion following vascular surgery is no longer supported because of high rate 30 days adverse events in these group of patients (death, myocardial infarction, renal failure, infection). Transfusion above a hemoglobin of 9 gm/dL is not advocated by most of the authors. Transfusion burden may in future be interpreted as a quality indicator in vascular surgery.[48,49]

The standard guidelines for red cell transfusion are available on several websites such as http//transfusion guidelines.org.uk and all follow the general recommendations given in Box 13.2.

| Box 13.2 | Guide lines for red cell transfusion· |
|---|---|

- No transfusion if Hb >10 gm/dl
- Transfuse if Hb <7 gm/dl
- Hb 8–10 gm/dl, is safe if euvolaemic, even in patients with cardiopulmonary disease
- Transfuse to the symptomatic anemic patients

## Fluid Transfusion

If large volume is required for volume transfusion, the usual recommendation is that, a balanced solution such as Lactated Ringers to be administered instead of normal saline to reduce the development of iatrogenic hyperchloremic metabolic acidosis. Most of the centers follow restricted fluid management regime to reduce postoperative morbidity. Commonly, most authors favor administrating intravenous fluids in the last operative period at a low maintenance rate of 75–100 ml/hr and giving small boluses' of crystalloid (500–1000 ml) as needed, with titration to blood pressure increased heartrate, or low urine output. Colloids are commonly used for fluid resuscitation because they have the theoretical benefit of expanding intravascular volume and because their osmotic activity reduces third spacing. However, there appears to be no survival benefit when using albumin in severely ill patients, as well as no difference among the difference types of colloid use.[50]

## Transfusion of Blood Products

*Platelets:* The decision to transfuse platelet concentrate must not be based exclusively on platelet count, but must also take into account the patients clinical condition, in particular fever above 38.5°C, presence of coagulation disorders, prolonged CPB ongoing oozing. Mean dose of platelet for each transfusion is about $3 \times 10''$ platelets (Platelet concentrate from aphaeresis or platelet concentrate from pool of 5–8 platelet concentrate from whole blood or from buffy coat pools.

Calculation of the dose of platelets to transfuse:

Platelet dose ($\times 10^{11}$) = (P × BV × 1.5)/100

P = desired platelet increment ($\times 10^{9/L}$)

BV = Patients blood volume (L) body surface area in $m^2 \times 2.5$

1.5 = correction factor.

Splenic sequestration, nonhemolytic transfusion reactions (shivering, fever, urticaria, sepsis may occur due to platelet transfusion and should be taken care.

## Fresh Frozen Plasma (FFP)

The main indication for transfusion of FFP is correction of deficiencies of clotting factors for which a specific concentrate is not available, in patients with ongoing bleeding. The recommended initial dose of FFP is 10–15 ml/kg of body weight. A maximum dose up to 30 ml/kg can be administered depending on the patients' clinical situation and laboratory parameters. The most inappropriate indication for using FFP in postoperative vascular surgery patients is as a blood volume expander. The absolute contraindications are:

documented intolerance to plasma or its components and congenital deficiency of immunoglobin (IgA) in the presence of anti IgA antibodies. Adverse reaction to FFP can happen, which can be manifested in the form of mild allergic reaction or severe anaphylaxis, citrate toxicity circulatory overload.

## Cryoprecipitate

Its can be givenn in the presence of severe hypofibrinogenemia despite treatment with FFP, and in the presence of clinically relevant chest tube drainage.[51]

## Adverse Events due to Hyperglycemia and Glycemic Control

The prevalence of diabetes and postoperative hyperglycemia is high among vascular surgery patients. Although the potential benefit of close glycemic control on incidence of long term complications of hyperglycemia has been known for sometime, it has been increasingly clear that acute hyperglycemia can have short term detrimental effects on postoperative patients. Krinsley in one of his retrospective review demonstrated that hospital mortality was directly related to the mean glucose value and nearly doubled between those with mean glucose level of 80–99 mg/dl and those with a mean glucose level of 140–159 mg/dl.[52] Thirty percent of patients presenting for vascular surgery are diabetics, and these patients have an average length of stay in hospital that is 3.5 days longer in comparison with the nondiabetic patient. Studies of glucose levels on the first postoperative day following peripheral vascular surgery demonstrate that they are an independent risk factor for infection and graft failure. Postoperative hyperglycemia occurs in 21 to 34% of patients within 72 hours of surgery. It has been shown that every 40 mg/dl increase in postoperative glucose measurement leads to a 30% increased risk of postoperative infection and longer length of stay.[53]

Glycemic control in the preoperative period has been variably managed for decades. Perioperative management has followed the trend of under-management of hyperglycemia in hospitalized patients in general.[54] Multiple factors contribute to practice inertia regarding perioperative hyperglycemia, including: variable study results; hyperglycemia being a secondary concern to other surgical conditions; overwhelming fear of hypoglycemia; and persistent use of ineffective sliding-scale coverage based on historical practice patterns. Sliding-scale insulin coverage has been discounted as an effective management technique to treat hyperglycemia, but preoperative use remains common. Harbin et al in one of their retrospective single center study demonstrated that a structured and proactive approach to management of hyperglycemia in vascular surgical patient is more effective in term of reduced mean daily blood glucose and severe hyperglycemic episodes and safer (no increase in incidence of hypoglycemia).[54]

Postoperative management of vascular surgery patients with diabetes or stress induced hyperglycemia should be based on defined guidelines. The American Association of Clinical Endocrinologists and American Diabetes Association issued a consensus statement in 2005 regarding inpatient glycemic control, and defined hyperglycemia as a blood glucose value greater than 140 mg/dl and hypoglycemia as a blood glucose value less than 70 mg/dl. Treatment of hyperglycemia in the ICU should begin with an intravenous insulin infusion with a starting threshold no higher than 180 mg/dl, although some benefit may be realized with lower target levels.[55]

In the non-ICU patient population, premeal glucose targets should be less than 140 mg/dl in conjunction with random blood glucose levels less than 180 mg/dl. Scheduled subcutaneous administration of insulin is preferred for achieving and maintaining glycemic control in non-ICU patients. The three recommended components of therapy include a basal, nutritional, and supplemental (correction) element to the insulin therapy. Attention should focus on eliminating sliding-scale insulin coverage, which has been proved to be ineffective.

Supplemental (correction) insulin dosing should be used to treat blood glucose levels that are off-target between the scheduled insulin. An insulin infusion may become necessary to provide tighter control for patients who remain hyperglycemic despite close attention to dosing in the 3-component format. The use of oral noninsulin agents to treat blood glucose is not indicated for hospitalized patients because of the potential complications. Greater attention need to be focused on perioperative glycemic control to optimize outcomes. Hospital-based improvement processes focused exclusively on inpatient glycemic control are cost-effective and should be replicated at more institutions. Physician and nurse champions, staff education, protocols, order sets, and system based improvement processes are needed to combat this persistent issue.

No randomized trials specifically addressing the monitoring and treatment of postoperative hyperglycemia during major vascular surgery have been performed. Therefore, results of studies in comparable patient groups usually translated for the management of current population. The usual advice is moderate tight glucose control with a target blood glucose level of 110 to 140 mg/dl could be more beneficial. In addition, there is an increased risk of both hyperglycemia and the prevention of hypoglycemia during major vascular surgery.

## RENAL COMPLICATIONS AND MANAGEMENT

Among the renal problems acute renal failure (ARF), remains as a major complication after extensive vascular surgery. Because TAAs involve variable parts of aorta, repair of such aneurysms, with or without adjuncts, is fraught with potential complications of severe ischemia to the spinal cord, kidneys and other intraoperative organs.[56] The total interruption of blood flow can result in postoperative ARF necessitating dialysis. Even if the incidence of this complication has fallen over time; it still remains as a major cause of mortality in these groups of patients. The term acute renal failure is used to describe an abrupt rise in serum creatinine and/or blood urea nitrogen (BUN) with or without oliguria (urine output <400 ml/day). The incidence of ARF is highest in ruptured AAA (20–29%) and lowest in infrarenal AAA (0–13.9%).[57,58] The occurrence of ARF increases with the addition of the following inciting factors: urgent or emergency surgery, proximal aortic repair, preoperative renal dysfunction, adverse intraoperative and postoperative events and co-morbidities (e.g. diabetes, hepatic disorder or coronary artery disease). The mortality of ARF requiring renal replacement therapy after repair of intact or ruptured AAA in 58–86% and likely represents the mortality list associated with ARF as a part of multiorgan dysfunction.

Kidney serves as a dominant site for maintenance of normal intravascular volume and composition. Under normovolumic unstressed conditions, the kidney receive approximately 25% of the cardiac output based on a cardiac output of 5 L/minute. Given the fact that the glomeruli filter 20% of the renal plasma flow and that the normal 24 hour urinary output for a 70 kg man is <1.8 L, the kidney's tabular system must reabsorb more than 99% of the 180 L/day of plasma to maintain the homeostasis. Moreover, the initial composition of the ultrafiltrate is the electrolyte and solute concentration of the plasma. Therefore, electrolytes and other solutes such as glucose must also be almost totally absorbed.

A major fluid shift associated with vascular surgery, lead to inappropriate fluid and electrolyte administration and subsequent risk of ARF during the postoperative period. The usual causes of fluid shifts include tissue trauma during surgical dissection, hemodynamic response to arterial clamping, and operative blood loss. The movement of water and electrolytes from the intravascular to the extravascular space normally takes place at the precapillary level due to increase hydrostatic pressure. The reentry of fluid into the intravascular space in the distal capillaries results from the oncotic pressure gradient of the intravascular proteins. Surgical dissection and disruption of lymphatic channels combined with inflammatory mediators causing alterations in tissue perfusion results in increased capillary membrane permeability to albumin. Reduced plasma albumin concentration leads to decrease water reabsorption into the intravascular space. The resulting decreased intravascular volume cause activation of neuroendocrine mechanisms that decrease renal excretion of sodium and free water. In addition ischemia reperfusion injury and/or shock secondary to blood loss causes changes in the cellular transmembrane potential with movement of sodium and water into intracellular space from extravascular space. The normal response to decrease intravascular volume is mobilization of extracellular fluid. Because of the increased oncotic pressure after vascular surgery, the extravascular fluid in less available for expansion of the intravascular space. Finally anesthesia may cause decrease in renal blood flow through reduction in effective blood volume and reduced MAP. The net result of these mechanisms is potential for renal hypoperfusion and ARF.[58] Table 13.3 depicts the potential causes of ARF following vascular surgery.

Presence of hypovolemia and extravascular fluid shift can lead to determination of intravascular volume and electrolyte difficult which is again a major determinant of postoperative ARF. The primary hormonal regulators of fluid and electrolyte balance are aldosterone, cortisol, vasopressin and angiotensin. However, the intractions between insulin, epinephrine, plasma glucose concentration, acid–base balance of plasma, and other resulting from inadequate replacement of intraoperative or postoperative fluid losses. Less commonly, it is caused by reduction in cardiac performance triggering neurohormonal mechanisms that lead to increased loss of sodium and water.[58,59]

In general, these two causes of reduced renal function are clinically distinguishable. Hypovolemia is associated with flat neck veins, dry mucous membranes, and reduced pulmonary artery end-diastolic wedge pressure whereas renal dysfunction from poor cardiac performance is manifest by distended neck veins, clinical fluid overload and elevated pulmonary artery wedge pressure. ARF patients with hypovolemia are resuscitated with isotonic crystalloid (along with blood and blood products if required), while those with ARF of cardiogenic origin require improvement in myocardial performance (management of preload and afterload). Most of the patients undergoing vascular surgery has associated coronary artery disease and improved ventricular systolic and diastolic function. Distinction between ARF of hypovolumic/cardiogenic origin is difficult in these groups of patients. These patients have raised base line total blood volume with associated higher central filling pressures. A normal or low normal filling pressure in this condition may actually reflect relative hypovolemia.

In patients with diastolic dysfunction normal or low normal filling pressures may actually reflect relative hypovolumia. In this situation, maintenance of a constant infusion of both after load-reducing and inotropic agents along with cautiously administration of small boluses of isotonic crystalloid while monitoring cardiac output, pulmonary artery wedge pressure and right ventricular end diastolic volume of urine volume is negligible once filling pressures, begin to rise diuretic therapy may be required. The frequent presence of ventricular dysfunction in patients undergoing vascular reconstruction requires that measures of cardiac function and filling pressures be established before starting diuretic or isotropic therapy.

Renal parechymal dysfunction caused by injury of renal tubules by ischemia or toxins. The common causes of renal ischemia after vascular surgery include suprarenal aortic cross clamping and systemic inflammatory response associated with multisystem to set organ dysfunction, hypovolemia, shock or atheroembolism. Aminoglycoside therapy, myoglobinuria, and radiological contrasts are the common causes of toxic injury in patients with vascular reconstruction.

Postrenal dysfunction is an uncommon cause of renal dysfunction after vascular surgery. The usual site of obstruction is at urethra or urinary catheter or rarely at ureter. Traumatic catheter insertion/hematuria may lead to catheter obstruction. Abrupt decline in urine output occurs in this situation which can lead to ARF. Immediate catheter irrigation/replacement has to be done in such cases. Iatrogenic injury to ureter, extrinsic compression of ureter by a graft limb/fibrotic reaction to surgery can lead to ARF during postoperative period.

**Table 13.3:** Potential causes of ARF following vascular surgery

| Prerenal | Renal parenhymal | Postrenal |
|---|---|---|
| Nephrotoxic drugs | Low cardiac output | Catheter kinking |
| Acute tabular necrosis | Increase intravascular space | Catheter clot |
| Radiological contrast | Septic shock | Bladder clot |

These conditions can be diagnosed by renal ultrasound and confirmed by retrograde urography. Therapy may require placement of ureteral stents or percutaneous nephrostomy. Patients with prostatic hypertrophy or with an epidural catheter for pain control may have acute urinary retention leading to obstruction uropathy leading to removal of a bladder catheter difficult. To avoid urinary retention in such cases 6-12 hour time is allowed to elapse after epidural analgesia is discontinued prior to removal or urinary catheters.

Vascular surgery complicated by sepsis, myocardial dysfunction, or reperfusion injury may cause renal ischemia leading to ARF. When it is a part of the systemic inflammatory response syndrome, ARF may be mediated by increases in proinflammatory mediators such as endotoxin, tumor necrosis factor, interleukin (1L-1), 1L-6, 1L-8, prostaglandins, or leukotrienes. Recovery of renal function is dependent upon maintenance of adequate renal function and requires prompt elimination of the septic focus and improvement in left ventricular performance.

Hypotension secondary to blood loss, myocardial dysfunction or sepsis can also diminish renal blood flow and incite acute ischemic injury. Myoglobinuria is an important cause of ARF in patients undergoing vascular surgery. A prolonged period of muscle ischemia in these patients leads to myoglobin release from the ischemic muscle, which subsequently cause direct tubular injury and abnormal renal blood flow. Myoglobinuria is suggested when the urine is dipstick-positive for blood but no red cells are present on microscopic analysis. Once diagnosed, myoglobinuria induced renal injury may be ameliorated alkalizing the urine with sodium bicarbonate and maximizing the urine output with crystalloid infusion and mannitol administration. Endovascular approaches to elective AAA repair may have lower rates of postoperative acute renal failure although the literature varies on this issue owing to differences in study design.

## Diagnosis and management of postoperative renal dysfunction

It is always ideal to prevent the development of ARF with some preoperative and intraoperative measures especially in the patients who are particularly at more risk. The diagnosis of ARF is based on an acute rise of serum creatinine and BUN with or without a concomitant decrease in urine output. However, creatinine and BUN are relatively insensitive markers of excretory renal function. The glomerular filtration rate may fall by 50% before a rise in serum creatinine can happen due to kidney's compensatory increase in creatinine excretion. Conversely, creatinine and BUN may rise without an associated decrease in glomerular filtration rate. The common causes of isolated increased in serum creatinine without an associated renal dysfunction include increased release from muscles and decreased secretion from proximal tubule (Trimethoprim and cephalosporine therapy). Increased protein intake, infusion of amino acids, gastrointestinal bleeding and steroid therapy causes rise in BUN without worsening renal function. Despite these limitations, serial determinations of serum creatinine and BUN, calculation of EGFR, and measurement of urine output are the main stage of renal function monitoring. Table 13.4 narrates the urinary and blood parameters that may aid in evaluation of the patient with ARF:

Postoperative care should focus on adequate renal perfusion to prevent further insult to the kidney following major vascular surgery. An organized plan of diagnosis and treatment is important while dealing with the patients with ARF after vascular surgery.[60,61] As prerenal causes are most frequent source of ARF in the early postoperative period, the patients' intravascular volume status and cardiac performance should be evaluated. Patients with sign of volume defection require fluid resuscitation with isotonic crystalloid potassium containing solutions and blood products until adequate renal function is confirmed. Patients with

| Table 13.4: Urinary and blood chemistry for evaluation of renal failure | | | |
|---|---|---|---|
| Variable | Prerenal dysfunction | Renal parenchyma dysfunction | Postrenal dysfunction |
| Urine specific gravity | >1.20 | <1.020 | <1.020 |
| Urine osmolality | >400 | <400 | <400 |
| Urine/plasma osmolality(mosm/L) | >15 | –1 | –1 |
| Urine Na(mEq/L) | <20 | >30 | <30 |
| Fractional excretion of Na | <1% | >1% | <1% |
| Blood urea nitrogen | >20 | <10 | 10–20 |
| Urine/plasma creatinine | >40 | <20 | <20 |

inadequate cardiac performance require judicious inotropic support. If correction of filling pressures or myocardial performance fails to improve urinary output, evaluation of other causes of oliguria should be done (Table 13.3). The conversion of oliguric renal failure to a nonoliguric state may delay the need for renal replacement therapy and simplify fluid management. It may also be associated with fewer complications and improved survival although prospective data to support this notion is lacking.

Patients with radio contrast induced ARF require supportive care. Renal perfusion should be optimized with fluid administration for patients with hypovolemia and diuresis of those with fluid overload. If required, myocardial performance can be enhanced with inotrope and/or vasodilator medications. One should not forget to avoid nephrotoxic drugs at the same time.[62]

Vascular surgery patients requiring chronic renal replacement therapy also have a grave prognosis. We use continuous veno-venous hemofiltration and dialysis until patient's hemodynamic status is stabilized. Continuous hemodialysis reduces hemodynamic instability, allows better control of fluid and metabolic status, removes the deleterious cytokines and thereby affects the outcome. The dose of renally excreted medications should be adjusted.[63,64] Nutritional support of the patients with ARF is important as protein-calorie malnutrition in common in these patients. Finally a frank discussion regarding the prognosis of these patients with their family member is essential.

## NUTRITION MANAGEMENT

Thoracoabdominal/abdominal aneurysms requiring extensive laparotomy or a retroperitoneal exposure involves extensive mobilization of viscera. Routine nasogastric tube drainage is required for such cases for several days postoperatively.[65,66] Patients undergoing elective EVAR would not be expected to have an ileus or require nasogastric decompression. Preoperative malnutrition can adversely affect the outcome in major vascular surgical patients. However, perioperative total parenteral nutrition is of benefit only if support is continued for several weeks. Patients undergoing elective EVAR would not be expected to have an ileus or require nasogastric decompression.

Major vascular surgery involving thoracoabdominal aorta, those requiring CPB, enhances the release of series of inflammatory mediators and stress hormones. Release of these mediators alters body metabolism and catabolism causing release of glucose, amino acid and free fatly acids to the circulation so that substrates are in pant diverted from the purpose they serve in non stressed state to the task of raising an adequate healing response.[67] For a better wound healing, the body needs to be well nourished to mobilize adequate substrates, largely derived from muscle and adipose tissue, with nutritional support to allow synthesis of acute phase proteins, white cells, fibroblasts, collagen and other tissue components in the wounded area. This group of patients usually needs large volume of crystalloids and colloids during an immediate postoperative period, resulting in substantial weight gain and edema. This overload is also a major cause of paralytic ileus and delayed gastric emptying. Restriction of fluid to the amount needed to maintain salt, electrolyte and water balance, gastric emptying returned sooner and patients can be capable of tolerating normal food and normal bowel movements several days earlier than those in positive balance. However, this claim has not been consistently supported by later studies. Preoperative carbohydrate loading to combat the fasting state has been shown to enhance postoperative recovery by causing improved protein balance, improved preservation of lean body mass and length of stay in general surgical patients. However, literature is missing for major vascular surgical cases in this context.

The main goal of nutritional support in vascular surgery patients is to minimize negative nitrogen balance by avoiding starvation, with the purpose of maintaining muscle, immune and cognitive function and to enhance postoperative recovery. Oral feeding should be started as soon as possible after surgery provided that there are no signs of ileus. After elective thoracoabdominal aneurysm repair, gastric emptying has been shown to return by 18 hours and normalization of small bowel function by 47 hours. If oral feeding is not possible for 7 days, other means of nutrition should be implemented. Management of nutrition is a major concern especially for the patients who undergoes AAA repair, needs prolonged mechanical ventilation due to several reasons. It has also been suggested that routine fluid and carbohydrate loading 2 hour before surgery can attenuate postoperative insulin resistance and patient well being. Uses of high dose of opioid analgesia contribute to increased incidence of postoperative ileus, nausea and vomiting. Patients frequently have a 'nil by mouth' sign pasted above their bed for 3–4 day in the postoperative period and during this period they receive maintenance fluids via the intravenous route. Some authors suggested that excess of intravenous fluids in particular normal saline may contribute to postoperative gastrointestinal tract dysfunction, prolong postoperative stay and averse clinical outcome.[68] Some patients also undergo enforced bed rest, not only as a part of traditional care, but also because of the presence of drips, catheters and drains. Within this pattern of postoperative care patients are subject to a period of starvation and immobilization that may last for minimum of 4–5 days. In order to combat the nutritional consequences of such starvation oral supplementation has been tested in order to try to enhance normal food intake following recommencement or oral nutrition. Nasogastric/naso-enteric nutrition is preferred because it is associated with fewer infections and metabolic complications (e.g. hyperglycemia) than parenteral nutrition. However, the major disadvantage of this route includes intolerance, risk of aspiration and diarrhea. Enteral mode is contra-indicated in the presence of associated bowel obstruction. Most of the time oral feeding is restricted until the bowel sound returned, the patient is usually allowed to sip water and have liquid diet within three hours of extubation. Removal of nasogastirc tube follows at the commence-ment of oral feeding. Routine metoclopramide intravenous injection every six hours can assist the movement of the bowel. The regular diet can be started as soon as possible once there is no vomiting or sensation of nausea. Parenteral nutrition is indicated if the gut cannot be used or the patient failed enteral nutrition despite the use of pro kinetic agents. Supplemental parenteral nutrition may consider in patients who receives inadequate enteral nutrition. However, parenteral nutrition when administered to patients who also tolerate to enteral nutrition to certain extent or who are not malnourished causes more harm than benefit.

## PAIN MANAGEMENT

Management of postoperative pain following vascular surgery is necessary not only to keep the patient comfortable but also to reduce the postoperative complications. The effective control of acute surgical pain may decrease the like hood of a patient developing a chronic pain syndrome. Intravenous opioid are the cornerstone of postoperative pain management after major vascular surgery, but are associated with well known complication including nausea, vomiting, respiratory depression and decreased gastrointestinal motility. The increase in prevalence of obesity and sleep apnea has also led to increase risk of respiratory complications in patients receiving intravenous opioids. Concern over the side effects, especially potential respiratory depression and hypotension, continue to be a barrier to adequate pain management during major vascular surgery procedures. Epidural analgesia is an effective method of pain control especially after

thoracoabdominal incision, but hard to use because of existing postoperative coagulopathy and avoidance of spinal cord ischemia. A Cochrane review reports a meta analysis of 13 randomized trials involving 1224 patients having abdominal aortic surgery 597 of whom were treated using systemic opioides. Those receieiving epidural anesthesia had significantly fewer overall cardiovascular complications and renal insufficiency. They too spent 20% less time intubated and reported less subjective pain, especially with movement. No mortality difference was reported. However, those potential benefits are associated with increased costs and increased risk of epidural hematoma.[74]

Neurologic assessment after major vascular surgery is important for detecting and treating latest onset of paraplegia. Routine used method of analgesia and epidural analgesia usually interfere with neurologic assessment. Use of paravetebral analgesia has been described by a few authors, which provides unilateral analgesia and hemodynamic side effects.

In a meta-analysis which involved 10 trials David RG et al compared the analgesic efficacy and side effects of paravetebral versus epidural blockade. They concluded that there was no significant difference between paravetebral block and epidural block for pain scores. However, the incidence of pulmonary complications, urinary retention, nausea and vomiting and hypotension was less common among the patients who received paravetebral block.

Because of the difficulty in pain control, multimodal therapeutic strategy provides central or peripheral block with nonsteroidal antiinflammatory drugs (NSAID) and adjuvant drugs is now the cornerstone of treatment, offering the possibility of reducing opioid requirement and side effects. Use of NSAID as an adjunct to opioid may decrease the postoperative morphine consumption by 30–50%. Marret and colleague in a meta-analysis demonstrated that there can be a reduction in some opioid related complications with NSAIDs use. These investigations found that there is a reduction in nausea and vomiting by 29%, however, the incidence of respiratory depression remains the same. Concern over bleeding, gastrointestinal ulceration, renal injury, cardiac ischemia/infarction, stroke, and bone and wound healing have limited the widespread utilization of NSAIDS in vascular surgery. Other multimodal adjuncts include but not limited to ketamine, pregaba-line, and gabapentin. Addition of low dose of ketamine (0.1–0.2 mg/kg) reduces opioid consumption and decreased opioid related complications postoperatively.

Though various dosing regimens of these adjuncts have been narrated for postoperative analgesia, no single standard has been defined. The use of pregabaline and gabapentin in major vascular surgery is yet to be reported.

Peripheral vascular surgeries, especially carotid surgery lend itself to the use of regional analgesia either alone or in combination with general anesthesia or sedation. Nerve blocks can avoid many disadvantages of neuroaxial analgesia. The technique choosen will depend upon the site of surgery. There is no overall benefit from regional analgesia, in comparison to opioid and neuroaxial blockade. Likewise, there is little evidence to demonstrate a reduction in phantom limb pain by using epidural analgesia for peripheral vascular surgery.

Early extubation, better ventilator mechanics and gas exchange, decrease incidence in atelectasis, pneumonia, and chronic postoperative pain are the major advantages of thoracic epidural analgesia with a local analgesic or opioid. In conditions where epidural analgesia is contraindicated, other regional technique of analgesia can be used. Continuous paravetebral infusion of local anesthetic can be used in patients who have a contra-indication for epidural block. Intercostals and intra-pleural blocks are mainly utilized, whereas a single shot of intrathecal injection of a hydrophilic opioid, such as morphine appear to be effective. Cryoanalgesia which is successful in the immediate postoperative period, has been abounded for its brief duration and increase incidence of chronic pain.

Finally there is continued interest regarding opioid, neuroaxial and peripheral nerve blocks to reduce postoperative pain in vascular surgery patients. A concern for these groups of patients is mainly around the use of anticoagulant and antiplatelet agents. The decision making process about optimal approach should be a combine one between surgeons, anesthesiologist and cardiologists.

## DEEP VEIN THROMBOSIS (DVT) PROPHYLAXIS

As most vascular surgery patients already receive intraoperative heparin, it has been suggested that the risk of DVT among these patients is lower than any other surgical patients. A Cochrane analysis of all nonrando-mized prospective studies in aortic surgeries identified an incidence of all DVT that ranged between 0 and 20.5%, averaging 9.2% among patients without DVT prophylaxis. Though the risk is low after EAVR, the incidence of femoral/popliteal DVT after EVAR, was 6% in one of the study as examined by Duplex ultrasono-graphy. Prophylaxis is generally given until patients became ambulatory and mobile.[76–79]

| Box 13.3 | Vascular disease patients who are at more risk of DVT |

- Age 60–74 year
- Surgery lasting >60 minutes
- Morbid obesity (BMI >40)
- Family history of DVT/PE/SVT (superficial venous thrombosis)
- Positive factor V Leiden
- Positive prothrombin 20210A
- Elevated serum homcysteine
- Heparin induce thrombocytopenia
- Abnormal pulmonary function
- Congestive cardiac failure
- Acute myocardial infarction
- Serious lung disease including pneumonia (<1 month)

The following measures to be taken during the post-operative period to reduce the incidence of taken DVT[80,81] (Box 13.4).

| Box 13.4 | Deep vein thrombosis prophylaxis measures |

| General measures | Elevation of leg |
|---|---|
| | Early ambulation |
| | Leg exercises |
| | Graduated compression stocking |
| | Intermittent pneumatic compression |

Extensively used method. It avoids venous stasis by intermittent pumping of the leg veins. The maximum pressure in 35–55 mmHg and the inflation time varies from 10–35 sec with a deflation period of maximum 1 minute to allow the veins to fill.

- Venous foot pumps

Foot compression pumps are usually foot slipper/boots with an air bladder in the area of the sole of the foot. The air chamber in rapidly inflated to a pressure up to 200 mmHg over 3 sec periods over every 20 sec. This planter compression increases venous flow and there by decreases the risk of DVT

| Pharmacologic method | Subcutaneous unfractionated heparin |
|---|---|
| | Low molecular weight heparin |
| | Aspirin |
| | Dextrans |
| | Oral vitamin K antagonist |
| | Factor X a inhibitor |

## Unfractionated Heparin

Several meta-analyses have confirmed that UFH reduces the rate of postoperative DVT in general surgical patients with minor bleeding complications by more than 50%. The usual dose is 5000 units 2 hrs before surgery followed by 10,000–15,000 U/24 hr. This treatment is however associated with heparin induced thrombocytopenia in up to 5% of patients receiving heparin. Twenty percent of people with heparin induced thrombocytopenia (HIT) have thrombin that may lead to ischemic complication. The short half life of UFH (0.5-2 hrs) is another limitation to make more frequent dosing necessary. This short half life the however is advantageous in the case of bleeding complications or patients with renal failure.

## Low Molecular Weight Heparin

The results of survival meta-analysis showed that UFH and LMWH has similar efficacy in DVT. Prophylaxis dose depends upon patients' weight and existing renal dysfunction.

## Oral Vitamin K Antagonist

The most commonly used drug is warfarin. This is mostly administered as orally/fixed low doses and doses not need any laboratory monitoring or at adjusted doses with the goal of achieving a therapeutic level of anticoagulation by using the international normalization ratio (INR). A prolongation of prothrombin time corresponding to an INR between 2.0 and 3.0 is considered adequate for DVT prophylaxis following vascular surgery.

## Aspirin

Aspirin (acetyl salicylic acid) inhibits platelet function through irreversible inhibition of the enzyme cyclo-oxygenase-1 and thereby blocks the production of thromboxane-A2, which induces platelet aggregation and vaso-constriction. The effect of aspirin lasts for the duration of the life span of platelets, around 10 days. The role of aspirin however remains controversial. Aspirin, used alone is not recommended for DVT prophylaxis during the postoperative period.

## Factor Xa Inhibitors

Fondaparinus and idraparinus are the systematic polysaccharides that selectively inhibits factor Xa by producing conformational change in the natural anticoagulant antihrombin molecule. The clinical half life of fondaparinus is 17 hours and contrary to heparin it does not cause thrombocytopenia. Idraparinus has a half-life of 130 hours and can be administered once a week.

## Direct Factor Xa Inhibitor

Rivaroxiban is currently under phase III trial.

### Direct thrombin Inhibitors (DTI)

i. *Hirudin*: This is the first available DTI, given subcutaneously, is more effective them LMWH for prophylaxis of postoperative DVT, but is associated with more risk of the bleeding.

ii. *Dabigatran etexilate*: It is an orally available DTI, reaches a peak plasma concentration within 2 hrs with a terminal half life of 8–10 hrs after single administration and 14–17 hrs after multiple administration.

The use of combination of mechanical and pharma-cologic methods improves the efficacy of these methods used separately. These two methods are complementary rather than competitive.

All the vascular surgery patients often receive several antithrombotic agents including one or more platelet agents or at least one anticoagulant the incidence of DVT is low in vascular surgery patients because of the above said reason. The latest while waiting for the results to detect HIT, all the heparin should be discontinued. The goal is to reduce platelet activation and thereby reduce the risk for thrombosis. If suspicious for HIT in high, alternative anticoagulation with direct thrombin inhibitors/heparinoids is too started. In the presence of isolated thrombocytopenia without thrombin, anti-coagulation should be continued for 2–4 weeks once platelet count recover to a stable pattern become of the risk of thrombin remain high in this period. If the patient had thrombosis transition to warfarin should occur once patient counts have recovered above 150,000/mm$^3$ and treatment should be maintained for 3–6 months. Despite systemic heparinization postoperative vascular surgery patients have a high incidence of DVT. A strict vigilance about DVT in essential in particular to the patients with fresh frozen plasma infusion.

## Heparin Induced Thrombocytopenia and Thrombosis

The risk of thrombosis remains high days to 4 weeks after discontinuation of heparin. Thrombosis can occur at venous or arterial system and commonly occurs at the site of vascular surgery.

The diagnosis of this problem in postoperative patients should be considered if there is presence of new or progressive thrombotic complications, even in the

212
Textbook of Vascular Anesthesia

absence of thrombocytopenia. This lethal disorder is caused by the development of antibodies against complexes of platelet factor 4 and heparin, exposure to UFH and LMWH are the main cause. A low platelet count ($<150,000$ /mm$^3$) or a drop in the platelet count of greater than 50% from the baseline is common in these patients. HIT usually begins 5 and 10 days after exposure. Thrombocytopenia most often proceeds thrombosis. However, platelet will rarely drop below 10,000/mm$^3$ in HIT patients, and therefore these patients will rarely suffer from thrombosis. The confirmed diagnosis of HIT is made by using either a serologic assay or a functional assay for heparin dependent antibodies. Because of a high sensitivity and low specificity this assay should not be used in patients with low clinical suspicion of HIT because they can defect heparin antibodies without the presence of HIT. Functional assays to measure platelet activation and defect, platelet antibody have a sensitivity of 90% and specificity of 77–100% and are helpful in patients with low/intermediate clinical suspicion of HIT. Consensus guidelines suggest that special prophylaxis has to be given to these patients unless additional risk factors are present. There are no firm data regarding the length of anticoagulation or low long extended prophylaxis should be used. The problem of selecting prophylaxis method and duration of its use should be guided by individual risk assessment. The risk and benefits of each approach should be carefully evaluated and communicated to the patient and family members before its use.

## RESPIRATORY MANAGEMENT

Pulmonary complications are a significant cause of morbidity after major vascular surgery and cause significant prolongation of hospital stay. Inadequate ventilation and insufficient oxygenation are the major cause of respiratory failure. Mechanical ventilation is to be continued following any major vascular surgery. The regulation of tidal volume, respiratory rate, FiO$_2$ and PEEP defends open the age, weight and respiratory status of the patient. Volume controlled/pressure controlled modes accounts for majority of modes with which patients are ventilated. Hemodynamically unstable patients/patients with severe respiratory distress should be continued with a controlled mode (volume/pressure) of ventilation to limit their work of breathing. Pressure controlled modes are usually used for the patient who are more stable and do not require full ventilator support. A lung protective strategy to be used to reduce ventilator-induced lung injury that can occur through two main mechanisms. It can be due to over distention of alveoli because of high tidal volume and high tidal pressure (volutrauma) and subsequent barotrauma. Secondly, it can happen due to shear forces on the alveolar endothelium. These forces are created in the alveoli by cyclic opening and closing, and the resultant injury is called "atelectatic trauma". Benefits of application of PEEP is unknown. The accepted range depending on the clinical situation, is 5–15 cm H$_2$O.[82]

A lung protection strategy should be applied for the patients who are at risk of volutrauma. Use of pressure control mode of ventilation to reduce peak airway pressure is most appropriate. In this mode inspiratory time can be lengthed to allow increased alveolar recruitment, and alveolar distending plateau pressure and transpulmonary pressure are to be kept below 30 cm H$_2$O be using low tidal volumes (6–8 ml/kg body weight). The main disadvantage of low tidal ventilation is decrease clearance of carbon dioxide and respiratory acidosis, but this permissive hypercapnia and acidosis are well tolerated if the pH is above 7.2. One cavet is that permissive hypercapnia is contraindicated in patients with cerebral edema.

These factors (Box 13.5) predispose to early airway closure and atelectasis, leading to V/Q mismatch, hypoxemia, retained secretion and respiratory failure. Deep breathing exercise and pulmonary hygiene are important postoperative considerations for impending pulmonary complications. Several techniques for lung expansion are available including intermittent positive pressure breathing (IPPB), incentive spirometry, continuous positive airway pressure (CPAP) and others.

| Box 13.5 | Predicting factors for postoperative respiratory dysfunction after vascular surgery |
| --- | --- |

- Advanced age
- Smoking history
- Pre existing COPD
- Obesity
- Poor general health
- Abnormal pulmonary function test
- Extensive thoracoabdominal incision
- Prolonged surgical time and CPB time
- Type of anesthesia—use of long acting muscle relaxant
- Postoperative hypothermia (this causes vasocontriction, reduced tissue perfusion, resulting in metabolic acidosin and hypercapnic respiratory failure
- Prolonged postoperative sedation and muscle relaxant use
- Improper postoperative analgesia
- Inadequate lung expansion due to extensive incision
- Bronchospasm
- Fluid overload
- Airway secretion

## Prevention of Respiratory Complication during Postoperative Period

Special precaution should be taken for the patients with COPD, obesity and elderly age group. Apart from the preoperative preparation, the following care should be imported during postoperative period.

1. *Lung expansion maneuvers*:

    Incentive spirometory
    - Deep breathing.
    - Continuous positive airway pressure.

2. *Antibiotic prophylaxis*: Decontamination of the nasopharynx with chlorhexidine glutamate can significantly decrease the risk of lower respiratory tract infection. De contamination should be considered in all patients who remain mechanically ventilated for more than one day.

3. *Pain control*: Pain control strategies including epidural analgesia, and intercostals nerve blocks, reduce splinting and promote the ability to take deep breaths after thoracic abdominal incision.

4. *Pneumonia*: The most important risk factor for development of this complication is prolonged mechanical ventilation, however, elderly age, comorbid conditions and presence of nasogastric tube are some other predisposing factor. A patient maintained on mechanical ventilation should be formally assessed for suitability for weaning and extubation on a daily basis. This assessment is best performed by a daily spontaneous breathing trial, usually as T-piece trial for 30–120 minutes. The longer time interval is best for marginal patients, however, both the time periods can predict the success or failure of extubation in most of the patients. Patient should be kept in upright position unless there in specific contra-indication. Tight glucose control (80–110 mg/dl) is again important to prevent nosocomial pneumonia. Selective decontamination of the digestive tracts and drainage of subglottic secretion may lessen the incidence of pneumonia.

## Weaning from Mechanical Ventilation

Daily assessment to be done before taking out of the patient from ventilator. Interruption of sedation is important before starting the weaning process. The usual approach to weaning is to reduce the ventilatory support progressively. The second approach is to use spontaneous breathing trials without progressive with drawl of ventilatory support. This may associated with earlier extubation. During the gradual reduction of ventilator support, patients are switched off from controlled to a spontaneous mode of ventilation such as pressure support ventilation. A gradual reduction of ventilator support and PEEP is done according to the oxygen saturation, respiratory rate and tidal volume. During spontaneous breathing trials, patients are allowed to breath spontaneously with little or no assistance. At times minimal pressure support of 5–10 cm $H_2O$ and PEEP at 5 cm $H_2O$ for 30 minutes to 2 hours is required. A successful trial is evidenced by the absence of respiratory distress (respiratory rate >35 minute for >5 minutes oxygen desaturation <90% for > 10 seconds), increase or decrease in heart rate ($\pm$ 20% for >5 minutes), SBP higher than 180 mm Hg or lower than 90mmHg, or other signs of agitation and distress.

## Extubation

The universal criterion for extubation is also followed for these patients. Patients who requires sedation, has inability to protect the airway, because of the presence of copious secretion or absence of cough reflex are not suitable for extubation. A patient with the presence of a difficult airway needs special attention. Failure to extubation is associated with increased mortality and need for long term ventilation.

## Tracheostomy

It is reserve for the patients who require prolonged ventilatory support due to the presence of some postoperative complications (e.g. pneumonia, severe cardiovascular instability neurological deficit patients with absence of cough reflex. Tracheostomy relieves the patient of the portion of work of breathing required to overcome the resistance of endotracheal tube and upper airway. It improves patients 'comport, allows better oral hygiene and secretion management. However, it is not free for complications like bleeding, procedure related complication, infection and tracheo-innominate fistula or tracheoesophageal fistula. Early tracheostomy within the first week is associated with short in length of hospital stay.

Tracheostomy can be done by open surgical method or percutaneously. Percutaneous tracheostomy is as safe as open surgical method; with the added advantage that patient does not require transport to the operating room. Percutaneous tracheostomy is however contraindicated in patients who are hypoxic and have high PEEP requirements, obese patients with short neck, presence of coagulopathy and in those with a recent (< 10 days) cervical spine fixation.

## NEUROLOGICAL COMPLICATIONS AND MANAGEMENT

Neurological injury resulting from spinal cord ischemia or cerebral ischemia is not uncommon after major vascular surgery on aorta. Permanent neurological deficit are major cause of morbidity and mortality and may shorten long term survival. Factors associated with neurological dysfunction are previous aortic surgery, preoperative renal dysfunction, elderly age, prolonged aortic cross clamp tme, emergency repair and repair of extensive aneurysm.[83,84] Some of the causes of neurologic dysfunction following vascular surgery are described below and in Box 13.6.

*Subdural hematoma:* At times it occurs during postoperative period especially in patients who undergoes drainage of cerebrospinal fluid (CSF). The patient often complaints of severe headache and brain computed tomography (CT) and brain magnetic resonance imaging (MRI) may show a high density shadow at any site of the brain. The treatment is usually conservative, though craniotomy a ventricular drain is essential at times. In a prospective randomized trial Coselli et al showed that perioperative CSF drainage up to 10 mmHg reduces the rate of paraplegia after repair of Crawford extent I and II TAAs. A spinal drain is usually inserted (L4-L5 intervertebral space, Fig. 13.2) by many anesthesiologists for continuous drainage of CSF and monitoring of CSF pressure during the perioperative period.

The CSF drain manometer tubings should be colour coaded and to be separate from other invasive monitoring lines to avoid inadvertent spinal injections. The CSF drain is attached to a three-way tap that allows connection directly to the pressure transducers via one limb of the three-way tap, and to a sterile drainage system via the other limb (Fig. 13.3).

The three way tap is kept routed so that the spinal drain is connected to the pressure transducer. In this position there will be no drainage of CSF and the patient can easily change the position. While not in use the ports are covered with sterile gauze to prevent inadvertent use, with labels stating "spinal drain". While monitoring the CSF pressure care should be taken when connecting the transducer plug to the socket in the back of the plate

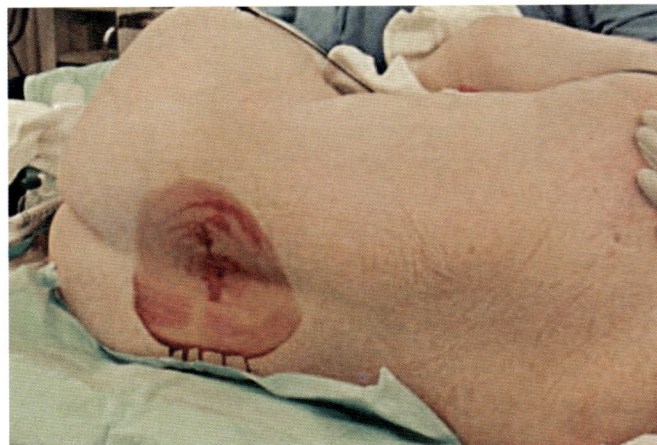

Fig. 13.1: Position of placement of spinal drain

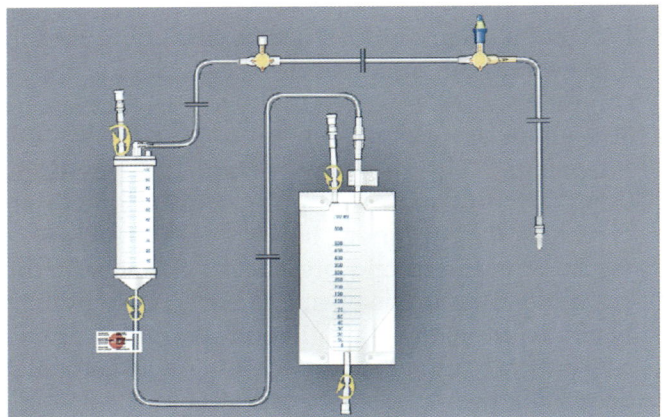

Fig. 13.2: External CSF drainage set

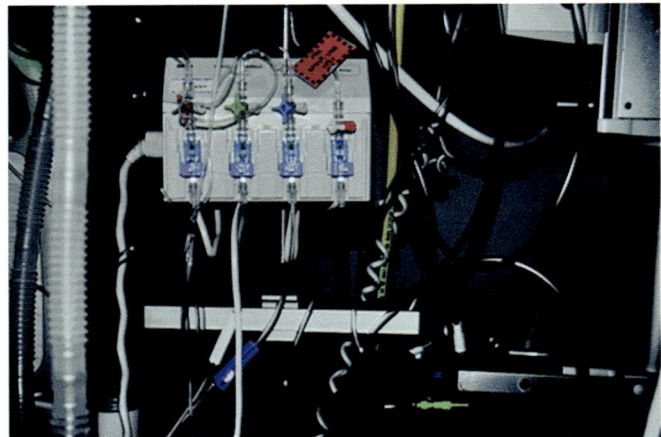

Fig. 13.3: Arrangement of pressure transducers for spinal drain

| Box 13.6 | Neurologic dysfunction following vascular surgery |
| --- | --- |

- Subdural hematoma
- Paraplegia
- Headache
- Altered mental status
- Cerebrovascular accident
- Cerebral hyperperfusion syndrome
- Vertebral artery occlusion with brain stem infarction
- Impaired binocular vision
- Sensory and motor deficit in left arm and hand due to over stenting of left subclavian artery

as there is no danger of cross connection to any other line. For maintain the CSF pressure, the line is calibrated and zeroed independently of all the pressure transducers and the plug connection is double checked. The spinal drain should never be left open to the collecting bag as the inadvertent sudden drainage of a large volume of CSF may cause precipitous fall in intracranial pressure and lead to tearing of subdural vessels within patients' skull, leading to cerebral damage from subdural hematoma. If the pressure exceeds a certain level than a three way tap is turned on the drainage line to allow a controlled release of CSF into the drainage reservoir before turning the tap back again so that the spinal drain is again open only to the transducer. The roller clamp on the line that delivers flush to the transducer is closed and the tap warped around this clamp to prevent it being rolled open. In addition, a second clamp is applied to the flush line and labeled to that specifically says "Do Not Flush." In case of suspicion, CSF drainage should be stopped immediately. To reduce the risk of hematoma, CSF drain placement should be done before systemic heparinization and management should be exercised with ultimate care, diligence and caution. CSF is generally drain in 10 ml increments with a goal of CSF pressure of less than 10 mmHg and the drainage is continued for at least 48–72 hours postoperatively to minimize neurological deficits. During the drainage of CSF, the MAP is usually maintained between 80 and 100 mmHg. If the CSF pressure exceeds 10 mmHg, it is drained to a limit of 15 ml/hour when the patient is neurologically intact. If delayed, neurologic deficit occurs; CSF is drained without limit to maintain pressure 5 mmHg, provided there is no visible blood in CSF.

The incidence of *postoperative delirium* is approximately 22% in vascular surgery patients according to one group of authors. Patients who developed delirium were older, and more likely had a history of transient ischemic attack or cerebrovascular accident, depression and CAD. These were the patients, who received preoperative beta blockers, which doubled the risk of delirium during the postoperative period. Statin administration reduced the risk by 44% in these patients. β-blockers interact with serotonin sensitive adenylate cyclase system and melantonin secretion mechanisms, which are part of neurotransmitter network involved in the pathogenesis of delirium. Cerebral hypoperfusion syndrome, characterized by hypertension, seizures, and neurologic deficits, can be observed in patients after carotid surgery and described elsewhere in this chapter. cerebrovascular accidents can occur following vascular surgery and mirror the occurrence of cardiac events, owing to similar underlying risk factors for patients undergoing vascular surgery.

*Paraplegia* is recognized as a devastating complication especially after thoracic aortic surgery. It is usually develop by postoperative day 1–3. Apart from certain intraoperative precautions, e.g. manipulation of perfusion pressure, sequential clamping/minimization of duration of cross clamp, intercostals reattachment, hypothermia, continuation of CSF drainage and manipulation of spinal cord perfusion pressure with a lumbar spinal drain insertion is becoming a standard of postoperative care in patients undergoing thoracic aortic intervention. However, cannulation of subarachonoid space is not without risks including meningitis, fistulation, epidural hematoma, and even subarachnoid hemorrhage.

## SPECIAL CARE FOR PATIENTS WITH CAROTID SURGERY

Every arrangement should be made for 4–6 hour observation in a suitable environment with continued close invasive hemodynamic and neurological monitoring. Immediate attention should be given to the patient developing neurological deficit. Prompt assessment of carotid artery patency with carotid duplex scanning help to assess the cause of neurological deterioration and suitability for re-exploration. In case of nonavailability of carotid scanning, patient should be assumed to have developed carotid artery occlusion and taken back to operating room without any delay. Overnight oxygenation is important.

### Hyperfusion Syndrome

Control of postoperative hypertension is important as uncontrolled BP may lead to **hyperperfusion syndrome**. Hyperperfusion syndrome can occur because in the preoperative state, the cerebral circulation has adapted to a significant carotid stenosis by maximal dilation and loss of autoregulation. Following restoration of carotid patency, the abnormal vasculature is susceptible to damage from excessive flow and pressure. This complication is manifested as occiputo-frontal headache which may progress to seizure and fatal cerebral hemorrhage. Blood pressure should be kept below the preoperative level as the cerebral vasculature becomes exposed to increased pressure and flow postoperatively. Use of short acting antihypertensive agent, e.g. labetolol (5 mg increments up to 100 mg maximum) have a role.[85]

### Bleeding and Hematoma

*Bleeding and hematoma* at the site may lead to progressive airway obstruction in the postoperative period. At times severe supraglottic edema due to venous congestion may lead to visualization of the larynx difficult. In this event patient should be returned to the OT for a re-exploration under local anesthesia/regional block. Wound Hematoma following carotid surgery require emergency treatment when large or expand precipitously. If there is no loss of airway, patient should undergo emergency evacuation of the hematoma in the operating room. In case of airway obstruction, it is better to open the wound in the ICU at bedside. In the early postoperative period special attention should be paid to detect neck discomfort and expansion of the wound.

## Hypertension

During postoperative period increases the risk of complication, including wound hematoma and hyper perfusion syndrome and neurological deficit. Towne and Bernhard reportedthat the incidence of preoperative hypertension in patients who developed postoperative hypertension was 79.6% with 57.4% in patients who did not develop this complication. Postoperative hypertension following carotid surgery also lead to intracerebral hemorrhage. About 21% of the normotensive patients also develop hypertension following carotid end arterectomy with highest peak in the first 48 hours of surgery. Surgically induced carotid baroreceptor sensitivity is responsible for this problem. Keeping the blood pressure within the accepted range for the patient solves this problem.

## Hypotension

*Hypotension,* following carotid surgery occurs in 5% of patients and responded well to low dose phenylephrine infusion and usually resolve within 24–48 hours. Significant and prolonged hypotension if non respondent to vasopressure in the presence of adequate filling pressure may warrant the possibility of development of myocardial infarction.

## Intracerebral Hemorrhage

All the patients undergoing carotid surgery should be strictly monitored for a normal range of blood pressure and development of intracerebral hemorrhage. The incidence of this complication as reported by various authors varies from 50 to 93%.

## Seizures

Though uncommon, the reported incidence is 3% especially the patients who are hemodynamically compromised 5–7 days after carotid endarterectomy. Brain edema due to cerebral hyperperfusion syndrome is another important cause of seizure. In series of 2439 patients reported by Reigel et al, 10 cases developed seizure and showed a significant increase in cerebral blood flow after surgery.[86] The authors concluded that the events were part of a hyperfusion syndrome. Even if there are no controlled studies that evaluate the

efficacy of ICU administration after carotid surgery, short term admission to ICU for close monitoring of neurological and vital signs has been recommended for these patients. Careful postoperative evaluation is essential for patients those with pre-existing hypertension, advanced age, previous MI, high grade ipsilateral carotid stenosis with or without contralateral occlusion and poor collateral flow or slow flow in the middle cerebral territory should need careful supervision at least during first 48 hours of surgery. For the patients who are hemodynamically and neurologically stable during first 24 hours, early discharge is possible.

## SPECIAL CARE FOR PREGNANT PATIENTS

Vascular disease in pregnant patients though rare is not uncommon. The postoperative care for these patients is a bit different and special compared to the nonpregnant cases. Pregnant patients and postparturient undergoes related physiological changes which demands extra care when these patients undergo vascular surgery especially that involves aorta and major vessels.[87] Acute aortic dissection may occur in association with severe hypertension due to pre-ecampcia, coartation of aorta and connective tissue disorders such as Marfans' syndrome. The postoperative risk doubles in these patients. An experienced team of surgeons and anesthesiologist should accept the responsibility of entire postoperative course too. Shu C et al. managed three cases of type B aortic dissection treated with endovascular stent repair of thoracic aorta either before/after delivery. All mothers and children were followed by outpatient observation. One of the patient developed type II endovascular leak who required a left common carotid artery stent.[88]

## DISCHARGE FROM ICU

Mortality is increased significantly (up to 40% according to various studies) in patients discharged prematurely from ICU and needing re-admission. Most of the units have their own discharge policies but suggested criteria's include:

- Hemodynamic stability without the need for vasoactive drugs
- Adequate analgesia to make patient comfort including mobilization and coughing
- Stable hemoglobin (more than 8 gm/dl)
- No indication for further surgical intervention
- Urine output >0.5 mL/kg/hr with normal or improving renal biochemistry
- Stable and predictable fluid requirement

All the major vascular surgical patients should be monitored using standardized physiological scores, e.g. early warning score (EWS) or modified EWS (MEWS). A high score is associated with an increased risk of clinical deterioration and should prompt early intervention to prevent readmission to intensive care unit.

## POSTOPERATIVE AREAS THAT NEED FURTHER RESEARCH

Despite advance in technology, a number of areas of uncertainty still exists in the care of vascular surgery cases. Future research should consider addressing the following segments:

1. Improved strategies to identify the patients at risk for postoperative myocardial infarction or cardiovascular related death.

2. Optional fluid management regimen especially for patients with pre-existing anemia.

3. Management of psychological aspect of patients and relative during their prolonged hospital stay.

4. Development of cost effective CU stay in patients with open repair.

## REFERENCES

1. Raval MV, Eskandari MK. Outcomes of elective abdominal aortic aneurysm repair among the elderly: Endovascular versus open repair. Surgery 2012 Feb;151:245–60.

2. de Maistre E, Terriat B, Lesne-Padieu AS, Abello N, Bouchot O, Steinmetz EF. High incidence of venous thrombosis after surgery for abdominal aortic aneurysm. J Vasc Surg 2009 Mar; 49:596–601.

3. Wolters U, Mannheim S, Wassmer G, Brunkwall J. What is the value of available risk-scores in predicting postoperative complications after aorto-iliac surgery? A prospective non randomized study. J Cardiovasc Surg (Torino) 2006 Apr; 47:177–85.

4. Panaretou V, Toufektzian L, Siafaka I, Kouroukli I, Sigala F, Vlachopoulos C, Katsaragakis S, Zografos G, Filis K. Postoperative pulmonary function after open abdominal aortic aneurysm repair in patients with chronic obstructive pulmonary disease: Epidural versus intravenous analgesia. Ann Vasc Surg 2012 Feb;26:149–55.

5. Barakat HM, Shahin Y, Barnes R, Gohil R, Souroullas P, Khan J, McCollum PT, Chetter IC. Supervised exercise program improves aerobic fitness in patients awaiting abdominal aortic aneurysm repair. Ann Vasc Surg 2014 Jan;28:74–9.

6. Chinsakchai K, Hongku K, Hahtapornsawan S, Wongwanit C, Ruangsetakit C, Sermsathanasawadi N, Mutirangura P. Outcomes of abdominal aortic aneurysm with aortic neck thrombus after endovascular abdominal aortic aneurysm repair. J Med Assoc Thai 2014 May;97:518–24.

7. Waiting J, Dias A, Patel T, Pencavel T, Rosenfeld K, Sarin S. Successful thrombolysis of a late acute thrombotic occlusion of an aortic prosthesis after endovascular aneurysm repairs. Ann Vasc Surg 2014 Oct;28:1791.e1–4.

8. Landesberg G, Mosseri M, Wolf Y, Vesselov Y, Weissman C. Perioperative myocardial ischemia and infarction: identification by continuous 12-lead electrocardiogram with online ST-segment monitoring. Anesthesiology 2002 Feb; 96:264–70.

9. Landesberg G, Shatz V, Akopnik I, Wolf YG, Mayer M, Berlatzky Y, Weissman C, Mosseri M. Association of cardiac troponin, CK-MB, and postoperative myocardial ischemia with long-term survival after major vascular surgery. J Am Coll Cardiol 2003 Nov;42:1547–54.

10. Marston N, Sandoval Y, Zakharova M, Brenes-Salazar J, Santili S, Adabag S, McFalls EO, Garcia S. Troponin elevations following vascular surgery in patients without preoperative myocardial ischemia. South Med J 2013 Nov; 106:612–7.

11. Kim SH, Lilot M, Sidhu KS, Rinehart J, Yu Z, Canales C, Cannesson M. Accuracy and precision of continuous non-invasive arterial pressure monitoring compared with invasive arterial pressure: A systematic review and meta-analysis. Anesthesiology 2014 May;120:1080–97.

12. Amar D, Melendez JA, Zhang H, Dobres C, Leung DH, Padilla RE. Correlation of peripheral venous pressure and central venous pressure in surgical patients. J Cardiothorac Vasc Anesth 2001 Feb;15:40–3.

13. McLemore EC, Tessier DJ, Rady MY, Larson JS, Mueller JT, Stone WM, Fowl RJ, Patel BM. Intraoperative peripherally inserted central venous catheter central venous pressure monitoring in abdominal aortic aneurysm reconstruction. Ann Vasc Surg 2006 Sep;20:577–81.

14. Greason KL, Kim S, Suri RM, Wallace AS, Englum BR. Hypothermia and operative mortality during on-pump coronary artery bypass grafting. J Thorac Cardiovasc Surg 2014 Dec;148:2712–8.

15. Conti CR. Hypothermia: Is it good for the brain and not for the arteries? J Am Coll Cardiol 2013 May;61:2113–4.

16. Karski JM. Transesophageal echocardiography in the intensive care unit. Semin Cardiothorac Vasc Anesth 2006 Jun;10:162–6.

17. Kauffman KE. Newer trends in monitoring: the esophageal Doppler monitor. AANA J 2000 Oct;68:421–8.

18. Valentine RJ, Duke ML, Inman MH, Grayburn PA, Hagino RT, Kakish HB, Clagett GP. Effectiveness of pulmonary artery catheters in aortic surgery: A randomized trial. J Vasc Surg 1998 Feb;27:203–11.

19. Isaacoson IJ, Lowdon JD, Berry AJ, et al. The value of pulmonary artery and central venous monitoring abdominal aortic reconstructive surgery: a comparative study of two selected, randomized groups. J Vasc Surg 1990 Dec;12: 754–60.

20. Björck M, Wanhainen A, Djavani K, Acosta S. The clinical importance of monitoring intra-abdominal pressure after ruptured abdominal aortic aneurysm repair. Scand J Surg 2008;97:183–90.

21. Papavassiliou V, Anderton M, Loftus IM, Turner DA, Naylor AR, London NJ, Bell PR, Thompson MM. The physiological effects of elevated intra-abdominal pressure following aneurysm repair. Eur J Vasc Endovasc Surg 2003 Sep;26: 293–8.

22. Cade R, Wagemaker H, Vogel S, Mars D, Hood-Lewis D, Privette M, Peterson J, Schlein E, Hawkins R, Raulerson D, et al. Hepatorenal syndrome. Studies of the effect of vascular volume and intraperitoneal pressure on renal and hepatic function. Am J Med 1987 Mar;82:427–38.

23. Järvinen O, Laurikka J, Salenius JP, Lepäntalo M. Mesenteric infarction after aortoiliac surgery on the basis of 1752 operations from the National Vascular Registry. World J Surg 1999 Mar;23:243–7.

24. Bruggink JL, Tielliu IF, Zeebregts CJ, Pol RA. Mesenteric ischemia after abdominal aortic aneurysm repair: A systemic review. J cardiovasc Surg (Torino) 2014 Dec;55:759–65.

25. Ayad M, Senders ZJ, Ryan S, Abai B, DiMuzio P, Salvatore DM. Chronic mesenteric ischemia after partial coverage of the celiac artery during TEVAR, case report, and review of the literature. Ann Vasc Surg 2014 Nov;28:1935.e1–6.

26. Mallick IH, Yang W, Winslet MC, Seifalian AM. Ischemia-reperfusion injury of the intestine and protective strategies against injury. Dig Dis Sci 2004 Sep;49:1359–77.

27. Neary P, Hurson C, Briain DO, Brabazon A, Mehigan D, Keaveny TV, Sheehan S. Colonic infarction following endovascular AAA repair: a multifactorial complication. J Endovasc Ther 2002;95:54–8.

28. Acosta S, Björck M. Modern treatment of acute mesenteric ischaemia. Br J Surg 2014 Jan;101:e100–8.

29. Bobadilla JL. Mesenteric ischemia. Surg Clin North Am 2013 Aug;93:925–40.

30. Lee ES1, Pevec WC, Link DP, Dawson DL. Use of T-Stat to predict colonic ischemia during and after endovascular aneurysm repair: a case report. J Vasc Surg 2008 Mar;47: 632–4.

31. Ziemann C, von Heesen M, Sperling J, Maßmann A, Jeanmonod P, Glanemann M, Moussavian MR. Successful management of postoperative necrotizing pancreatitis after infrarenal abdominal aortic aneurysm repair. Ann Vasc Surg 2013 Nov;27:1184.

32. Olthof E, Blankensteijn JD, Akkersdijk GJ. Chyloperitoneum following abdominal aortic surgery. Vascular 2008 Sep-Oct;16:258–62.

33. Scher KS, Sarap MD, Jaggers RL. Acute acalculous cholecystitis complicating aortic aneurysm repair. Surg Gynecol Obstet 1986 Nov;163:475–8.

34. Cadot H, Addis MD, Faries PL, Carroccio A, Burks JA Jr, Gravereaux EC, Morrissey NJ, Teodorescu V, Sparacino S, Hollier LH, Marin ML. Abdominal aortic aneurysmorrhaphy and cholelithiasis in the era of endovascular surgery. Am Surg. 2002 Oct;68:839–43.

35. Borrero E, Aylward CA, Logan WD. Aortoesophageal fistula: early postoperative complication at the distal anastomosis of an aortic graft. South Med J 1989 Jul;82:927–30.

36. Chiesa R, Melissano G, Marone EM, Marrocco-Trischitta MM, Kahlberg A. Aorto-oesophageal and aortobronchial fistulae following thoracic endovascular aortic repair: A national survey. Eur J Vasc Endovasc Surg 2010 Mar;39: 273–9.

37. Sprung J, Tabares AH, Gottlieb A, Schoenwald PK, Olin JW. Ischemic liver dysfunction after elective repair of infrarenal aortic aneurysm: incidence and outcome. J cardiothorac Vasc Anesth 1998 Oct;12:507–11.

38. Varon J, Marik PE. Perioperative hypertension management. Vasc Health Risk manag 2008;4:651–27.

39. Varon J, Strikman WE. Diagnosis and management of hypertensive crisis in the elderly patients. J of Geriat Cardiol 2007;491:50–5.

40. Singh A, Antognini JF. Perioperative hypotension and myocardial ischemia: Diagnostic and therapeutic approaches. 2011 May-Aug;14:127–32.

41. Ms Sabina A, Murphy C, Gibson M. Metoprolol after vascular surgery. The Amer Coll of Cardiol Cardio Source 2006.

42. Heintz KM, Hollenberg SM. Perioperative cardiac issues: postoperative arrhythmias. Surg Clin North Am 2005 Dec; 85:1103–14.

43. Noorani A, Stewart RW, Tjun YT, et al. Atrial fibrillation following elective abdominal aortic repair. Int J of Surg 2009 Feb;7:24–7.

44. Le Manach Y, Perel A, Coriat P, et al. Early and delayed myocardial infarction after abdominal aortic surgery. Anesthesiology 2005 May;102:885–91.

45. Bryce GJ, Payne CJ, Gibson SC, Kingsmore DB, Byrne DS. The prognostic value of raised preoperative cardiac troponin I in major vascular surgery. Br J Cardiol 2009 May;16: 147–50.

46. Kertai MD, Boersma E, Westerhout CM, Klein J, Van Urk H, Bax JJ, Roelandt JR, Poldermans D. A combination of statins and beta-blockers is independently associated with a reduction in the incidence of perioperative mortality and nonfatal myocardial infarction in patients undergoing abdominal aortic aneurysm surgery. Eur J Vasc Endovasc Surg 2004 Oct;28:343–52.

47. Rawn JD. Blood transfusion in cardiac surgery: A silent epidemic revisited. Circulation 2007 Nov;116:2523–4.

48. Bursi F, Barbieri A, Politi L, Di Girolamo A, Malagoli A, Grimaldi T, Rumolo A, Busani S, Girardis M, Jaffe AS, Modena MG. Perioperative red blood cell transfusion and outcome in stable patients after elective major vascular surgery. Eur J Vasc Endovasc Surg 2009 Mar;37:311–8.

49. Liumbruno GM, Bennardello F, Lattanzio A, Piccoli P, Rossetti G. Italian Society of Transfusion Medicine and Immunohaematology Working Party. Recommendations for the transfusion management of patients in the perioperative period. III. The postoperative period. Blood Transfus 2011 Jul;9:320–35.

50. Moskowitz DM, Shander A, Javidroozi M, Klein JJ, Perelman SI, Nemeth J, Ergin MA. Postoperative blood loss and transfusion associated with use of Hextend in cardiac surgery patients at a blood conservation center. Transfusion 2008 Apr;48:768–75.

51. Liumbruno GM, Bennardello F, Lattanzio A, Piccoli P, Rossetti G; Italian Society of Transfusion Medicine and Immunohaematology (SIMTI) Working Party. Recommendations for the transfusion management of patients in the perioperative period. II. The intraoperative period. Blood Transfus 2011 Apr;9:189–217.

52. Krinsley JS. Association between hyperglycemia and increased hospital mortality in a heterogeneous population of critically ill patients. Mayo Clin Proc 2003 Dec;78:1471–8.

53. Serio S, Clements JM, Grauf D, Merchant AM. Outcomes of diabetic and nondiabetic patients undergoing general and vascular surgery. ISRN Surg 2013 Dec;2013:963930.

54. Hogwoerf BJ. Postoperative Management of diabetic patient. Med Clin North Am 2001 Sep;85:1213–28

55. Harbin M, Dossa A, de Lemos J, Drummond I, Paty B, Taylor B. Evaluation of protocol-guided scheduled Basal-nutritional-correction insulin over standard care for vascular surgery patients. Can J Diabetes 2015 Jun;39:210–5.

56. Hirsch AT, Haskal ZJ, Hertzer NR, Bakal CW, Creager MA, Halperin JL, Hiratzka LF, Murphy WR, Olin JW, Puschett JB, Rosenfield KA, Sacks D, Stanley JC, Taylor LM Jr, White CJ, White J, White RA, Antman EM, Smith SC Jr, Adams CD, Anderson JL, Faxon DP, Fuster V, Gibbons RJ, Hunt SA, Jacobs AK, Nishimura R, Ornato JP, Page RL, Riegel B; American Association for Vascular Surgery; Society for Vascular Surgery; Society for Cardiovascular Angiography and Interventions; Society for Vascular Medicine and Biology; Society of Interventional Radiology; ACC/AHA Task Force on Practice Guidelines Writing Committee to Develop Guidelines for the Management of Patients With Peripheral Arterial Disease; American Association of Cardiovascular and Pulmonary Rehabilitation; National Heart, Lung, and Blood Institute; Society for Vascular Nursing; TransAtlantic Inter-Society Consensus; Vascular Disease Foundation. ACC/AHA 2005 Practice Guidelines for the management of patients with peripheral arterial disease (lower extremity, renal, mesenteric, and abdominal aortic): a collaborative report from the American Association for Vascular Surgery/Society for Vascular Surgery, Society for Cardiovascular Angiography and Interventions, Society for Vascular Medicine and Biology, Society of Interventional Radiology, and the ACC/AHA Task Force on Practice Guidelines (Writing Committee to Develop Guidelines for the Management of Patients With Peripheral Arterial Disease): endorsed by the American Association of Cardiovascular and Pulmonary Rehabilitation; National Heart, Lung, and Blood Institute; Society for Vascular Nursing; TransAtlantic Inter-Society Consensus; and Vascular Disease Foundation. Circulation. 2006 Mar;113: e463–654.

57. Schepens MA, Defauw JJ, Hamerlijnck RP, Vermeulen FE. Risk assessment of acute renal failure after thoraco abdominal aortic aneurysm surgery. Ann Surg. 1994 Apr; 219:400–7.

58. Gornick CC Jr, Kjellstrand CM. Acute renal failure complicating aortic aneurysm surgery. Nephron 1983;35:145–57.

59. Barratt J, Parajasingam R, Sayers RD, Feehally J. Outcome of acute renal failure following surgical repair of ruptured abdominal aortic aneurysms. Eur J Vasc Endovasc Surg 2000 Aug;20:163–8.

60. Safi HJ, Harlin SA, Miller CC, Iliopoulos DC, Joshi A, Mohasci TG, Zippel R, Letsou GV. Predictive factors for acute renal failure in thoracic and thoracoabdominal aortic aneurysm surgery. J Vasc Surg 1996 Sep; 24:338–44.

61. Aftab M, Coselli JS. Reprint of: Renal and visceral protection in thoracoabdominal aortic surgery. J Thorac Cardiovasc Surg 2015 Feb;149:S130–3.

62. Wish JB, Moritz CE. Preventing radiocontrast-induced acute renal failure. J Crit Illness 1990;5:16–25.

63. Bang JY, Lee JB, Yoon Y, Seo HS, Song JG, Hwang GS. Acute kidney injury after infrarenal abdominal aortic aneurysm surgery: a comparison of AKIN and RIFLE criteria for risk prediction. Br J Anaesth 2014 Dec;113:993–1000.

64. Chaikof EL, Brewster DC, Dalman RL, Makaroun MS, Illig KA, Sicard GA, Timaran CH, Upchurch GR Jr, Veith FJ; Society for Vascular Surgery. The care of patients with an abdominal aortic aneurysm: the Society for Vascular Surgery practice guidelines. J Vasc Surg 2009 Oct;50:S2–49.

65. Ko PJ, Hsieh HC, Liu YH, Liu HP. Experience with early postoperative feeding after abdominal aortic surgery. Chang Gung Med J 2004 Mar;27:210–6.

66. Fearon KC, Luff R. The nutritional management of surgical patients: enhanced recovery after surgery. Proc Nutr Soc 2003 Nov;62:807–11.

67. Singh S, Maldonado Y, Taylor MA. Optimal perioperative medical management of the vascular surgery patient. Anesthesiol Clin 2014 Sep;32:615–37.

68. Braga M, Ljungqvist O, Soeters P, Fearon K, Weimann A, Bozzetti F; ESPEN. ESPEN Guidelines on Parenteral Nutrition: surgery. Clin Nutr 2009 Aug;28:378–86.

69. Nishimori M, Ballantyne JC, Low JH. Epidural pain relief versus systemic opioid-based pain relief for abdominal aortic surgery. Cochrane Database Syst Rev. 2006 Jul 19;(3): CD005059.

70. Shine TS, Greengrass RA, Feinglass NG. Use of continuous paravertebral analgesia to facilitate neurologic assessment and enhance recovery after thoracoabdominal aortic aneurysm repair. Anesth Analg 2004 Jun;98:1640–3.

71. Davies RG, Myles PS, Graham JM. A comparison of the analgesic efficacy and side-effects of paravertebral vs epidural blockade for thoracotomy—a systematic review and meta-ana lysis of randomized trials. Br J Anaesth 2006 Apr;96:418–26.

72. Sato N, Sugiura T, Takahashi K, Kato G, Kamada T, Mori Y, Kobayashi Y. [Analgesia with paravertebral block for postoperative pain after thoracic or thoracoabdominal aortic aneurysm repair]. Masui. 2014 Jun;63:640–3.

73. Marret E, Kurdi O, Zufferey P, Bonnet F. Effects of non-steroidal antiinflammatory drugs on patient-controlled analgesia morphine side effects: Meta-analysis of randomized controlled trials. Anesthesiology 2005 Jun;102:1249–60.

74. Savage C, McQuitty C, Wang D, Zwischenberger JB. Post-thoracotomy pain management. Chest Surg Clin N Am 2002 May;12:251–63.

75. De Cosmo G, Aceto P, Gualtieri E, Congedo E. Analgesia in thoracic surgery: review. Minerva Anestesiol 2009 Jun;75: 393–400.

76. de Maistre E, Terriat B, Lesne-Padieu AS, Abello N, Bouchot O, Steinmetz EF. High incidence of venous thrombosis after surgery for abdominal aortic aneurysm. J Vasc Surg 2009 Mar;49:596–601.

77. Eagleton MJ, Grigoryants V, Peterson DA, Williams DM, Henke PK, Wakefield TW, Stanley JC, Upchurch GR Jr. Endovascular treatment of abdominal aortic aneurysm is associated with a low incidence of deep venous thrombosis. J Vasc Surg 2002 Nov;36:912–6.

78. Ameli FM. Regarding "The incidence of deep venous thrombosis in patients undergoing abdominal aortic aneurysm resection". J Vasc Surg 1995 Mar;21:540–1.

79. Olin JW, Graor RA, O'Hara P, Young JR. The incidence of deep venous thrombosis in patients undergoing abdominal aortic aneurysm resection. J Vasc Surg 1993 Dec;18:1037–41.

80. Wilson NV, Melissari E, Standfield NJ, Kakkar VV. Intra-operative antithrombotic therapy with low molecular weight heparin in aortic surgery. How should heparin be administered? Eur J Vasc Surg 1991 Oct;5:565–9.

81. Davenport DL, Xenos ES. Deep venous thrombosis after repair of nonruptured abdominal aneurysm. J Vasc Surg 2013 Mar;57:678–83.

82. Postoperative management recommendations for patients at risk for postoperative pulmonary dysfunction, pre-existing diabetes, patients with renal insufficiency ...???

83. Coselli JS, Bozinovski J, LeMaire SA. Open surgical repair of 2286 thoracoabdominal aortic aneurysms. Ann Thorac Surg 2007 Feb;83:S862–4.

84. Singh S, Maldonado Y, Taylor MA. Optimal perioperative medical management of the vascular surgery patient. Anesthesiol Clin 2014 Sep;32:615–37.

85. Biller J, Feinberg WM, Castaldo JE, Whittemore AD, Harbaugh RE, Dempsey RJ, Caplan LR, Kresowik TF, Matchar DB, Toole JF, Easton JD, Adams HP Jr, Brass LM, Hobson RW 2nd, Brott TG, Sternau L. Guidelines for carotid endarterectomy: A statement for healthcare professionals from a Special Writing Group of the Stroke Council, American Heart Association. Circulation 1998 Feb 10;97: 501–9.

86. Reigel MM, Hollier LH, Sundt TM Jr, Piepgras DG, Sharbrough FW, Cherry KJ. Cerebral hyperperfusion syndrome: a cause of neurologic dysfunction after carotid endarterectomy. J Vasc Surg 1987 Apr;5:628–34.

87. Jalalian R, Saravi M, Banasaz B. Aortic dissection and postpartum cardiomyopathy in a postpartum young woman: a case report study. Iran Red Crescent Med J 2014 Apr;16:e9849.

88. Shu C,Fang K,Dardik A,Li X,Li M. Pregnancy associated type B dissection treated with thoracic endovascular aneurysm repair. Ann Thorac Surg 2014 Feb;97:582–7.

# CHAPTER 14

# Anesthesia Management for Endovascular Repair of Aortic Aneurysm in Cardiac Catheterization Laboratory

Sambhunath Das

## INTRODUCTION

Aortic aneurysm (AA) repair by open surgical methods has postoperative problems like bleeding, renal, neurological, pulmonary and gastrointestinal complications.[1] Many patients are associated with comorbidities like diabetes, hypertension, chronic obstructive pulmonary diseases, renal disease, neurological sequel, skeletal deformity and very old age. These situations predispose for poor post-surgery outcome for AA patients. Percutaneous endovascular aneurysm repair (EVAR) for AA treatment is a promising better alternative at present in selected patients.[2] The procedure is performed in cardiac or radiology catheterization laboratory and sometime in hybrid operation room.[3] The EVAR procedures produce complications like hemodynamic alterations, vascular injury, bleeding and embolic events.[4] Anesthetists are not much familiar to administer anesthesia and to manage the patient in the radiological suit.[5] This chapter will highlight the different aspects of anesthesia management for endovascular graft placement to treat AA.

## EPIDEMIOLOGY

The number of patients undergoing endovascular grafting for AA are more than 50% at present. In a survey, 84% patients prefer to undergo EVAR for treatment of AA.[6] EVAR is preferred in elderly.[7] The failure rate of EVAR for abdominal aortic aneurysm (AAA) is 8.3–10.7% compared to 15–30% in open surgery.[8]

## TECHNIQUE AND PROCEDURE

In 1991, the first published report of stent graft implantation for AAA in humans suggested that this approach was feasible.[9] Subsequent a greater degree of improvement has emerged in both the number of EVAR performed and technological improvements in stent graft design. Before the procedure CT and MRI evaluation for the shape, size, extension and involvement of branch arteries by the aneurysm are checked. The condition of the vessel at the site of insertion is to be assessed. The presence of thrombus and calcification inside aneurysm is to be evaluated and necessary precautions to be adopted. The guideline for EVAR has been formed by a task force committee in 2010.[10]

The procedure is performed in well-equipped bigger catheterization laboratory with facility to anesthesia, monitoring, radiology and resuscitation (Fig. 14.1). The stent graft consist of 3 components (i) delivery system for graft introduction and deployment, (ii) self-expandable metallic stent frame work and (iii) fabric that separates the aneurysm and serve as a conduit for blood flow. The catheter is passed through femoral artery. The catheter is placed under fluoroscope guide. The collapsible stent is introduced through the catheter and deployed in the aneurysm site. The endo-graft is self-expandable or expanded by introducing a balloon (Fig. 14.2). The proximal and distal landing zones are checked for correct placement by fluoroscope. The endo-graft is checked for any leak by injecting dye. The stent fabric interrupts disease progression and reverses the natural growth resulting in shrinkage of the aneurysmal sac around the stent (Fig. 14.3). In aortic dissections, the area of the primary tear is covered so flow is redirected to the true lumen and thrombosis of the false lumen and aortic remodeling occur.

Wherever the aneurysm includes critical vessels, hybrid procedures, combine open and endovascular

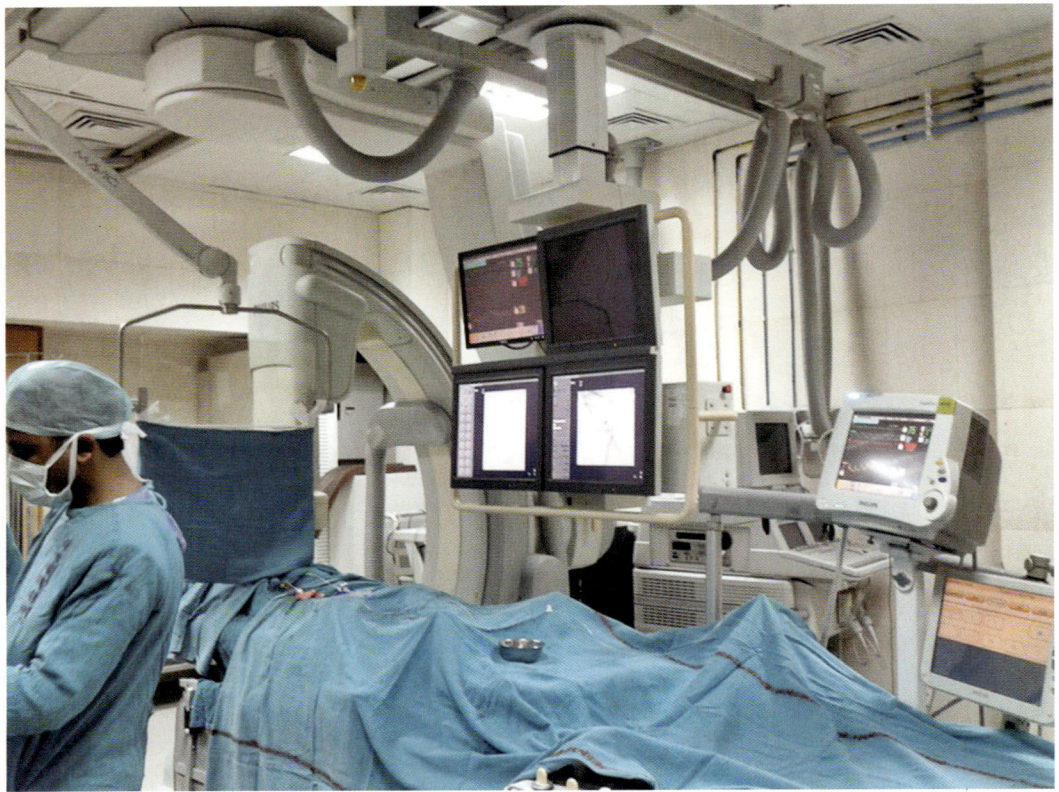

Fig. 14.1: Setup of a catheterization laboratory with an ongoing stenting procedure

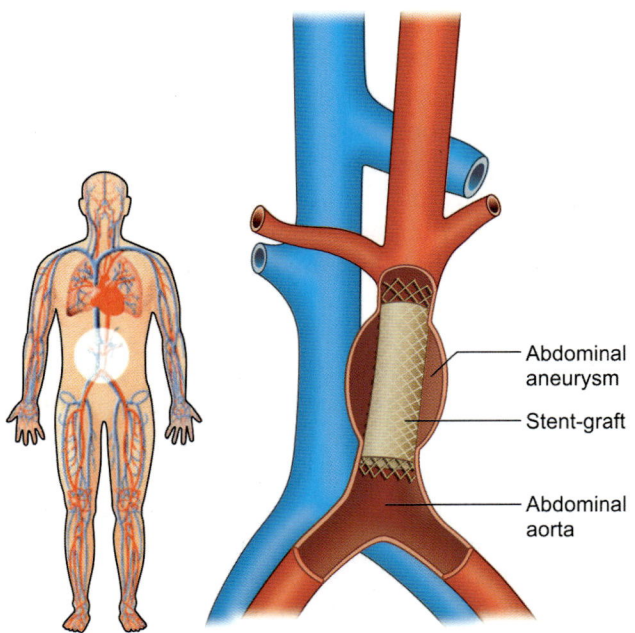

Fig. 14.2: Diagram of endovascular graft for AAA

**Advantages of EVAR over open surgical repair**

1. Less surgical transgression
2. Less blood loss
3. Fewer transfusions
4. Less fluid shifts
5. Less hemodynamic perturbations
6. Less distal tissue ischemia
7. Less end-organ damage
8. Less aggressive anesthetic management
9. Less intraoperative stress intraoperative
10. Fewer complications related to cardiac, pulmonary, renal system
11. Shorter recovery times
12. Lower mortality
13. May be suitable for patients otherwise considered inoperable

approaches to assure branch perfusion is planned.[11] The aortic visceral debranching allows for endovascular stenting of AA that involve major visceral branches (celiac, SMA, renal, IMA) can be performed just before EVAR or as a first part of a "staged" procedure (Figs 14.4 and 14.5). Requires a midline laparotomy and systemic heparinization to activated clotting time >300 seconds. A custom designed fenestrated or multibranched graft with distal anastomoses to the left renal artery, SMA, celiac axis, and right renal artery (Fig. 14.6). Inflow for visceral debranching is typically performed via a single proximal anastomosis from iliac, infrarenal aorta or existing infrarenal aortic graft.

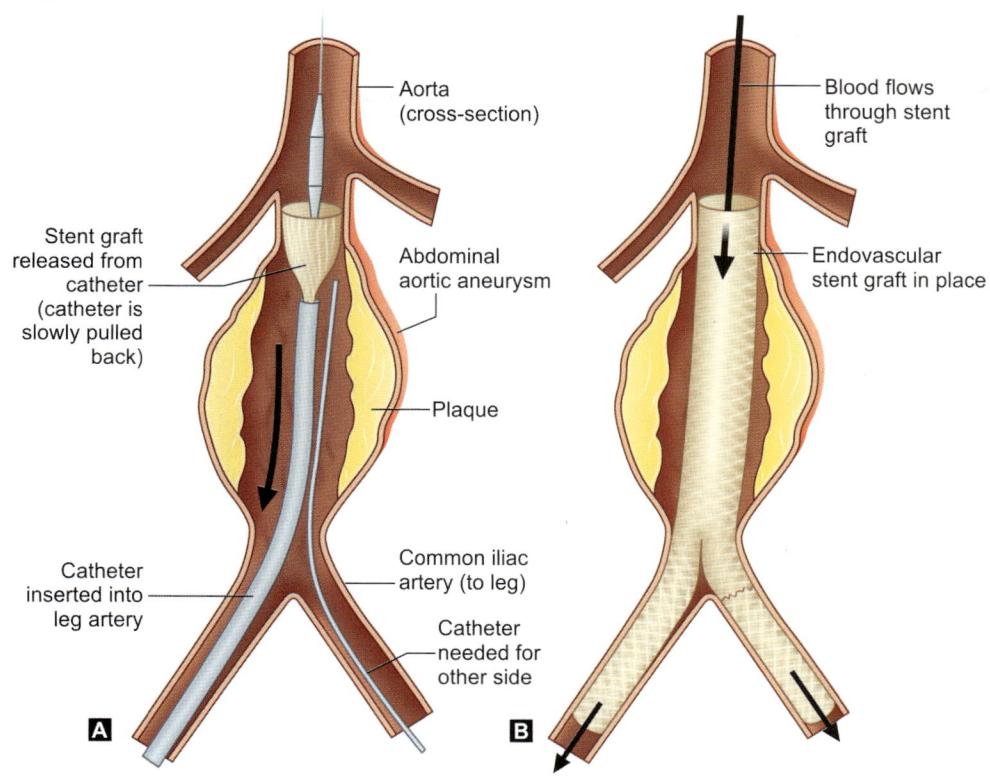

**Figs 14.3A and B:** Diagram of EVAR procedure for abdominal aortic aneurysm

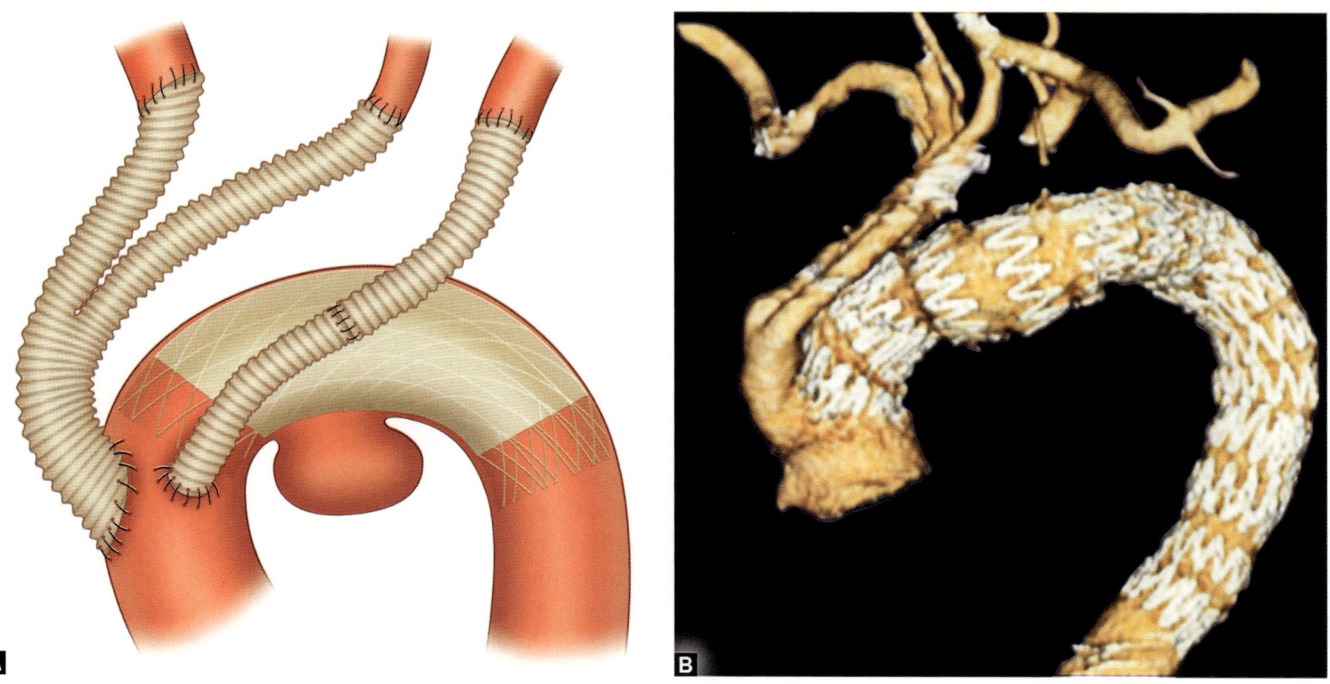

**Figs14.4A and B:** Debranching of aortic arch vessels

## PREANESTHETIC PREPARATIONS

The patients posted for EVAR must be empty stomach for more than 8 hours for solid foods. All the cardiac medications in the form of antihypertensive, beta blockers, aspirin and statins are to be continued. Anxiolytic in the form of benzodiazepines are to be

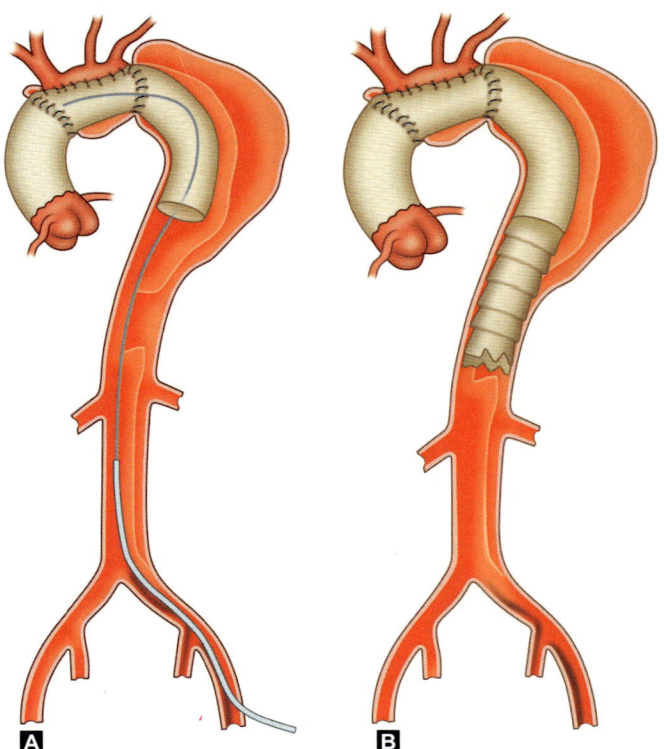

**Figs 14.5A and B:** Staging of open surgery and EVAR of elephant trunk by staged procedure

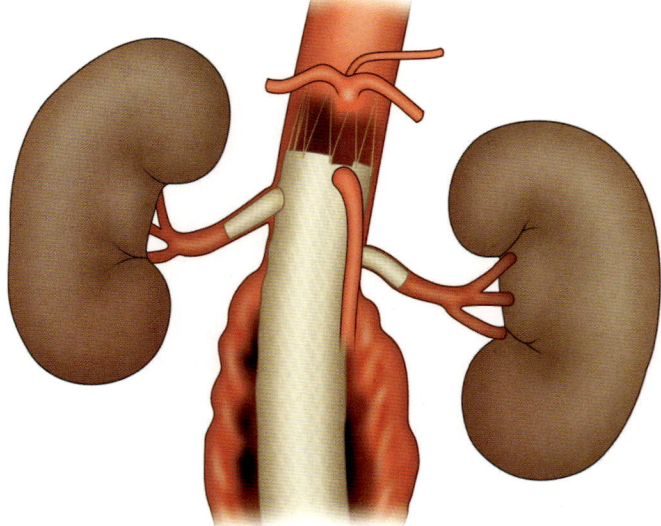

**Fig. 14.6:** Endovascular graft of abdominal aortic aneurysm with fenestrated branch graft

advised at bed time and on day of the procedure. Mild sedation with promethazine and morphine will help to reduce procedural pain and discomfort.

Special precaution is to be adopted in patients with prior cerebrovascular accidents and neurological injury. CT scan and TEE will identify mobile atheroma. Peripheral vascular disease is at risk of vascular injury and bleeding. Large bore IV access and blood are to be available prior to surgery. High risk of acute kidney injury (AKI) is aggravated with hypoperfusion, mechanical encroachment of stent on renal vessels and renal emboli.

Patients with preoperative renal insufficiency (creatinine >1.5 mg% or GFR of ≤60 mL) are at especially high risk for 4 fold more risk for AKI. AKI-risk reduction strategies should ensure perioperative euvolemia, maintain cardiac output and blood pressure and limit contrast dye exposure, when possible. Use iso-osmolar non-ionic contrast dye, pharmacologic strategies especially in patients with baseline chronic kidney disease with N-acetylcysteine, hydration with sodium bicarbonate containing solution and statin drugs.

## ANESTHESIA MANAGEMENT DURING THE PROCEDURE

The choice of anesthesia for EVAR is decided by hospital policy and all the techniques have some merits and demerits.[12] Anesthesia delivery during EVAR can be established with four techniques like

i.   Monitored anesthesia care
ii.  Total intravenous anesthesia
iii. Endotracheal intubation general anesthesia
iv.  Neuroaxial block or regional anesthesia.

*Monitored anesthesia care:* Local anesthetic drug like lignocaine or ropivacaine was infiltrated at the site of puncture for vascular assess in the groin. After numbness at the part the EVAR procedure is started with constant monitoring of vitals.[13] Mild sedation in the form of fentanyl or midazolam may be added for patient's comfort. Patient cooperation and understanding that a deep anesthesia is not being feasible as there is a need for periodic breath holding during angiography.

*Total intravenous anesthesia:* In this method of anesthesia, propofol, dexmedetomidine with fentanyl are infused and patient's respiration, hemodynamic parameters are monitored.

*Endotracheal intubation general anesthesia:* Here anesthesia is induced with sedation, analgesia and muscle relaxant. After tracheal intubation the lungs are mechanically ventilated. The options for fast track are kept in mind. The respiration of the patient is controlled so it helps during deployment of endovascular graft.

*Neuroaxial block or regional anesthesia:* Regional anesthesia with epidural or spinal is occasionally adopted for EVAR procedure.[14] The chance of spinal hematoma and long hospital stay limit its use. This technique is never used in emergency rupture aneurysm cases.

| Anesthetic Goals in EVAR |
| --- |
| i. Maintain hemodynamic stability, and preserve perfusion to vital organs including the brain, heart, spinal cord, kidney and splanchnic vessels. |
| ii. Avoid imbalance in myocardial oxygen supply/demand relationship and avoid the resultant ischemic acute coronary events. |
| iii. Reducing dp/dt in patients with both aortic aneurysms and dissections (avoidance of hypertension and tachycardia). |
| iv. Maintenance of intravascular volume and early identification and management of bleeding. |

During the placement of graft the need *for transient cessation of blood flow by using adenosine 6–18 mg, overdrive ventricular pacing (180–220 rate/min)* is mandatory. The chance of hypotension and bleeding is present at this period. Risk of cerebral emboli is common when EVAR is performed for aortic arch and descending thoracic aorta. Prior AAA or stent covering T6 diaphragm are at risk of spinal cord ischemia.

During EVAR the risk of *radiation hazards* is present. All the medical personnel have to use lead apron and thyroid collar to minimize radiation. The catheterization lab is a remote and less familiar area for anesthetist. All anesthetic equipment and drugs may not be available. Anesthetist is to be prepared prior to administering anesthesia.

## MONITORING DURING EVAR

The monitoring that used during the procedure are as follows:

| Monitoring |
| --- |
| a. ECG with automated ST segment analysis |
| b. Right radial Artery-line (left brachial often used for surgical access) |
| c. Central access with large bore multiple access catheter |
| d. Femoral Artery pressure |
| e. CSF pressure |
| f. Bispectral index[R] |
| g. SSEP, EEG (limit inhalation to MAC, avoid hypothermia) |
| h. MEP (limit inhalation, avoid muscle relaxant, avoid hypothermia) |
| i. TEE (transesophageal echocardiography)—Transesophageal echocardiography has promising role in assessing the cardiac function and the size as well as the extension of aneurysm or dissection. The presence of thrombus can be also evaluated with TEE at the ascending, arch, descending and upper part of abdominal aorta |
| j. NIRS (near infrared spectroscopy) |

## POSTPROCEDURAL COMPLICATIONS AND CARE

The postimplantation period of EVAR is not free of complication. The common complications are as follows:[15]

i. Risk of spinal cord ischemia and paraplegia is 1–8%. Biggest risk factor is the amount of collateral circulation that is sacrificed, extent of the aorta covered by the graft and critical intercostals T6–T12 supply anterior spinal artery that are involved.

ii. Hypotension, severe atherosclerosis of the thoracic aorta and injury to external iliac artery are responsible for high patient's morbidity.

iii. Endoleak from the graft

iv. Infection

v. Limb vessel occlusion

vi. Device migration

Patients who undergo EVAR need regular clinical follow-up with appropriate imaging for the remaining part of their life because of the potential for stent graft migration and other causes like sac repressurization that will put the patient at risk of aneurysm rupture.[16] CT is the gold standard for follow-up imaging. Concerns with this method include the cumulative effects of radiation exposure and the effect of repetitive administration of intravenous contrast on renal function.[17] Magnetic resonance imaging/angiography is an alternative for follow-up of most devices but is costly, time consuming, and not universally available.

## TREATMENT OF ENDOLEAK AFTER EVAR

There are five categories of leak through the endovascular graft which are as follows:

| Types of endoleak | |
| --- | --- |
| Type I: | Incompetent proximal or distal seal |
| Type II: | Backflow from collaterals |
| Type III: | Disassociation where modular components overlap |
| Type IV: | Leaks through porous graft of fabric |
| Type V: | Leak without any obvious cause |

Endoleak is defined as a persistant blood flow outside the lumen of the endoluminal graft but within an aneurysm sac or adjacent vascular segment being treated by the device. Endoleaks are due to incomplete sealing, or exclusion of the aneurysm sac, and thus cause reflux of blood flow in the sac. Four types of endoleaks are currently known and labeled (Figs 14.7A to D).

*Type I endoleak:* Blood flow in to the aneurysm sac due to incomplete seal or ineffective seal at the end of the graft. This type of endoleak usually occurs later.

*Type II endoleak:* Blood flow into the aneurysm sac due to (retrograde) blood flow from collateral vessels. In some circumstance when there are two or more patent vessels a situation of inflow and outflow develops creating an active blood flow within channel created within the aneurysm sac.

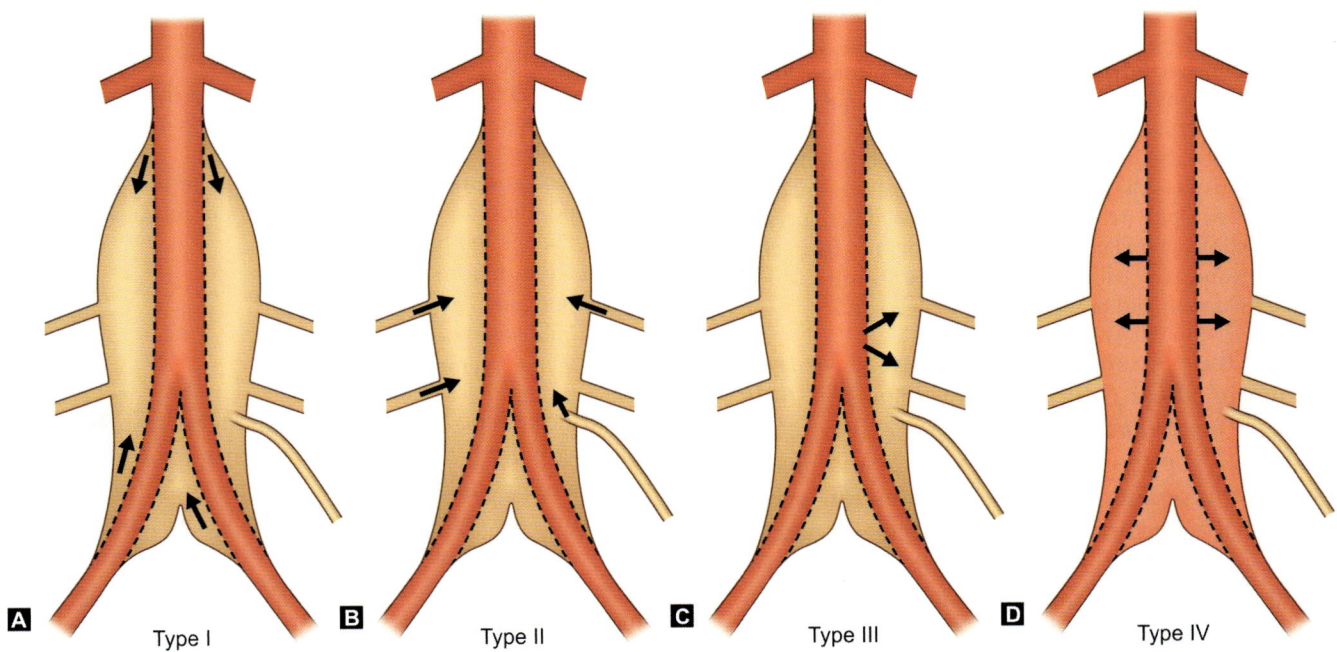

**Figs 14.7A to D:** Endoleak—types I to IV

*Type III endoleak:* Blood flow into the aneurysm sac due to inadequate or ineffective sealing of overlapping graft joints rupture of the graft fabric. Again, this endoleak usually occure early after treatment, due to technical problems, or later due to device break down.

*Type IV endoleak:* Blood flow into the aneurysm sac due to the porosity of the graft fabric, causing blood to pass through from the graft and into the aneurysm sac.

Endoleak is the major cause of complications, and thus failure in endoluminal treatment of AAA. When an endoleak occurs, it causes continued pressurization of the aneurysm sac and may leave the patient at risk of an AAA rupture. As a result of the major complications that endoleaks cause, one may consider endovascular treatment of AAA is still an evolving field.

I and type III endoleaks are treated with immediate intervention to halt perigraft flow or flow between modular components. Type II endoleaks are typically managed expectantly with intervention reserved for persistent endoleaks in the presence of aneurysm sac enlargement. The presence of a persistent type II endoleak for 6 months, however, has been associated with aneurysm enlargement, increased rate of secondary interventions, and even aneurysm rupture.[18] Type IV endoleaks rarely occur with modern stent graft design, and type V endoleaks (endotension), although still reported, are much less frequent after modification of the graft materials. Secondary interventions occur in a spectrum ranging from diagnostic angiography to endograft removal with conversion to open repair, although the majority are percutaneous treatment of type II endoleaks with source embolization.

A related cause of endoleak and potential complication of EVAR is device failure. The integrity of stent graft materials and maintenance of proper positioning within the aneurysm are critical in preventing pressurization of the aneurysm sac and rupture. Material failure includes fracture of any of the metallic components of the stent graft, including stents, hooks, or barbs, or tears in the fabric component of the stent graft. Loss of proper stent graft position can occur for many reasons. Material failure, inadequate proximal or distal seal zone, aneurysm remodeling after EVAR, or features of the vessel, such as thrombus or calcium, that limit stent purchase, have all been implicated in the migration of stent grafts. Each of these modes of failure needs to be analyzed within the context of their clinical significance. A stent fracture that leaves the graft fabric intact and is not in a critical region for maintaining fixation would likely need only follow-up, whereas modular component separation resulting in a large type III endoleak will require urgent intervention to restore stent graft integrity.

## HYBRID PROCEDURE

This is a combination of percutaneous technique (radiology suit) and open surgical repair (operation room).[19] Both the pieces of equipment of cath lab and operation room are available with proper anesthesia work station (Figs 14.8 to 14.10). Merits of hybrid procedure (OR + CATH Lab) are:

1. The aortic angiography → endovascular graft
2. Better control of emergency events by hybrid procedure
3. Anesthesia—LA, monitored anesthesia (MAC), GA.

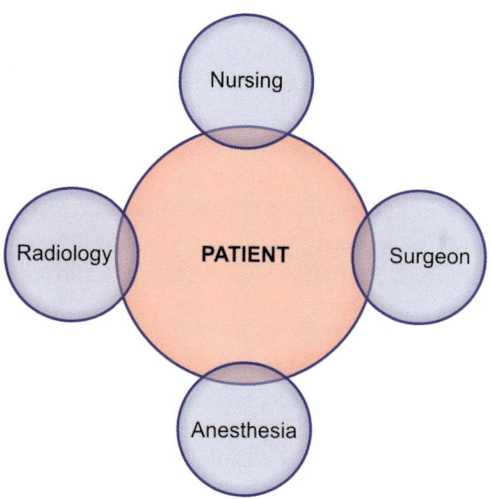

**Fig. 14.8:** Design of hybrid operation room

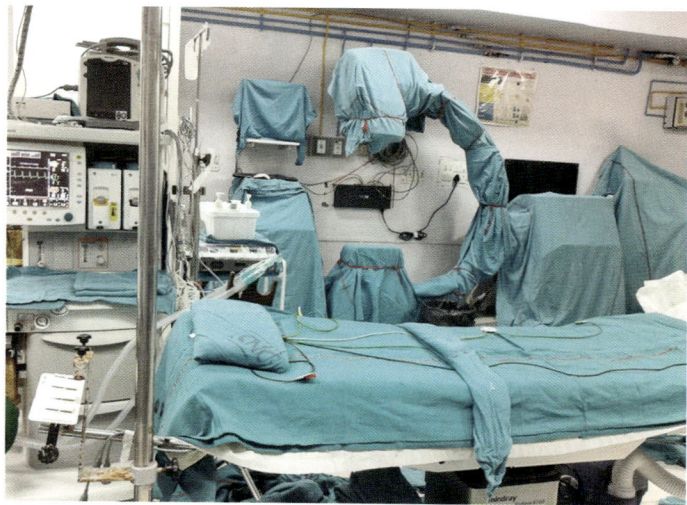

**Fig. 14.9:** The setup of hybrid operation room with operation table, C-arm and anesthesia machine

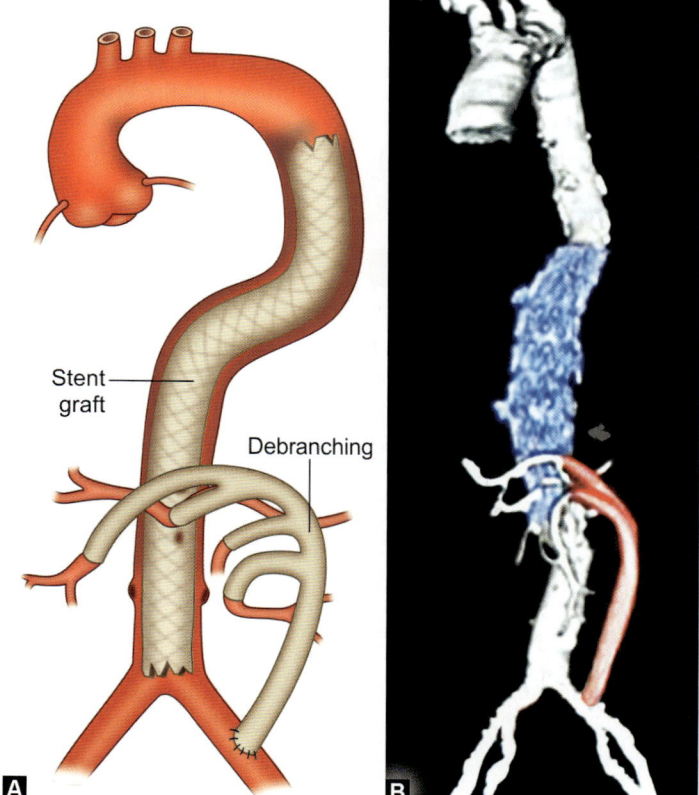

**Figs 14.10A and B:** (A) Hybrid procedures: Thoracoabdominal stent and debranching, (B) stenting and debranching

## SUMMARY

Endovascular aneurysm repair is a procedure for treatment of all types of aortic aneurysm. In the coming years the number of EVAR will dramatically increase due to less time consuming, less early morbidity and shorter hospital stay. More involvement of anesthetist will be required in EVAR management. The anesthetic considerations are related to the patients' coexisting morbidity, choice of anesthesia, radiation safety, control of hemodynamic stability and continuous monitoring to prevent graft related complication.

## Key Notes

i. Endovascular aneurysm repair (EVAR) is a percutaneous route of placing a biocompatible stent fabric material into the lumen of aortic aneurysm. EVAR is performed in the radiological or cardiological catheterization laboratory.

ii. Anaesthetist is less familiar to the radiological suit area. The thorough understanding of the steps of EVAR is essential to deliver a better care.

iii. Monitored anesthesia care is commonly used for shorter period EVAR. Longer duration procedure requires general or continuous epidural anesthesia.

iv. Control of heart rate between 50 and 60 per minute, transient asystole by adenosine, overdrive pacing at fast rate and reduction of blood pressure facilitate the easy placement of endovascular graft.

v. Neurological monitoring with BIS, NIRS, SSEP, MEP and CSF pressure is helpful in detecting the neurological complications related to EVAR.

vi. Transesophageal echocardiography has promising role in assessing the cardiac function and the size as well as the extension of aneurysm or dissection. The presence of thrombus can be also evaluated with TEE.

vii. Hybrid operation room with both provision of surgical and catheterization facility for EVAR and open surgical procedure has a promising role to avoid the problems related to both techniques. The patient can be better managed with stable vital parameters combined by anesthetist, surgeon and interventional radiologist.

## REFERENCES

1. Selman AR, Kursbaum EA, Ubilla SM, Turner GE, Espinoza SC, Espinoza HJ, González FR, Villavicencio TM, Valladares JE, Naranjo TL, Oppliger PE. Surgical results among 100 patients with type A aortic dissection: retrospective review. Rev Med Chil 2010 Aug;138:982–7.

2. Matsumura JS, Brewster DC, Makaroun MS, Naftel DC. A multicenter controlled clinical trial ofopen versus endovascular treatment of abdominal aortic aneurysm. J Vasc Surg 2003;37:262–71.

3. Cazavet A, Alacoque X, Marcheix B, Chaufour X, Rousseau H, Glock Y, et al. Aortic arch aneurysm: short- and mid-term results comparing open arch surgery and the hybrid procedure. Eur J Cardiothorac Surg. 2016 Jan; 49(1):134–40.

4. Bryce Y, Rogoff P, Romanelli D, Reichle R. Endovascular Repair of Abdominal Aortic Aneurysms: Vascular Anatomy, Device Selection, Procedure, and Procedure-specific Complications. Radiographics 2015 Mar-Apr;35:593–615.

5. Hamid A. Anesthesia for cardiac catheterization procedures. Heart, Lung and Vessels 2014;6:225–31.

6. Timaran CH, Rosero EB, Smith ST, Moderall JG, Valentine RJ, Clagett GP. Influence of age, aneurysm size, and patient fitness on suitability for endovascular aneurysm repair. Ann Vasc Surg 2008; 22:730–5.

7. Dardik A, Lin JW, Gordon TA, Williams GM, Perler BA. Results of elective abdominal aortic aneurysm repair in the 1990s: A population-based analysis of 2335 cases. J Vasc Surg 1999;30:985–95.

8. Dattilo JB, Brewster DC, Fan CM, et al. Clinical failures of endovascular abdominal aortic aneurysm repair: incidence, causes, and management. J Vasc Surg 2002;35:1137–44.

9. Veith FJ1, Marin ML, Cynamon J, Schonholz C, Parodi J. 1992: Parodi, Montefiore, and the first abdominal aortic aneurysm stent graft in the United States. Ann Vasc Surg. 2005 Sep;19:749–51.

10. Walker TG, Kalva SP, Yeddula K, et al. Clinical practice guidelines for endovascular abdominal aortic aneurysm repair: Written by standards of practice committee for the society of interventional radiology society and endorsed by the cardiovascular and interventional radiology society of Europe and the Canadian interventional radiological society. J Vasc Interven Radiol 2010;21:1632–55.

11. Donas KP1, Torsello G, Lazaridis K. Current status of hybrid procedures for thoracoabdominal and pararenal aortic aneurysm repair: Techniques and considerations.J Endovasc Ther 2010 Oct;17:602–8.

12. Sadat U, Cooper DG, Gillard JH, Walsh SR, Hayes PD. Impact of the type of anesthesia on outcome after elective endovascular aortic aneurysm repair: Literature review. Vascular 2008 Nov-Dec;16:340–5.

13. Elisha S, Nagelhout J, Heiner J, Gabot M. Anesthesia case management for endovascular aortic aneurysm repair. AANA J 2014 Apr;82:145–52.

14. Flaherty J, Horn JL, Derby R. Regional anesthesia for vascular surgery. Anesthesiol Clin 2014 Sep;32:639–59.

15. Stather PW, Sidloff D, Dattani N, Choke E, Bown MJ, Sayers RD. Systematic review and meta-analysis of the early and late outcomes of open and endovascular repair of abdominal aortic aneurysm. Br J Surg 2013 Jun;100:863–72.

16. Chang RW, Goodney P, Tucker LY, Okuhn S, Hua H, Rhoades A, Sivamurthy N, Hill B. Ten-year results of endovascular abdominal aortic aneurysm repair from a large multicenter registry. J Vasc Surg 2013 Aug;58:324–32.

17. Von Tengg-Kobligk H, Correa Londono M, Von Allmen R, Heverhagen JT, Van Den Berg JC. State-of-the-art of imaging detecting endoleaks post-EVAR with special focus on low-flow endoleaks. J Cardiovasc Surg (Torino) 2014 Oct;55:563–79.

18. Van Strijen MJ, Vos JA. Experience with new techniques for the treatment of type II endoleaks post-EVAR. J Cardiovasc Surg (Torino) 2014 Oct;55:581–92.

19. Rosset E, Ben Ahmed S, Galvaing G, Favre JP, Sessa C, Lermusiaux Pea, et al. Association Universitaire de Rechercheen Chirurgie. Editor's choice—hybrid treatment of thoracic, thoracoabdominal, and abdominal aortic aneurysms: A multicenter retrospective study. Eur J Vasc Endovasc Surg 2014 May;47:470–8.